Contagious Diseases
SOURCEBOOK

FOURTH EDITION

Contagious Diseases
SOURCEBOOK

FOURTH EDITION

Basic Consumer Health Information about Diseases Spread from Person to Person through Direct Physical Contact, Airborne Transmissions, Sexual Contact, or Contact with Blood or Other Body Fluids, Including Pneumococcal, Staphylococcal, and Streptococcal Diseases, Colds, Influenza, Lice, Measles, Mumps, Tuberculosis, and Others

Along with Information about Self-Care and Over-the-Counter Medications, Antibiotics and Drug Resistance, Disease Prevention, Vaccines, and Bioterrorism, a Glossary, and a Directory of Resources for More Information

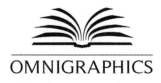

OMNIGRAPHICS

615 Griswold, Ste. 520, Detroit, MI 48226

Table of Contents

Preface xiii

Part I: What You Need to Know about Germs

Chapter 1 — Understanding Microbes 3

    Section 1.1 — What Are Microbes? 4

    Section 1.2 — Microbes Can Cause
    Different Kinds of Infections 8

    Section 1.3 — Preventing Microbial
    Diseases 11

    Section 1.4 — General Symptoms,
    Diagnosis, and Treatment
    of Microbial Diseases 15

Chapter 2 — Immunity: An Overview 21

    Section 2.1 — The Immune System 22

    Section 2.2 — Immune System Response
    to Infection 24

Chapter 3 — Immunodeficiency and Contagious
Diseases 33

Chapter 4 — Transmission of Contagious Disease 39

    Section 4.1 — Transmission of Microbes
    That Cause Contagious
    Disease 40

Section 4.2 — Preventing the Transmission
of Sexually Transmitted
Disease 44

Section 4.3 — Risk of Infectious Disease
from Blood Transfusion 46

Section 4.4 — Contagious Disease
Transmission on Airplanes
and Cruise Ships........................ 54

Chapter 5 — Screening Internationally Adopted
Children for Contagious Diseases........................... 65

Chapter 6 — Bioterrorism: Disease Used as a
Weapon 71

Section 6.1 — Bioterrorism Overview 72

Section 6.2 — Strategic National
Stockpile of Medicine................. 74

Section 6.3 — U.S. Preparedness for
Health Emergencies from
Bioterrorism (Anthrax).............. 79

Part II: Viral Contagious Diseases

Chapter 7 — Adenovirus 85

Chapter 8 — Avian Flu... 89

Chapter 9 — Chickenpox (Varicella) and Shingles..................... 93

Chapter 10 — Common Colds 103

Chapter 11 — Conjunctivitis....................................... 107

Chapter 12 — Ebola Virus Disease.............................. 117

Chapter 13 — Epstein-Barr Virus and Infectious
Mononucleosis....................................... 125

Chapter 14 — Fifth Disease (*Parvovirus B19*)........................ 131

Chapter 15 — Genital Herpes...................................... 135

Chapter 16 — Gonorrhea 143

Chapter 17 — Hand, Foot, and Mouth Disease 149

Chapter 18—Hepatitis: A through E and Beyond 155

Chapter 19—Human Immunodeficiency Virus and
Acquired Immunodeficiency Syndrome 161

Chapter 20—Human Papillomavirus 169

Chapter 21—Influenza 175

Section 21.1—Seasonal Flu 176

Section 21.2—Pandemic Flu 182

Section 21.3—H1N1 Flu 187

Chapter 22—Measles 193

Chapter 23—Viral Meningitis 199

Chapter 24—Mumps 205

Chapter 25—Nonpolio Enterovirus 209

Chapter 26—Norovirus 213

Chapter 27—Polio 219

Chapter 28—Respiratory Syncytial Virus Infection 223

Chapter 29—Rubella 227

Chapter 30—Smallpox 231

Chapter 31—Zika Virus 237

Part III: Bacterial Contagious Diseases

Chapter 32—Chancroid 247

Chapter 33—Chlamydia and Lymphogranuloma
Venereum 251

Chapter 34—Cholera 263

Chapter 35—*Clostridium difficile* Infection 269

Chapter 36—Diphtheria 277

Chapter 37—Hansen Disease (Leprosy) 281

Chapter 38—Hib Disease 287

Chapter 39—Impetigo 291

Chapter 40—Bacterial Meningitis 295

Chapter 41—Methicillin-Resistant *Staphylococcus
   aureus* 301

Chapter 42—Pneumonia 307

Chapter 43—Shigellosis 321

Chapter 44—Staph Infections: Group A................... 327

   Section 44.1—Staphylococcal Infections 328

   Section 44.2—*Staphylococcus aureus* and
      Pregnancy................................. 331

   Section 44.3—Vancomycin-Intermediate/
      Resistance *Staphylococcus
      aureus* 335

Chapter 45—Streptococcal Infections: Group A..................... 339

   Section 45.1—Strep Throat........................... 340

   Section 45.2—Scarlet Fever........................... 344

Chapter 46—Streptococcal Infections: Group B..................... 349

   Section 46.1—*Streptococcus pneumoniae*........ 350

   Section 46.2—Group B Strep in
      Pregnancy and Newborns......... 356

Chapter 47—Syphilis................................... 361

Chapter 48—Tuberculosis 369

Chapter 49—Typhoid Fever 377

Chapter 50—Vaginal and Reproductive Tract
   Infections... 381

Chapter 51—Vancomycin-Resistant Enterococci..................... 391

Chapter 52—Whooping Cough............................... 395

Part IV: Parasitic and Fungal Contagious Diseases

Chapter 53—Amebiasis 405

Chapter 54—Cryptosporidiosis 409

Chapter 55—Lice 417

    Section 55.1—Body Lice 418

    Section 55.2—Head Lice 420

    Section 55.3—Pubic Lice 425

Chapter 56—Parasitic, Amebic, and Fungal Meningitis 431

Chapter 57—Pinworms 439

Chapter 58—Scabies 443

Chapter 59—Tinea Infections 451

Chapter 60—Trichomoniasis 459

Part V: Self-Treatment for Contagious Diseases

Chapter 61—Self-Care for Colds or Flu 467

    Section 61.1—What to Do for Colds
                and Flu 468

    Section 61.2—Cold, Flu, or Allergy?
                Know the Difference 471

    Section 61.3—Antibiotics Do Not Work
                for a Cold or the Flu 473

    Section 61.4—Healthy Habits to Help
                Prevent Flu 474

    Section 61.5—Taking Care of Yourself
                When You Have
                Seasonal Flu 476

Chapter 62—Sore Throat Care 479

Chapter 63—Fever: What You Can Do 483

Chapter 64—Mouth Sores: Causes and Care 489

Chapter 65—Over-the-Counter Medications 495

    Section 65.1—Over-the-Counter
                Medications and How
                They Work 496

    Section 65.2—Kids Are Not Just Small
                Adults: Tips on Giving
                Over-the-Counter Medicine
                to Children 499

Section 65.3—Over-the-Counter Cough
and Cold Products for
Children 502

Chapter 66—Avoiding Drug Interactions 505

Chapter 67—Complementary and Alternative
Medicine for Contagious Diseases 511

Section 67.1—Complementary and
Alternative Medicine for
Flu and Colds 512

Section 67.2—Getting to Know "Friendly
Bacteria"—Probiotics 519

Section 67.3—Herbal Supplements 522

Section 67.4—Dietary Supplements 533

Section 67.5—Hepatitis C and
Complementary and
Alternative Medicine 536

Part VI: Medical Diagnosis and Treatment of Contagious Diseases

Chapter 68—Diagnostic Tests for Contagious Diseases 543

Section 68.1—Medical Tests That
Diagnose Infection 544

Section 68.2—Testing for Influenza 546

Section 68.3—Strep Throat Testing and
Treatment 552

Section 68.4—Rapid and Home Tests for
Human Immunodeficiency
Virus 556

Chapter 69—Prescription Medicines That Treat
Contagious Diseases (Antibiotics,
Antivirals, and Other Prescription
Medicines) 561

Chapter 70—Antiviral Drugs for Seasonal Flu 567

Chapter 71—Drug Resistance 571

Section 71.1—Antibiotic Safety and Drug
Resistance 572

Section 71.2—Antimicrobial (Drug)
Resistance 575

Section 71.3—Surveillance of
Antimicrobial Resistance
Patterns and Rates 580

Section 71.4—Influenza Antiviral Drug
Resistance 583

Part VII: Preventing Contagious Diseases

Chapter 72—Handwashing Prevents the Spread of
Germs 591

Chapter 73—Vaccines: What They Are and How
They Work 597

Section 73.1—Understanding How
Vaccines Work 598

Section 73.2—Making the Vaccine
Decision 601

Chapter 74—Vaccine Types and Ingredients 605

Chapter 75—Childhood Immunizations: Ten
Vaccines for Fourteen Diseases 613

Chapter 76—Questions and Answers about
Immunizations 621

Chapter 77—Facts about Adolescent Immunization 629

Chapter 78—Adult Immunization Recommendations 633

Chapter 79—Possible Side Effects from Vaccines 645

Chapter 80—Vaccine Adverse Event Reporting
System 665

Chapter 81—Vaccination Records 669

Chapter 82—Vaccine Misinformation May Have
Tragic Consequences 673

Chapter 83—What Would Happen If We Stopped
Vaccinations? 677

Chapter 84—Preventing Transmission of Infections
            in Hospitals and Nursing Homes......................... 681

        Section 84.1—Tips for Patients to Prevent
                        Healthcare-Associated
                        Infections................................... 682

        Section 84.2—Prevention and Control of
                        Influenza in Healthcare
                        Settings 683

Chapter 85—Legal Authorities for Isolation and
            Quarantine to Control the Spread of
            Contagious Diseases... 697

Chapter 86—U.S. Nationally Notifiable Infectious
            Diseases: Protecting the Public Health............... 701

Chapter 87—Countering Bioterrorism and
            Emerging Infectious Diseases........................... 705

Part VIII: Additional Help and Information

Chapter 88—Glossary of Terms Related to
            Contagious Diseases... 711

Chapter 89—Directory of Organizations with
            Information about Contagious
            Diseases... 717

Index.. 727

Preface

About This Book

Contagious diseases occur when microbes—bacteria, viruses, and fungi—are passed from person to person. Vaccination programs and other prevention measures have been successful in reducing the number of new cases of many contagious diseases. However, in many industrialized countries where communicable disease mortality has greatly decreased over the past century, the return of old communicable diseases, the emergence of new ones, and the evolution of antimicrobial resistance continue to present a challenge, and infectious diseases remain a major public-health concern in the United States and around the world.

Contagious Diseases Sourcebook, Fourth Edition provides updated information about microbes that are spread from person to person and the diseases they cause, including influenza, lice infestation, pneumonias, staphylococcal and streptococcal infections, tuberculosis, and others. The types of diagnostic tests and treatments available from medical professionals are explained, and self-care practices for familiar symptoms—such as fever and sore throat that often accompany the common cold—are described. Other topics addressed include antibiotic resistance, the role of handwashing in preventing the spread of disease, and recommendations and controversies surrounding vaccination programs. The book concludes with a glossary of related terms and a directory of additional resources.

How to Use This Book

This book is divided into parts and chapters. Parts focus on broad areas of interest. Chapters are devoted to single topics within a part.

Part I: What You Need to Know about Germs describes various types of microbes and different kinds of infections. It explains how the immune system responds to germs and how diseases can be transmitted from one person to another. Public health issues are also discussed, including the practice of screening internationally adopted children for contagious diseases and the threat of bioterrorism.

Part II: Viral Contagious Diseases provides information about the causes, transmission, symptoms, diagnosis, treatment, and prevention of various diseases caused by viruses such as chickenpox, gonorrhea, influenza, measles, polio, rubella, and other diseases.

Part III: Bacterial Contagious Diseases discusses in detail about the diseases and infections caused by bacteria such as chancroid, diphtheria, impetigo, pneumonia, streptococcal infections, tuberculosis, and so on.

Part IV: Parasitic and Fungal Contagious Diseases provides information about the contagious diseases caused by parasites and fungi including amebiasis, cryptosporidiosis, lice, meningitis, pinworms, scabies, tinea infections, and trichomoniasis.

Part V: Self-Treatment for Contagious Diseases discusses frequently used remedies for common illnesses and disease symptoms. Facts about the proper use of over-the-counter (OTC) medications are included along with a chapter focusing on the dangers associated with drug interactions. The part concludes with information about the use of probiotics, herbal and dietary supplements, and other forms of complementary and alternative medicine.

Part VI: Medical Diagnosis and Treatment of Contagious Diseases explains the tests and procedures used to identify the presence of microbial infection, colds, influenza, and other diseases. Antibiotic and antiviral medications are discussed, and the growing problem of antimicrobial resistance—the way microbes change to counteract the effectiveness of drug treatments—is explained.

Part VII: Preventing Contagious Diseases begins with information about a simple practice that is a key element in the fight against the spread of germs—handwashing. It continues with facts about vaccines, another effective tool for halting the proliferation of disease. Information about vaccine recommendations for children, adolescents, and adults is included, and this part also addresses problems associated with vaccines, the vaccine adverse event reporting system, and the difficulties that can arise as a result of vaccine misinformation.

Part VIII: Additional Help and Information provides a glossary of terms related to contagious diseases and a directory of resources for additional information.

Bibliographic Note

This volume contains documents and excerpts from publications issued by the following U.S. government agencies: Centers for Disease Control and Prevention (CDC); National Center for Complementary and Integrative Health (NCCIH); National Heart, Lung, and Blood Institute (NHLBI); National Institute of Allergy and Infectious Diseases (NIAID); National Institute of Diabetes and Digestive and Kidney Diseases (NIDDK); National Institute on Aging (NIA); National Institute on Drug Abuse (NIDA); National Institutes of Health (NIH); *NIH News in Health*; Office of Adolescent Health (OAH); Office of the Assistant Secretary for Preparedness and Response (ASPR); Office on Women's Health (OWH); U.S. Department of Health and Human Services (HHS); and U.S. Food and Drug Administration (FDA).

It may also contain original material produced by Omnigraphics and reviewed by medical consultants.

About the Health Reference Series

The *Health Reference Series* is designed to provide basic medical information for patients, families, caregivers, and the general public. Each volume takes a particular topic and provides comprehensive coverage. This is especially important for people who may be dealing with a newly diagnosed disease or a chronic disorder in themselves or in a family member. People looking for preventive guidance, information about disease warning signs, medical statistics, and risk factors for health problems will also find answers to their questions in the *Health Reference Series*. The *Series*, however, is not intended to serve as a tool for diagnosing illness, in prescribing treatments, or as a substitute for the physician/patient relationship. All people concerned about medical symptoms or the possibility of disease are encouraged to seek professional care from an appropriate healthcare provider.

A Note about Spelling and Style

Health Reference Series editors use *Stedman's Medical Dictionary* as an authority for questions related to the spelling of medical terms and the *Chicago Manual of Style* for questions related to grammatical structures, punctuation, and other editorial concerns. Consistent adherence is not always possible, however, because the individual volumes within the *Series* include many documents from a wide variety of different producers, and the editor's primary goal is to present material from each source as accurately as is possible. This sometimes means that information in different chapters or sections may follow other guidelines and alternate spelling authorities. For example, occasionally a copyright holder may require that eponymous terms be shown in possessive forms (Crohn's disease vs. Crohn disease) or that British spelling norms be retained (leukaemia vs. leukemia).

Medical Review

Omnigraphics contracts with a team of qualified, senior medical professionals who serve as medical consultants for the *Health Reference Series*. As necessary, medical consultants review reprinted and originally written material for currency and accuracy. Citations including the phrase "Reviewed (month, year)" indicate material reviewed by this team. Medical consultation services are provided to the *Health Reference Series* editors by:

Dr. Vijayalakshmi, MBBS, DGO, MD
Dr. Senthil Selvan, MBBS, DCH, MD
Dr. K. Sivanandham, MBBS, DCH, MS (Research), PhD

Our Advisory Board

We would like to thank the following board members for providing initial guidance on the development of this series:

- Dr. Lynda Baker, Associate Professor of Library and Information Science, Wayne State University, Detroit, MI

- Nancy Bulgarelli, William Beaumont Hospital Library, Royal Oak, MI

- Karen Imarisio, Bloomfield Township Public Library, Bloomfield Township, MI

- Karen Morgan, Mardigian Library, University of Michigan-Dearborn, Dearborn, MI

- Rosemary Orlando, St. Clair Shores Public Library, St. Clair Shores, MI

Health Reference Series *Update Policy*

The inaugural book in the *Health Reference Series* was the first edition of *Cancer Sourcebook* published in 1989. Since then, the *Series* has been enthusiastically received by librarians and in the medical community. In order to maintain the standard of providing high-quality health information for the layperson the editorial staff at Omnigraphics felt it was necessary to implement a policy of updating volumes when warranted.

Medical researchers have been making tremendous strides, and it is the purpose of the *Health Reference Series* to stay current with the most recent advances. Each decision to update a volume is made on an individual basis. Some of the considerations include how much new information is available and the feedback we receive from people who use the books. If there is a topic you would like to see added to the update list, or an area of medical concern you feel has not been adequately addressed, please write to:

Managing Editor
Health Reference Series
Omnigraphics
615 Griswold, Ste. 520
Detroit, MI 48226

Part One

What You Need to Know about Germs

Chapter 1

Understanding Microbes

Chapter Contents

Section 1.1—What Are Microbes? 4

Section 1.2—Microbes Can Cause Different Kinds
of Infections 8

Section 1.3—Preventing Microbial Diseases 11

Section 1.4—General Symptoms, Diagnosis, and
Treatment of Microbial Diseases 15

Section 1.1

What Are Microbes?

This section includes text excerpted from "Understanding Microbes in Sickness and in Health," National Institute of Allergy and Infectious Diseases (NIAID), January 2006. Reviewed July 2019.

Microbes are tiny organisms—too tiny to see without a microscope, yet they are abundant on Earth. They live everywhere—in air, soil, rock, and water. Some live happily in searing heat, while others thrive in freezing cold. Some microbes need oxygen to live, but others do not. These microscopic organisms are found in plants and animals, as well as in the human body.

Some microbes cause disease in humans, plants, and animals. Others are essential for a healthy life, and we could not exist without them. Indeed, the relationship between microbes and humans is delicate and complex. Some microbes keep us healthy, while others can make us sick.

Most microbes belong to one of four major groups: bacteria, viruses, fungi, or protozoa. A common word for microbes that cause disease is "germs." Some people refer to disease-causing microbes as "bugs." "I have got the flu bug," for example, is a phrase you may hear during the wintertime to describe an influenza virus infection.

Since the 19th century, we have known that microbes cause infectious diseases. Near the end of the 20th century, researchers began to learn that microbes also contribute to many chronic diseases and conditions. Mounting scientific evidence strongly links microbes to some forms of cancer, coronary artery disease, diabetes, multiple sclerosis, and chronic lung diseases.

Bacteria

Microbes belonging to the bacteria group are made up of only 1 cell. Under a microscope, bacteria look like balls, rods, or spirals. Bacteria are so small that a line of 1,000 could fit across the eraser of a pencil. Life in any form on Earth could not exist without these tiny cells.

Scientists have discovered fossilized remains of bacteria that date back more than three and a half billion years, placing them among the oldest living things on Earth. Bacteria can inhabit a variety of environments, including extremely hot and cold areas.

- Psychrophiles, or cold-loving bacteria, can live in the subfreezing temperature of the Arctic.

- Thermophiles are heat-loving bacteria that can live in extreme heat, such as in the hot springs in Yellowstone National Park.

- Extreme thermophiles, or hyperthermophiles, thrive at 235 degrees Fahrenheit near volcanic vents on the ocean floor.

Many bacteria prefer the milder temperature of the healthy human body

As with humans, some bacteria (aerobic bacteria) need oxygen to survive. Others (anaerobic bacteria), however, do not. Amazingly, some can adapt to new environments by learning to survive with or without oxygen.

As with all living cells, each bacterium requires food for energy and building materials. There are countless numbers of bacteria on Earth—most are harmless, and many are even beneficial to humans. In fact, less than one percent of bacteria cause diseases in humans. For example, harmless anaerobic bacteria, such as *Lactobacillus acidophilus*, live in our intestines, where they help to digest food, destroy disease-causing microbes, fight cancer cells, and give the body needed vitamins. Healthy food products, such as yogurt, sauerkraut, and cheese, are made using bacteria.

Some bacteria produce poisons called "toxins," which also can make us sick.

Are Toxins Always Harmful?

Certain bacteria give off toxins that can seriously affect your health. Botulism, a severe form of food poisoning, affects the nerves and is caused by toxins from Clostridium botulinum bacteria. Under certain circumstances, however, bacterial toxins can be helpful. Several vaccines that protect us from getting sick are made from bacterial toxins. One type of pertussis vaccine, which protects infants and children from whooping cough, contains toxins from *Bordetella pertussis* bacteria. This vaccine is safe and effective and causes fewer reactions than other types of pertussis vaccine.

Viruses

Viruses are among the smallest microbes, much smaller even than bacteria. Viruses are not cells. They consist of one or more molecules of deoxyribonucleic acid (DNA) or ribonucleic acid (RNA), which contain the virus's genes surrounded by a protein coat. Viruses can be rod-shaped, sphere-shaped, or multisided. Some viruses look like tadpoles.

Unlike most bacteria, most viruses do cause disease because they invade living, normal cells, such as those in your body. They then multiply and produce other viruses similar to themselves. Each virus is very particular about which cell it attacks. Various human viruses specifically attack particular cells in your body's organs, systems, or tissues, such as the liver, respiratory system, or blood.

Although types of viruses behave differently, most survive by taking over the machinery that makes a cell work. Briefly, when a piece of a virus, called a "virion," comes in contact with a cell it likes, it may attach to special landing sites on the surface of that cell. From there, the virus may inject molecules into the cell, or the cell may swallow the virion. Once inside the cell, viral molecules, such as DNA or RNA, direct the cell to make new virus offspring. That is how a virus infects a cell.

Viruses can even "infect" bacteria. These viruses, called "bacteriophages," may help researchers develop alternatives to antibiotic medicines for preventing and treating bacterial infections.

Many viral infections do not result in disease. For example, by the time most people in the United States become adults, they have been infected by cytomegalovirus (CMV). Most of these people, however, do not develop CMV-disease symptoms.

Other viral infections can result in deadly diseases, such as acquired immunodeficiency syndrome (AIDS) or Ebola hemorrhagic fever.

Fungi

A fungus is actually a primitive plant. Fungi can be found in the air, in soil, on plants, and in water. Thousands, perhaps millions, of different types of fungi exist on Earth. The most familiar ones to us are mushrooms, yeast, mold, and mildew. Some live in the human body, usually without causing illness. Fungal diseases are called "mycoses."

Mycoses can affect your skin; nails; body hair; internal organs, such as your lungs; and body systems, such as your nervous system. *Aspergillus fumigatus*, for example, can cause aspergillosis, a fungal infection in your respiratory system.

Some fungi have made our lives easier. Penicillin and other antibiotics, which kill harmful bacteria in our bodies, are made from fungi. Other fungi, such as certain yeasts, also can be helpful. For example, when a warm liquid, such as water, and a food source are added to certain yeasts, the fungus ferments. The process of fermentation is essential for making healthy foods, such as some breads and cheeses.

Protozoa

Protozoa are a group of microscopic one-celled animals. Protozoa can be parasites or predators. In humans, protozoa usually cause disease.

Some protozoa, such as plankton, live in water environments and serve as food for marine animals, such as some kinds of whales. Protozoa also can be found on land in decaying matter and in soil, but they must have a moist environment to survive. Termites would not be able to do such a good job of digesting wood without these microorganisms in their guts.

Malaria is caused by a protozoan parasite. Another protozoan parasite, *Toxoplasma gondii*, causes toxoplasmosis in humans. This is an especially troublesome infection in pregnant women because of its effects on the fetus and in people with human immunodeficiency virus (HIV) infection or other immune deficiency disorder.

Table 1.1. Microbes in the Healthy Human Body*

Found In	Microbes
Ear (outer)	*Aspergillus* (fungus)
Skin	*Candida* (fungus)
Small intestine	*Clostridium*
Intestines	*Escherichia coli*
Vagina	*Gardnerella vaginalis*
Stomach	*Lactobacillus*
Urethra	*Mycobacterium*
Nose	*Staphylococcus aureus*
Mouth	*Streptococcus salivarius*
Large intestine	*Trichomonas hominis* (protozoa)

* *A selection of usually harmless microbes, some of which help keep our bodies functioning normally. If their numbers become unbalanced, however, these microbes may make us sick. All are bacteria, unless otherwise noted.*

Section 1.2

Microbes Can Cause Different Kinds of Infections

This section includes text excerpted from "Understanding Microbes in Sickness and in Health," National Institute of Allergy and Infectious Diseases (NIAID), January 2006. Reviewed July 2019.

Microbes Infections

Some disease-causing microbes can make you very sick quickly and then not bother you again. Some can last for a long time and continue to damage tissues. Others can last forever, but you will not feel sick anymore, or you will feel sick only once in a while. Most infections caused by microbes fall into three major groups.

- Acute infections
- Chronic infections
- Latent infections

Acute Infections

Acute infections are usually severe and last a short time. They can make you feel very uncomfortable, with signs and symptoms such as tiredness, achiness, coughing, and sneezing. The common cold is such an infection. The signs and symptoms of a cold can last for 2 to 24 days (but usually a week), though it may seem such as a lot longer. Once your body's immune system has successfully fought off one of the many different types of rhinoviruses or other viruses that may have caused your cold, the cold does not come back. If you get another cold, it is probably because you have been infected with other cold-causing viruses.

Chronic Infections

Chronic infections usually develop from acute infections and can last for days to months to a lifetime. Sometimes, people are unaware they are infected but still may be able to transmit the germ to others. For example, hepatitis C, which affects the liver, is a chronic viral infection. In fact, most people who have been infected with the hepatitis C virus do not know it until they have a blood test that shows antibodies to the virus. Recovery from this infection is rare—about 85 percent of infected persons become chronic carriers of the virus. In addition, serious signs of liver damage, such as cirrhosis or cancer, may not appear until as long as 20 years after the infection began.

The Difference between Infection and Disease

A disease occurs when cells or molecules in your body stop working properly, causing symptoms of illness. Many things can cause a disease, including altered genes, chemicals, aging, and infections. An infection occurs when a microbe—such as a virus, bacterium, fungus, or parasite—enters your body and begins to reproduce. The invading microbe can directly damage cells, or the immune system can cause symptoms, such as fever, as it tries to rid your body of the invader. Some infections do not cause disease because the microbe is quickly killed or it remains dormant.

Latent Infections

Latent infections are "hidden" or "silent" and may or may not cause symptoms again after the first acute episode. Some infectious microbes, usually viruses, can "wake up"—become active again but not always causing symptoms—off and on for months or years. When these microbes are active in your body, you can transmit them to other people. Herpes simplex viruses, which cause genital herpes and cold sores, can remain latent in nerve cells for short or long periods of time, or for forever.

Chickenpox is another example of a latent infection. Before the chickenpox vaccine became available in the 1990s, most children in the United States got chickenpox. After the first acute episode, usually, when children are very young, the Varicella zoster virus goes into hiding in the body. In many people, it emerges many years later when they are older adults and causes a painful disease of the nerves called "herpes zoster," or "shingles."

Emerging and Reemerging Microbes

By the mid-20th century, some scientists thought that medicine had conquered infectious diseases. With the arrival of antibiotics and modern vaccines, as well as improved sanitation and hygiene, many diseases that formerly posed an urgent threat to public health were brought under control or largely eliminated.

The emergence of new microbes and the reemergence of old microbes has continued, however, as it has throughout history. Several pressures are contributing to the emergence of new diseases such as:

- Rapidly changing human demographics

- Rapid global travel

- Changes in land use patterns

- Ecological, environmental, and technological changes

Even public health practices, such as widespread antibiotic, use are contributing to this emergence. These pressures are both shaping the evolution of microbes and bringing people into closer and more frequent contact with microbes.

Table 1.2. Common Diseases and Infections and Their Microbial Causes

	Bacteria	Fungus	Protozoa	Virus
Athlete's foot		X		
Chickenpox				X
Common cold				X
Diarrheal disease	X		X	X
Flu				X
Genital herpes				X
Malaria			X	
Meningitis	X			X
Pneumonia	X	X		X
Sinusitis	X	X		
Skin diseases	X	X	X	X
Strep throat	X			
Tuberculosis	X			
Urinary tract infection	X			
Vaginal infections	X	X		
Viral hepatitis				X

Unsanitary conditions in animal agriculture and increasing commerce in exotic animals (for food and as pets) have also contributed to the rise in opportunity for animal microbes to jump from animals to humans. From time to time, with the right combination of selective pressures, a formerly harmless human or animal microbe can evolve into a pathogen that can cause a major outbreak of human disease. At times, changes in societal and environmental factors can also lead to the reemergence of diseases that were previously under control.

Section 1.3

Preventing Microbial Diseases

This section includes text excerpted from "Understanding Microbes in Sickness and in Health," National Institute of Allergy and Infectious Diseases (NIAID), January 2006. Reviewed July 2019.

You Can Prevent Catching or Passing on Germs
Handwashing

Handwashing is one of the simplest, easiest, and most effective ways to prevent getting or passing on many germs. Amazingly, it is also one of the most overlooked. Healthcare experts recommend scrubbing your hands vigorously for at least 15 seconds with soap and water, about as long as it takes to recite the English alphabet. This will wash away cold viruses and staph and strep bacteria, as well as many other disease-causing microbes.

It is especially important to wash your hands:

- Before preparing or eating food

- After coughing or sneezing

- After using the bathroom

- After changing a diaper

Healthcare providers should be especially conscientious about washing their hands before and after examining any patient. Workers in child care and elder care settings, too, should be vigilant about handwashing around those in their care.

Medicines

There are medicines on the market that help prevent people from getting infected by germs. For example, you can prevent getting the flu (influenza) by taking an antiviral medicine. Vaccines, however, are the best defense against influenza viruses.

Under specific circumstances, healthcare providers may prescribe antibiotics to protect people from getting certain bacteria, such as Mycobacterium tuberculosis, which causes tuberculosis (TB). Healthcare experts usually advise people traveling to areas where malaria is present to take antiparasitic medicines to prevent possible infection.

Vaccines

In 1796, Edward Jenner laid the foundation for modern vaccines by discovering one of the basic principles of immunization. He had used a relatively harmless microbe, cowpox virus, to bring about an immune response that would help protect people from getting infected by the related but deadly smallpox virus.

Dr. Jenner's discovery helped researchers find ways to ease human disease suffering worldwide. By the beginning of the 20th century, doctors were immunizing patients with vaccines for diphtheria, typhoid fever, and smallpox.

Nowadays, safe and effective vaccines prevent childhood diseases, including measles, whooping cough, chickenpox, and the form of meningitis caused by *Haemophilus influenzae type b* (Hib) virus.

Vaccines, however, are not only useful for young children. Adolescents and adults should get vaccinated regularly for tetanus and diphtheria. A vaccine to prevent meningococcal meningitis is now available and recommended for all adolescents. In addition, adults who never had diseases such as measles or chickenpox during childhood or those who never received vaccines to prevent them should consider being immunized. Childhood diseases can be far more serious in adults.

More people travel all over the world today. So, finding out which immunizations are recommended for travel to your destination(s) is even more important than ever. Vaccines also can prevent yellow fever, polio, typhoid fever, hepatitis A, cholera, rabies, and other bacterial and viral diseases that are more prevalent abroad than in the United States.

In the Fall, many adults and children may benefit from getting the flu vaccine. Your healthcare provider also may recommend immunizations for pneumococcal pneumonia and hepatitis B if you are at risk of getting these diseases.

Some Vaccine-Preventable Infectious Diseases

- Bacterial meningitis
- Chickenpox
- Cholera
- Diphtheria
- *Haemophilus influenzae type b*
- Hepatitis A
- Hepatitis B
- Flu
- Measles
- Mumps
- Pertussis (whooping cough)
- Pneumococcal pneumonia
- Polio
- Rabies
- Rubella
- Tetanus (lockjaw)
- Yellow fever

Some People Are Immune to Certain Diseases

We become immune to germs through natural and artificial means. As long ago as the 5th century B.C., Greek doctors noticed that people who had recovered from the plague would never get it again—they seemed to have become immune or resistant to the germ. You can become immune, or develop immunity, to a microbe in several ways.

The first time T cells and B cells in your immune system meet up with an antigen, such as a virus or bacterium, they prepare the immune system to destroy the antigen. Because the immune system often can remember its enemies, those cells become active if they meet that particular antigen again. This is called "naturally acquired immunity."

Another example of naturally acquired immunity occurs when a pregnant woman passes antibodies to the fetus. Babies are born with weak immune responses, but they are protected from some diseases for their first few months of life by antibodies received from their mothers before birth. Babies who are nursed also receive antibodies from breast milk that help protect their digestive tracts.

Artificial immunity can come from vaccines. Immunization with vaccines is a safe way to get protection from germs. Some vaccines contain microorganisms or parts of microorganisms that have been weakened or killed. If you get this type of vaccine, those microorganisms (or their parts) will start your body's immune response, which will demolish the foreign invader but not make you sick. This is a type of artificially acquired immunity.

Immunity can be strong or weak and short- or long-lived, depending on the type of antigen, the amount of antigen, and the route by which it enters your body. When faced with the same antigen, some people's immune system will respond forcefully, others feebly, and some not at all.

The genes you inherit also can influence your likelihood of getting a disease. In simple terms, the genes you get from your parents can influence how your body reacts to certain microbes.

Section 1.4

General Symptoms, Diagnosis, and Treatment of Microbial Diseases

This section includes text excerpted from "Understanding Microbes in Sickness and in Health," National Institute of Allergy and Infectious Diseases (NIAID), January 2006. Reviewed July 2019.

When You Should Go to the Doctor

You should call a healthcare provider immediately if:

- You have been bitten by an animal.
- You are having difficulty breathing.
- You have a cough that has lasted for more than a week.
- You have a fever higher than 100 degrees Fahrenheit.
- You have episodes of rapid heartbeat.
- You have a rash (especially if you have a fever at the same time).
- You have swelling.
- You suddenly start having difficulty with seeing (blurry vision, for example).
- You have been vomiting.

Generally, you should consult your healthcare provider if you have or think you may have an infectious disease. These trained professionals can determine whether you have been infected, determine the seriousness of your infection, and give you the best advice for treating or preventing disease. Sometimes, however, a visit to the doctor may not be necessary.

Some infectious diseases, such as the common cold, usually do not require a visit to your doctor. They often last a short time and are not life-threatening, or there is no specific treatment. We have all heard the advice to rest and drink plenty of liquids to treat colds. Unless there are complications, most victims of colds find that their immune systems successfully fight off the viral culprits. In fact, the coughing and sneezing that make you feel miserable are part of your immune system's way of fighting off the culprits.

If, however, you have other conditions in which your immune system does not function properly, you should be in contact with your healthcare provider whenever you suspect you have any infectious disease, even the common cold. Such conditions can include asthma and immune deficiency diseases, like human immunodeficiency virus (HIV) infection and acquired immunodeficiency syndrome (AIDS).

In addition, some common, usually mild infectious diseases, such as chickenpox or flu, can cause serious harm in very young children and the elderly.

Diagnosis of Microbial Diseases

Sometimes your healthcare provider can diagnose an infectious disease by listening to your medical history and doing a physical exam. For example, listening to you describe what happened and any symptoms you have noticed plays an important part in helping your doctor find out what is wrong.

Blood and urine tests are other ways to diagnose an infection. A laboratory expert can sometimes see the offending microbe in a sample of blood or urine viewed under a microscope. One or both of these tests may be the only way to determine what caused the infection, or they may be used to confirm a diagnosis that was made based on taking a medical history and doing a physical exam.

In another type of test, your healthcare provider will take a sample of blood or other body fluid, such as vaginal secretion, and then put it into a special container called a "Petri dish" to see if any microbe "grows." This test is called a "culture." Certain bacteria, such as chlamydia and strep, and viruses, such as herpes simplex, usually can be identified using this method.

X-rays, scans, and biopsies (taking a tiny sample of tissue from the infected area and inspecting it under a microscope) are among other tools the doctor can use to make an accurate diagnosis.

All of the above procedures are relatively safe, and some can be done in your doctor's office or a clinic. Others pose a higher risk to you because they involve procedures that go inside your body. One such invasive procedure is taking a biopsy from an internal organ. For example, one way a doctor can diagnose Pneumocystis carinii pneumonia, a lung disease caused by a fungus, is by doing a biopsy on lung tissue and then examining the sample under a microscope.

Treatment of Microbial Diseases

How an infectious disease is treated depends on the microbe that caused it and sometimes on the age and medical condition of the person affected. Certain diseases are not treated at all but are allowed to run their course, with the immune system doing its job alone. Some diseases, such as the common cold, are treated only to relieve the symptoms. Others, such as strep throat, are treated to destroy the offending microbe, as well as to relieve symptoms.

By Your Immune System

Your immune system has an arsenal of ways to fight off invading microbes. Most begin with B and T cells and antibodies whose sole purpose is to keep your body healthy. Some of these cells sacrifice their lives to rid you of disease and restore your body to a healthy state. Some microbes normally present in your body also help destroy microbial invaders. For example, normal bacteria, such as lactobacillus in your digestive system, help destroy disease-causing microbes.

Other important ways your body reacts to an infection include fever and coughing and sneezing.

Fever

Fever is one of your body's special ways of fighting an infectious disease. Many microbes are very sensitive to temperature changes and cannot survive in temperatures higher than normal body heat, which is usually around 98.6 degrees Fahrenheit. Your body uses fever to destroy flu viruses, for example.

Coughing and Sneezing

Another tool in your immune system's reaction to invading infection-causing microbes is mucus production. Coughing and sneezing help mucus move those germs out of your body efficiently and quickly.

Other methods your body may use to fight off an infectious disease include:

- Inflammation
- Vomiting
- Diarrhea

- Fatigue

- Cramping

By Your Healthcare Provider
For Bacteria

The last century saw an explosion in our knowledge about how microbes work and in our methods of treating infectious diseases. For example, the discovery of antibiotics to treat and cure many bacterial diseases was a major breakthrough in medical history. Doctors, however, sometimes prescribe antibiotics unnecessarily for a variety of reasons, including pressure from patients with viral infections. Patients may insist on being prescribed an antibiotic without knowing that it will not work on viruses. Colds and flu are two notable viral infections for which some doctors send their patients to the drugstore with a prescription for an antibiotic.

Because antibiotics have been overprescribed or inappropriately prescribed for many years, bacteria have become resistant to the killing effects of these drugs. This resistance, called "antibiotic resistance" or "drug resistance," has become a very serious problem, especially in hospital settings.

Bacteria that are not killed by the antibiotic become strong enough to resist the same medicine the next time it is given. Because bacteria multiply so rapidly, changed or mutated bacteria that resist antibiotics will quickly outnumber those that can be destroyed by those same drugs.

For Viruses

Viral diseases can be very difficult to treat because viruses live inside your body's cells where they are protected from medicines in the bloodstream. Researchers developed the first antiviral drug in the late 20th century. The drug, acyclovir, was first approved by the U.S. Food and Drug Administration (FDA) to treat herpes simplex virus infections. Only a few other antiviral medicines are available to prevent and treat viral infections and diseases.

Healthcare providers treat HIV infection with a group of powerful medicines that can keep the virus in check. Known as "highly active antiretroviral therapy" (HAART), this treatment has improved the lives of many suffering from this deadly infection.

Viral diseases should never be treated with antibiotics. Sometimes, a person with a viral disease will develop a bacterial disease as a complication of the initial viral disease. For example, children with chickenpox often scratch the skin lesions (sores) caused by the viral infection. Bacteria, such as staph, can enter those lesions and cause a bacterial infection. The doctor may then prescribe an antibiotic to destroy the bacteria. The antibiotic, however, will not work on the chickenpox virus. It will work only against staph.

Although safe and effective treatments and cures for most viral diseases have eluded researchers, there are safe vaccines to protect you from viral infections and diseases.

For Fungi

Medicines applied directly to the infected area are available by prescription and over-the-counter (OTC) for treating skin and nail fungal infections. Unfortunately, many people have had limited success with them. During the 1990s, oral prescription medicines became available for treating fungal infections of the skin and nails.

For many years, very powerful oral antifungal medicines were used only to treat systemic (within the body) fungal infections, such as histoplasmosis. Doctors usually prescribe oral antifungal medications cautiously because all of them, even the milder medicines for skin and nail fungi, can have very serious side effects.

For Protozoa

Diseases caused by protozoan parasites are among the leading causes of death and disease in tropical and subtropical regions of the world. Developing countries within these areas contain three-quarters of the world's population, and their people suffer the most from these diseases. Controlling parasitic diseases is a problem because there are no vaccines for any of them.

In many cases, controlling the insects that transmit these diseases is difficult because of pesticide resistance, concerns regarding environmental damage, and lack of adequate public health systems to apply existing insect control methods. Thus, disease control relies heavily on the availability of medicines. Healthcare providers usually use antiparasitic medicines to treat protozoal infections. Unfortunately, there are very few medicines that fight protozoa, and some of those are either harmful to humans or are becoming ineffective.

The fight against the protozoan Plasmodium falciparum, the cause of the most deadly form of malaria, is a good example. This protozoan has become resistant to most of the medicines currently available to destroy it. A major focus of malaria research is on developing a vaccine to prevent people from getting the disease. In the meantime, many worldwide programs hope to eventually control malaria by keeping people from contact with infected mosquitoes or preventing infection if contact cannot be avoided.

Chapter 2

Immunity: An Overview

Chapter Contents

Section 2.1—The Immune System 22

Section 2.2—Immune System Response to Infection 24

Section 2.1

The Immune System

This section includes text excerpted from "Overview of the Immune System," National Institute of Allergy and Infectious Diseases (NIAID), December 30, 2013. Reviewed July 2019.

Function

The overall function of the immune system is to prevent or limit infection. An example of this principle is found in immune-compromised people, including those with genetic immune disorders; immune-debilitating infections, such as human immunodeficiency virus (HIV); and even pregnant women, who are susceptible to a range of microbes that typically do not cause infection in healthy individuals.

The immune system can distinguish between normal, healthy cells and unhealthy cells by recognizing a variety of "danger" cues called "danger-associated molecular patterns" (DAMPs). Cells may be unhealthy because of infection or because of cellular damage caused by noninfectious agents, such as sunburn or cancer. Infectious microbes, such as viruses and bacteria, release another set of signals recognized by the immune system called "pathogen-associated molecular patterns" (PAMPs).

When the immune system first recognizes these signals, it responds to address the problem. If an immune response cannot be activated when there is sufficient need, problems arise, such as an infection. On the other hand, when an immune response is activated without a real threat or is not turned off once the danger passes, different problems arise, such as allergic reactions and autoimmune disease.

The immune system is complex and pervasive. There are numerous cell types that either circulates throughout the body or reside in a particular tissue. Each cell type plays a unique role, with different ways of recognizing problems, communicating with other cells, and performing their functions. By understanding all the details behind this network, researchers may optimize immune responses to confront specific issues, ranging from infections to cancer.

Location

All immune cells come from precursors in the bone marrow and develop into mature cells through a series of changes that can occur in different parts of the body.

Skin

The skin is usually the first line of defense against microbes. Skin cells produce and secrete important antimicrobial proteins, and immune cells can be found in specific layers of skin.

Bone Marrow

The bone marrow contains stems cells that can develop into a variety of cell types. The common myeloid progenitor stem cell in the bone marrow is the precursor to innate immune cells—neutrophils, eosinophils, basophils, mast cells, monocytes, dendritic cells, and macrophages—that are important first-line responders to infection.

The common lymphoid progenitor stem cell leads to adaptive immune cells—B cells and T cells—that are responsible for mounting responses to specific microbes based on previous encounters (immunological memory). Natural killer (NK) cells also are derived from the common lymphoid progenitor and share features of both innate and adaptive immune cells, as they provide immediate defenses similar to innate cells but also may be retained as memory cells like adaptive cells. B, T, and NK cells also are called "lymphocytes."

Bloodstream

Immune cells constantly circulate throughout the bloodstream, patrolling for problems. When blood tests are used to monitor "white blood cells" (WBCs), another term for immune cells, a snapshot of the immune system is taken. If a cell type is either scarce or overabundant in the bloodstream, this may reflect a problem.

Thymus

T cells mature in the thymus, a small organ located in the upper chest.

Lymphatic System

The lymphatic system is a network of vessels and tissues composed of lymph, an extracellular fluid, and lymphoid organs, such as lymph nodes. The lymphatic system is a conduit for travel and communication between tissues and the bloodstream. Immune cells are carried through the lymphatic system and converge in lymph nodes, which are found throughout the body.

Lymph nodes are a communication hub where immune cells sample information brought in from the body. For instance, if adaptive immune cells in the lymph node recognize pieces of a microbe brought in from a distant area, they will activate, replicate, and leave the lymph node to circulate and address the pathogen. Thus, doctors may check patients for swollen lymph nodes, which may indicate an active immune response.

Spleen

The spleen is an organ located behind the stomach. While it is not directly connected to the lymphatic system, it is important for processing information from the bloodstream. Immune cells are enriched in specific areas of the spleen, and upon recognizing blood-borne pathogens, they will activate and respond accordingly.

Mucosal Tissue

Mucosal surfaces are prime entry points for pathogens, and specialized immune hubs are strategically located in mucosal tissues, such as the respiratory tract and gut. For instance, Peyer's patches are important areas in the small intestine where immune cells can access samples from the gastrointestinal tract.

Section 2.2

Immune System Response to Infection

This section includes text excerpted from "Overview of the Immune System," National Institute of Allergy and Infectious Diseases (NIAID), December 30, 2013. Reviewed July 2019.

Features of an Immune Response

An immune response is generally divided into innate and adaptive immunity. Innate immunity occurs immediately, when circulating innate cells recognize a problem. Adaptive immunity occurs later, as it relies on the coordination and expansion of specific adaptive immune cells. Immune memory follows the adaptive response, when mature adaptive cells, highly specific to the original pathogen, are retained for later use.

Innate Immunity

Innate immune cells express genetically encoded receptors, called "Toll-like receptors" (TLRs), which recognize general danger- or pathogen-associated patterns. Collectively, these receptors can broadly recognize viruses, bacteria, fungi, and even noninfectious problems. However, they cannot distinguish between specific strains of bacteria or viruses.

There are numerous types of innate immune cells with specialized functions. They include neutrophils, eosinophils, basophils, mast cells, monocytes, dendritic cells, and macrophages. Their main feature is the ability to respond quickly and broadly when a problem arises, typically leading to inflammation. Innate immune cells also are important for activating adaptive immunity. Innate cells are critical for host defense, and disorders in innate cell function may cause chronic susceptibility to infection.

Adaptive Immunity

Adaptive immune cells are more specialized, with each adaptive B or T cell bearing unique receptors, B-cell receptors (BCRs) and T-cell receptors (TCRs), that recognize specific signals rather than general patterns. Each receptor recognizes an antigen, which is simply any molecule that may bind to a BCR or TCR. Antigens are derived from a variety of sources, including pathogens, host cells, and allergens. Antigens are typically processed by innate immune cells and presented to adaptive cells in the lymph nodes.

The genes for BCRs and TCRs are randomly rearranged at specific cell maturation stages, resulting in unique receptors that may potentially recognize anything. Random generation of receptors allows the immune system to respond to new or unforeseen problems. This concept is especially important because environments may frequently change, for instance when seasons change or a person relocates, and pathogens are constantly evolving to survive. Because BCRs and TCRs are so specific, adaptive cells may only recognize one strain of a particular pathogen, unlike innate cells, which recognize broad classes of pathogens. In fact, a group of adaptive cells that recognize the same strain will likely recognize different areas of that pathogen.

If a B or T cell has a receptor that recognizes an antigen from a pathogen and also receives cues from innate cells that something is wrong, the B or T cell will activate, divide, and disperse to address the problem. B cells make antibodies, which neutralize pathogens, rendering them harmless. T cells carry out multiple functions, including killing infected cells and activating or recruiting other immune cells. The adaptive response has a system of checks and balances to prevent unnecessary activation that could cause damage to the host. If a B or T cell is autoreactive, meaning its receptor recognizes antigens from the body's own cells, the cell will be deleted. Also, if a B or T cell does not receive signals from innate cells, it will not be optimally activated.

Immune memory is a feature of the adaptive immune response. After B or T cells are activated, they expand rapidly. As the problem resolves, cells stop dividing and are retained in the body as memory cells. The next time this same pathogen enters the body, a memory cell is already poised to react and can clear away the pathogen before it establishes itself.

Vaccination

Vaccination, or immunization, is a way to train your immune system against a specific pathogen. Vaccination achieves immune memory without an actual infection, so the body is prepared when the virus or bacterium enters. Saving time is important to prevent a pathogen from establishing itself and infecting more cells in the body.

An effective vaccine will optimally activate both the innate and adaptive response. An immunogen is used to activate the adaptive immune response so that specific memory cells are generated. Because BCRs and TCRs are unique, some memory cells are simply better at eliminating the pathogen. The goal of vaccine design is to select immunogens that will generate the most effective and efficient memory response against a particular pathogen. Adjuvants, which are important for activating innate immunity, can be added to vaccines to optimize the immune response. Innate immunity recognizes broad patterns, and without innate responses, adaptive immunity cannot be optimally achieved.

Immune Cells

Granulocytes include basophils, eosinophils, and neutrophils. Basophils and eosinophils are important for host defense against parasites. They also are involved in allergic reactions. Neutrophils, the most numerous innate immune cell, patrol for problems by circulating in the bloodstream. They can phagocytose, or ingest, bacteria, degrading them inside special compartments called "vesicles."

Mast cells also are important for defense against parasites. Mast cells are found in tissues and can mediate allergic reactions by releasing inflammatory chemicals, such as histamine.

Monocytes, which develop into macrophages, also patrol and respond to problems. They are found in the bloodstream and in tissues. Macrophages, which means "big eater" in Greek, are named for their ability to ingest and degrade bacteria. Upon activation, monocytes and macrophages coordinate an immune response by notifying other immune cells of the problem. Macrophages also have important nonimmune functions, such as recycling dead cells, like red blood cells (RBCs), and clearing away cellular debris. These "housekeeping" functions occur without activation of an immune response.

Neutrophils accumulate within minutes at sites of local tissue injury (center). They then communicate with each other using lipid and other secreted mediators to form cellular "swarms." Their coordinated movement and exchange of signals then instruct other innate immune cells called "macrophages" and "monocytes" to surround the neutrophil cluster and form a tight wound seal.

Dendritic cells (DC) are an important antigen-presenting cell (APC), and they also can develop from monocytes. Antigens are molecules from pathogens, host cells, and allergens that may be recognized by adaptive immune cells. Similar to DCs, APCs are responsible for processing large molecules into "readable" fragments (antigens) recognized by adaptive B or T cells. However, antigens alone cannot activate T cells. They must be presented with the appropriate major histocompatibility complex (MHC) expressed on the APC. MHC provides a checkpoint and helps immune cells distinguish between host and foreign cells.

Natural killer (NK) cells have features of both innate and adaptive immunity. They are important for recognizing and killing virus-infected cells or tumor cells. They contain intracellular compartments called "granules," which are filled with proteins that can form holes in the target cell and also cause apoptosis, the process for programmed cell death. It is important to distinguish between apoptosis and other forms of cell death, such as necrosis. Apoptosis, unlike necrosis, does not release danger signals that can lead to greater immune activation and inflammation. Through apoptosis, immune cells can discreetly remove infected cells and limit bystander damage. Recently, researchers have shown in mouse models that NK cells, similar to adaptive cells, can be retained as memory cells and respond to subsequent infections by the same pathogen.

Adaptive Cells

B cells have two major functions: They present antigens to T cells, and more importantly, they produce antibodies to neutralize infectious microbes. Antibodies coat the surface of a pathogen and serve three major roles: neutralization, opsonization, and complement activation.

Neutralization occurs when the pathogen, because it is covered in antibodies, is unable to bind and infect host cells. In opsonization, an antibody-bound pathogen serves as a red flag to alert immune cells, such as neutrophils and macrophages, to engulf and digest the pathogen. Complement is a process for directly destroying, or lysing, bacteria.

Antibodies are expressed in two ways. The B-cell receptor (BCR), which sits on the surface of a B cell, is actually an antibody. B cells also secrete antibodies to diffuse and bind to pathogens. This dual expression is important because the initial problem, for instance, a bacterium, is recognized by a unique BCR and activates the B cell. The activated B cell responds by secreting antibodies, essentially the BCR but in soluble form. This ensures that the response is specific against the bacterium that started the whole process.

Every antibody is unique, but they fall under general categories: IgM, IgD, IgG, IgA, and IgE. (Ig is short for immunoglobulin, which is another word for antibody.) While they have overlapping roles, IgM generally is important for complement activation; IgD is involved in activating basophils; IgG is important for neutralization, opsonization, and complement activation; IgA is essential for neutralization in the gastrointestinal tract; and IgE is necessary for activating mast cells in parasitic and allergic responses.

T cells have a variety of roles and are classified by subsets. T cells are divided into two broad categories: CD8+ T cells or CD4+ T cells, based on which protein is present on the cell's surface. T cells carry out multiple functions, including killing infected cells and activating or recruiting other immune cells.

CD8+ T cells also are called "cytotoxic T cells" or "cytotoxic lymphocytes" (CTLs). They are crucial for recognizing and removing virus-infected cells and cancer cells. CTLs have specialized compartments, or granules, containing cytotoxins that cause apoptosis, i.e., programmed cell death. Because of its potency, the release of granules is tightly regulated by the immune system.

The four major CD4+ T-cell subsets are TH1, TH2, TH17, and Treg, with "TH" referring to "T helper cell." TH1 cells are critical for coordinating immune responses against intracellular microbes, especially bacteria. They produce and secrete molecules that alert and activate other immune cells, such as bacteria-ingesting macrophages. TH2 cells are important for coordinating immune responses against extracellular pathogens, such as helminths (parasitic worms), by alerting B cells, granulocytes, and mast cells. TH17 cells are named for their ability to produce interleukin 17 (IL-17), a signaling molecule that activates immune and nonimmune cells. TH17 cells are important for recruiting neutrophils.

Regulatory T cells (Tregs), as the name suggests, monitor and inhibit the activity of other T cells. They prevent adverse immune activation and maintain tolerance or the prevention of immune responses against the body's own cells and antigens.

Communication

Immune cells communicate in a number of ways, either by cell-to-cell contact or through secreted signaling molecules. Receptors and ligands are fundamental for cellular communication. Receptors are protein structures that may be expressed on the surface of a cell or in intracellular compartments. The molecules that activate receptors are called "ligands," which may be free-floating or membrane-bound.

Ligand-receptor interaction leads to a series of events inside the cell involving networks of intracellular molecules that relay the message. By altering the expression and density of various receptors and ligands, immune cells can dispatch specific instructions tailored to the situation at hand.

Cytokines are small proteins with diverse functions. In immunity, there are several categories of cytokines important for immune cell growth, activation, and function.

- Colony-stimulating factors are essential for cell development and differentiation.

- Interferons are necessary for immune-cell activation. Type I interferons mediate antiviral immune responses, and type II interferon is important for antibacterial responses.

- Interleukins, which come in over 30 varieties, provide context-specific instructions, with activating or inhibitory responses.

- Chemokines are made in specific locations of the body or at a site of infection to attract immune cells. Different chemokines will recruit different immune cells to the site needed.

- The tumor necrosis factor (TNF) family of cytokines stimulates immune-cell proliferation and activation. They are critical for activating inflammatory responses, and as such, TNF blockers are used to treat a variety of disorders, including some autoimmune diseases.

Toll-like receptors are expressed on innate immune cells, such as macrophages and dendritic cells. They are located on the cell surface or in intracellular compartments because microbes may be found in the body or inside infected cells. TLRs recognize general microbial patterns, and they are essential for innate immune-cell activation and inflammatory responses.

B-cell receptors and T-cell receptors are expressed on adaptive immune cells. They are both found on the cell surface, but BCRs also are secreted as antibodies to neutralize pathogens. The genes for BCRs and TCRs are randomly rearranged at specific cell maturation stages, resulting in unique receptors that may potentially recognize anything. Random generation of receptors allows the immune system to respond to unforeseen problems. They also explain why memory B or T cells are highly specific and, upon re-encountering their specific pathogen, can immediately induce a neutralizing immune response.

Major histocompatibility complex (MHC), or human leukocyte antigen (HLA), proteins serve two general roles.

Major histocompatibility complex proteins function as carriers to present antigens on cell surfaces. MHC class I proteins are essential for presenting viral antigens and are expressed by nearly all cell types, except red blood cells. Any cell infected by a virus has the ability to signal the problem through MHC class I proteins. In response, CD8+ T cells (also called "CTLs") will recognize and kill infected cells. MHC class II proteins are generally only expressed by antigen-presenting cells, such as dendritic cells and macrophages. MHC class II proteins are important for presenting antigens to CD4+ T cells. MHC class II antigens are varied and include both pathogen- and host-derived molecules.

Major histocompatibility complex proteins also signal whether a cell is a host cell or a foreign cell. They are very diverse, and every person has a unique set of MHC proteins inherited from her or his parents. As such, there are similarities in MHC proteins between family members. Immune cells use MHC to determine whether or not a cell is friendly. In organ transplantation, the MHC or HLA proteins of donors and recipients are matched to lower the risk of transplant rejection, which occurs when the recipient's immune system attacks the donor tissue or organ. In stem cell or bone marrow transplantation, improper MHC or HLA matching can result in graft-versus-host disease, which occurs when the donor cells attack the recipient's body.

Complement refers to a unique process that clears away pathogens or dying cells and also activates immune cells. Complement consists of a series of proteins found in the blood that forms a membrane-attack complex. Complement proteins are only activated by enzymes when a problem, such as an infection, occurs. Activated complement proteins stick to a pathogen, recruiting and activating additional complement proteins, which assemble in a specific order to form a round pore or hole. Complement literally punches small holes into the pathogen, creating leaks that lead to cell death. Complement proteins also serve as signaling molecules that alert immune cells and recruit them to the problem area.

Immune Tolerance

Tolerance is the prevention of an immune response against a particular antigen. For instance, the immune system is generally tolerant of self-antigens, so it does not usually attack the body's own cells, tissues, and organs. However, when tolerance is lost, disorders such as autoimmune disease or food allergy may occur. Tolerance is maintained in a number of ways:

- When adaptive immune cells mature, there are several checkpoints in place to eliminate autoreactive cells. If a B cell produces antibodies that strongly recognize host cells, or if a T cell strongly recognizes self-antigen, they are deleted.

- Nevertheless, there are autoreactive immune cells present in healthy individuals. Autoreactive immune cells are kept in a nonreactive, or anergic, state. Even though they recognize the body's own cells, they do not have the ability to react and cannot cause host damage.

31

- Regulatory immune cells circulate throughout the body to maintain tolerance. Besides limiting autoreactive cells, regulatory cells are important for turning an immune response off after the problem is resolved. They can act as drains, depleting areas of essential nutrients that surrounding immune cells need for activation or survival.

- Some locations in the body are called "immunologically privileged sites." These areas, such as the eye and brain, do not typically elicit strong immune responses. Part of this is because of physical barriers, such as the blood-brain barrier, that limits the degree to which immune cells may enter. These areas also may express higher levels of suppressive cytokines to prevent a robust immune response.

Fetomaternal tolerance is the prevention of a maternal immune response against a developing fetus. Major histocompatibility complex proteins help the immune system distinguish between host and foreign cells. MHC also is called "human leukocyte antigen." By expressing paternal MHC or HLA proteins and paternal antigens, a fetus can potentially trigger the mother's immune system. However, there are several barriers that may prevent this from occurring: The placenta reduces the exposure of the fetus to maternal immune cells, the proteins expressed on the outer layer of the placenta may limit immune recognition, and regulatory cells and suppressive signals may play a role.

Transplantation of a donor tissue or organ requires appropriate MHC or HLA matching to limit the risk of rejection. Because MHC or HLA matching is rarely complete, transplant recipients must continuously take immunosuppressive drugs, which can cause complications such as higher susceptibility to infection and some cancers. Researchers are developing more targeted ways to induce tolerance to transplanted tissues and organs while leaving protective immune responses intact.

Chapter 3

Immunodeficiency and Contagious Diseases

Immunodeficiency is a disease wherein your body's immune system is either absent or not functioning properly. This disease impairs the immune system's ability to defend against foreign cells, such as cancer cells, bacteria, virus, and fungi, invading your body.

Types of Immunodeficiency Diseases

There are two types of immunodeficiency diseases:

- Primary immunodeficiency (PID)
- Secondary immunodeficiency (SID)

Primary Immunodeficiency

Primary immunodeficiency disorder is usually acquired from birth and is hereditary. Most PIDs manifest during childhood and infancy. There are many types of PIDs, and all are relatively rare.

Primary immunodeficiency disorders are sometimes caused by single-gene mutations, but mostly by the susceptibility of genes combined with environmental factors. Primary immunodeficiency

---

disorders are categorized based on the part of the immune system that is affected. Examples of PIDs are:

Common variable immune deficiency (CVID). Common variable immune deficiencies (CVIDs) are the most commonly diagnosed form of PIDs, especially in adults, and are characterized by low levels of antibodies and serum immunoglobins, causing more susceptibility to infections.

B cell immunodeficiencies. The main role of the B cells is to produce antibodies, which helps the immune system to detect and kill invading microbes. Mutations in the B cells, which control genes, can affect the production of antibodies, which can in turn result in severe recurrent bacterial infections.

T cell immunodeficiencies. One role of the T cells is to activate the B cells and to pass information about the identity of the microbe, so that the B cells can produce the right antibodies. Some T cells get involved in killing the invading microbes. Mutations in the genes that control T cells can result in fewer T cells or in ones that have low functionality. This can cause disruptions in their killing ability and can also affect B cell functions.

Secondary Immunodeficiency

Secondary immunodeficiency is normally acquired after birth and is more common than PID. Secondary immunodeficiency is commonly acquired from primary illnesses such as human immunodeficiency virus (HIV). Examples of secondary immunodeficiency disorders are:

Malnutrition. One of the most common causes of SID is protein-calorie malnutrition. Deficiency in protein can affect the production of T cells and their functions. This leaves you susceptible to diarrhea and infections related to the respiratory tract.

Drug regimens. Taking certain drugs used for other primary illness, such as an immunosuppressive drug in cancer treatment, may result in SID. The immunosuppressive drug usage is to prevent transplant rejection, wherein the drug is used to suppress the immune system of the transplant recipient and prevent the immune system from attacking the transplanted tissue. These drugs have significant side effects and can suppress more areas of the immune system, leading to susceptibility to infections.

Signs and Symptoms of Immunodeficiency Diseases

Having infections that are longer lasting, frequent, and harder to treat are the most common signs that denote the presence of immunodeficiency diseases. You may also get infections that healthy people could fight off. The signs and symptoms of immunodeficiency diseases include:

- Infection and inflammation of internal organs
- Blood disorders (anemia or low platelet counts)
- Delayed growth and development
- Autoimmune disorders (type 1 diabetes, lupus, or rheumatoid arthritis)
- Problems in the digestive system (cramping, loss of appetite, nausea, and diarrhea)
- Frequent and recurrent infections in the sinuses, ears, or skin.

Other signs and symptoms may include:

- Bacterial infections that may cause pus-filled sores
- Chronic gum disease (gingivitis)
- Frequent fever and chillness
- Infections in the ears, nose, and digestive tract

These symptoms vary based on the duration and severity of the infection.

Diagnosis of Immunodeficiency Diseases

The diagnosis of immunodeficiency diseases is as follows:

- Physical examination
- Blood tests
- Biopsy

Physical Examination

The doctor may conduct a physical examination to find the presence of immunodeficiency diseases by examining:

- Enlargement in spleen

- Problems with lymph nodes and tonsils

The doctor may ask questions about your history, such as drug usage for any previous illness, exposure to toxic substances, the possibility of family members with immunodeficiency disorder, use of intravenous drugs, and previous blood transfusions.

Blood Tests

The doctor will order blood tests, including a complete blood count (CBC). A CBC test can detect abnormalities in blood cells, which can help your doctor determine the presence of immunodeficiency disease. A blood sample is taken and tested to determine your white blood cell (WBC) count. The sample is observed under a microscope to check for abnormalities. The immunoglobin levels are also checked after vaccination.

Biopsy

A biopsy is performed to identify the type of immunodeficiency disease. The doctor takes a sample from bone marrow and/or lymph nodes. These samples are used to determine whether the immune cells are present.

Treatment of Immunodeficiency Diseases

The treatment for immunodeficiency diseases is based on specific conditions and involves immunoglobin therapy and antibiotics. Antiviral drugs, such as acyclovir and amantadine or a drug called "interferon," are used to treat viral infections caused by immunodeficiency disorders.

Your doctor may suggest an immune globulin injection to replace the missing antibodies in your body. If the severity of the immunodeficiency disease is high, the doctor may perform a stem-cell transplant.

The risk of contagious diseases is high if you have immunodeficiency diseases such as HIV or cancer.

References

1. "Primary Immunodeficiency," Mayo Clinic, September 14, 2018.

2. "Immunodeficiency," British Society for Immunology (BSI), November 2017.

3.   Fernandez, James. "Overview of Immunodeficiency Disorders," MSD and the MSD Manuals, June 2018.

4.   "Primary Immunodeficiency Disease," American Academy of Allergy, Asthma & Immunology (AAAAI), December 16, 2016.

5.   "Immunodeficiency Disorders," Healthline, August 30, 2016.

Chapter 4

Transmission of Contagious Disease

Chapter Contents

Section 4.1—Transmission of Microbes That Cause
Contagious Disease 40

Section 4.2—Preventing the Transmission of
Sexually Transmitted Disease 44

Section 4.3—Risk of Infectious Disease from
Blood Transfusion 46

Section 4.4—Contagious Disease Transmission on
Airplanes and Cruise Ships..................................... 54

Section 4.1

Transmission of Microbes That Cause Contagious Disease

This section includes text excerpted from "Understanding Microbes
in Sickness and in Health," National Institute of Allergy and
Infectious Diseases (NIAID), January 2006. Reviewed July 2019.

Microbes Can Make Us Sick

According to healthcare experts, infectious diseases caused by
microbes are responsible for more deaths worldwide than any other
single cause. They estimate the annual cost of medical care for treating
infectious diseases in the United States alone is about $120 billion.

The science of microbiology explores how microbes work and how to
control them. It seeks ways to use that knowledge to prevent and treat
the diseases microbes cause. The 20th century saw an extraordinary
increase in our knowledge about microbes. Microbiologists and other
researchers had many successes in learning how microbes cause certain infectious diseases and how to combat those microbes.

Unfortunately, microbes are much better at adapting to new environments than are people. Having existed on Earth for billions of
years, microbes are constantly challenging human newcomers with
ingenious new survival tactics.

- Many microbes are developing new properties to resist drug
  treatments that once effectively destroyed them. Drug resistance
  has become a serious problem worldwide.

- Changes in the environment have put certain human
  populations in contact with newly identified microbes that cause
  diseases we have never seen before or those that previously
  occurred only in isolated populations.

- Newly emerging diseases are a growing global health concern.
  Since 1976, scientists have identified approximately 30 new
  pathogens.

Microbes Can Infect Us

Below are some of the many different ways you can get infected
by germs.

Some Microbes Can Travel through the Air

You can transmit microbes to another person through the air by coughing or sneezing. These are common ways to get viruses that cause colds or the flu, or the bacteria that cause tuberculosis (TB). Interestingly, international airplane travel can expose you to germs not common in your own country.

Close Contact Can Pass Germs to Another Person

Scientists have identified more than 500 types of bacteria that live in our mouths. Some keep the oral environment healthy, while others cause problems such as gum disease. One way you can transmit oral bacteria is by kissing.

Microbes such as human immunodeficiency virus (HIV), herpes simplex virus (HSV), and gonorrhea bacteria are examples of germs that can be transmitted directly during sexual intercourse.

You Can Pick up and Spread Germs by Touching Infectious Material

A common way for some microbes to enter the body, especially when caring for young children, is through unintentionally passing feces from hand to mouth or the mouths of young children. Infant diarrhea is often spread in this way. Day care workers, for example, can pass diarrhea-causing rotavirus or *Giardia lamblia* (protozoa) from one baby to the next between diaper changes and other child care practices.

It also is possible to pick up cold viruses from shaking someone's hand or from touching contaminated surfaces, such as a handrail or telephone.

A Healthy Person Can Carry Germs and Pass Them onto Others

The story of "Typhoid Mary" is a famous example from medical history about how a person can pass germs on to others yet not be affected by those germs. The germs, in this case, were *Salmonella typhi* bacteria, which cause typhoid fever and are usually spread through food or water.

In the early 20th century, Mary Mallon, an Irish immigrant, worked as a cook for several New York City families. More than half of the first family she worked for came down with typhoid fever. Through a clever deduction, a researcher determined that the disease was caused by the family cook. He concluded that although Mary had no symptoms of the disease, she probably had a mild typhoid infection sometime in the past. Though not sick, she still carried the *Salmonella* bacteria and was able to spread them to others through the food she prepared.

Germs from Your Household Pet Can Make You Sick

You can catch a variety of germs from animals, especially household pets. The rabies virus, which can infect cats and dogs, is one of the most serious and deadly of these microbes. Fortunately, rabies vaccine prevents animals from getting rabies. Vaccines protect people from accidentally getting the virus from an animal. They also prevent people who already have been exposed to the virus, such as through an animal bite, from getting sick.

Dog and cat saliva can contain any of more than 100 different germs that can make you sick. *Pasteurella* bacteria, the most common, can be transmitted through bites that break the skin causing serious, and sometimes fatal, diseases such as blood infections and meningitis. Meningitis is an inflammation of the lining of the brain and spinal cord.

Warm-blooded animals are not the only ones that can cause you harm. Pet reptiles, such as turtles, snakes, and iguanas, can give *Salmonella* bacteria to their unsuspecting owners.

You Can Get Microbes from Tiny Critters

Mosquitoes may be the most common insect carriers, also called "vectors," of pathogens. *Anopheles* mosquitoes can pick up *Plasmodium*, which causes malaria, from the blood of an infected person and transmit the protozoan to an uninfected person.

Fleas that pick up *Yersinia pestis* bacteria from rodents can then transmit plague to humans. Ticks, which are more closely related to crabs than to insects, are another common vector. The tiny deer tick can infect humans with *Borrelia burgdorferi*, the bacterium that causes Lyme disease, which the tick picks up from mice.

Some Microbes in Food or Water Could Make You Sick

Every year, millions of people worldwide become ill from eating contaminated foods. Although many cases of foodborne illness or "food poisoning" are not reported, the Centers for Disease Control and Prevention (CDC) estimates that there are 76 million cases of such illnesses in the United States each year. In addition, the CDC estimates that 325,000 hospitalizations and 5,000 deaths are related to foodborne diseases each year. Microbes can cause these illnesses, some of which can be fatal if not treated properly.

Poor manufacturing processes or poor food preparation can allow microbes to grow in food and, subsequently, infect the consumer. *Escherichia coli (E. coli)* bacteria sometimes persist in food products such as undercooked hamburger 18 meat and unpasteurized fruit juice. These bacteria can have deadly consequences in vulnerable people, especially children and the elderly.

Cryptosporidia are bacteria found in human and animal feces. These bacteria can get into the lake, river, and ocean water from sewage spills, animal waste, and water runoff. Millions can be released from infectious fecal matter. People who drink, swim, or play in infected water can get sick.

People, including babies, with diarrhea caused by *Cryptosporidia* or other diarrhea-causing microbes, such as *Giardia* and *Salmonella*, can infect others while using swimming pools, waterparks, hot tubs, and spas.

Transplanted Animal Organs May Harbor Germs

Researchers are investigating the possibility of transplanting animal organs, such as pig hearts, into people. They, however, must guard against the risk that those organs also may transmit microbes that were harmless to the animal into humans, where they may cause disease.

Section 4.2

Preventing the Transmission of Sexually Transmitted Disease

This section contains text excerpted from the following sources: Text in this section begins with excerpts from "Sexually Transmitted Diseases," MedlinePlus, National Institutes of Health (NIH), October 23, 2017; Text beginning with the heading "Get the Facts" is excerpted from "How You Can Prevent Sexually Transmitted Diseases," Centers for Disease Control and Prevention (CDC), January 21, 2016.

Sexually transmitted diseases (STDs) are infections that are passed from one person to another through sexual contact. The causes of STDs are bacteria, parasites, yeast, and viruses. There are more than 20 types of STDs, including:

- Chlamydia

- Genital herpes

- Gonorrhea

- Human immunodeficiency virus/acquired immunodeficiency syndrome (HIV/AIDS)

- Human papillomavirus (HPV)

- Syphilis

- Trichomoniasis

Most STDs affect both men and women, but in many cases, the health problems they cause can be more severe for women. If a pregnant woman has an STD, it can cause serious health problems for the fetus.

Get the Facts

Arm yourself with basic information about STDs:

- How are these diseases spread?

- How can you protect yourself?

- What are the treatment options?

Take Control

You have the facts; now, protect yourself and your sexual partners.

Abstinence

The most reliable way to avoid infection is to not have sex (i.e., anal, vaginal or oral).

Vaccination

Vaccines are safe, effective, and recommended ways to prevent hepatitis B and HPV. HPV vaccines for males and females can protect against some of the most common types of HPV. It is best to get all 3 doses (shots) before becoming sexually active. However, HPV vaccines are recommended for all teen girls and women through age 26 and all teen boys and men through age 21 who did not get all 3 doses of the vaccine when they were younger. You should also get vaccinated for hepatitis B if you were not vaccinated when you were younger.

Reduce Number of Sex Partners

Reducing your number of sex partners can decrease your risk for STDs. It is still important that you and your partner get tested and that you share your test results with one another.

Mutual Monogamy

Mutual monogamy means that you agree to be sexually active with only one person who has also agreed to be sexually active only with you. Being in a long-term mutually monogamous relationship with an uninfected partner is one of the most reliable ways to avoid STDs. But, you must both be certain you are not infected with STDs. It is important to have an open and honest conversation with your partner.

Use Condoms

Correct and consistent use of the male latex condom is highly effective in reducing STD transmission. Use a condom every time you have anal, vaginal, or oral sex.

If you have latex allergies, synthetic nonlatex condoms can be used. But, it is important to note that these condoms have higher breakage rates than latex condoms. Natural membrane condoms are not recommended for STD prevention.

Put Yourself to the Test

Knowing your STD status is a critical step to stopping STD transmission. If you know you are infected, you can take steps to protect yourself and your partners.

Be sure to ask your healthcare provider to test you for STDs—asking is the only way to know whether you are receiving the right tests. And do not forget to tell your partner to ask a healthcare provider about STD testing as well.

Many STDs can be easily diagnosed and treated. If either you or your partner is infected, both of you need to receive treatment at the same time to avoid getting re-infected.

Section 4.3

Risk of Infectious Disease from Blood Transfusion

This section contains text excerpted from the following sources: Text under the heading "Blood Transfusion" is excerpted from "Blood Transfusion," National Heart, Lung, and Blood Institute (NHLBI), January 18, 2019; Text under the heading "Diseases and Organisms" is excerpted from "Diseases and Organisms," Centers for Disease Control and Prevention (CDC), January 31, 2019.

Blood Transfusion

A blood transfusion is a common, safe medical procedure in which healthy blood is given to you through an intravenous (IV) line that has been inserted in one of your blood vessels.

Your blood carries oxygen and nutrients to all parts of your body. Blood transfusions replace blood that is lost through surgery or injury or provide it if your body is not making blood properly. You may need a blood transfusion if you have anemia, sickle cell disease, a bleeding disorder such as hemophilia, or cancer. For people in critical condition, blood transfusions can be lifesaving.

Four types of blood products may be given through blood transfusions: whole blood, red blood cells, platelets, and plasma. Most of the blood used for transfusions comes from whole blood donations given by volunteer blood donors. A person can also have his or her own blood collected and stored a few weeks before surgery in case it is needed.

After a doctor determines that you need a blood transfusion, he or she will test your blood to make sure that the blood you are given matches your blood type. A small needle is used to insert an IV line in one of your blood vessels. Through this line, you receive healthy blood. Blood transfusions usually take 1 to 4 hours to complete. You will be monitored during and after the procedure.

Blood transfusions are usually very safe, because donated blood is carefully tested, handled, and stored. However, there is a small chance that your body may have a mild to severe reaction to the donor blood. Other complications may include fever, heart or lung complications, alloimmunization, and rare but serious reactions in which donated white blood cells attack your body's healthy tissues. Some people have health problems from getting too much iron from frequent transfusions. There is also a very small chance of getting an infectious disease such as hepatitis B or C or human immunodeficiency virus (HIV) through a blood transfusion. For HIV, that risk is less than one in 1 million. Scientific research and careful medical controls make the supply of donated blood very safe. Blood transfusions are among the most common medical procedures in the nation.

Diseases and Organisms

The U.S. blood supply is safer than it has ever been. However, any bloodborne pathogen has the potential to be transmitted by blood transfusion.

Transfusion-transmitted infections (TTIs) are infections resulting from the introduction of a pathogen into a person through blood transfusion. A wide variety of organisms, including bacteria, viruses, prions, and parasites can be transmitted through blood transfusions.

The use of a standard donor screening questionnaire, as well as laboratory tests, help to reduce the risk of an infectious organism being transmitted by blood transfusion.

Additionally, the introduction of pathogen reduction technology (PRT) may help to further reduce the risk of TTIs. PRT involves treating certain blood products with a pathogen-inactivating agent soon after collection. The use of PRT cannot only limit the number of TTIs but may also eliminate the need for irradiation to prevent transfusion-associated graft-versus-host diseases (TA-GVHD) and serologic testing for cytomegalovirus (CMV) for at-risk patients. Currently, this technology is approved for apheresis platelets and plasma products.

Bacterial Contamination of Blood Products

Bacterial contamination of blood products, especially in platelets that are stored at room temperature, is the most common infectious risk of blood transfusion, occurring in approximately 1 of 2,000 to 3,000 platelet transfusions. Transfusion-transmitted sepsis, while less common, can cause severe illness and death. Improved donor screening, as well as improved methods of collection, handling, and storing of blood products, has decreased bacterial contamination in recent years.

Gram-Positive Bacteria

Gram-positive bacteria normally found on the skin, such as *Staphylococcus epidermidis* or *Staphylococcus aureus*, are the most common bacterial contaminants of blood products. This type of contamination is thought to occur when the bacteria on the skin is passed into the collected blood through the collection needle.

Gram-Negative Bacteria

Gram-negative bacteria are part of normal flora in the gastrointestinal tract (intestines). This type of contamination is thought to occur when blood is collected from donors who have bacteria in the bloodstream but do not exhibit any symptoms. Examples include *Acinetobacter, Klebsiella,* and *Escherichia coli* (*E. coli*). Some gram-negative bacteria are resistant to multiple drugs and are increasingly resistant to many available antibiotics.

Anaplasmosis

Anaplasmosis is a tickborne disease caused by the bacterium *Anaplasma phagocytophilum*. It is transmitted to humans by tick bites, primarily from the black-legged tick and the western black-legged tick, and can be transmitted via blood product from an infected donor. Symptoms of anaplasmosis include fever, headache, chills, and muscle aches.

Brucellosis

Brucellosis is a disease caused by bacteria from the Brucella species, which is transmitted to humans from contact with infected animals, such as sheep, cattle, and dogs. Brucellosis has been previously described to be transmissible via blood product from an infected donor. Symptoms include fever, sweats, headache, and fatigue.

Ehrlichiosis

Ehrlichiosis is a group of tick-borne diseases caused by bacteria in the Ehrlichia species. It is transmitted to humans mainly from the lone star tick and the black-legged tick. Transmission via blood product from an infected donor has previously been documented. Symptoms include fever, chills, headache, and muscle ache.

Parasitic Diseases

Transmission of parasitic infections through blood donation is rare. To help minimize the risk of transfusion-transmitted illnesses, including parasitic infections, donors are asked questions to assist in determining if they are in good health. To reduce the risk of transmitting specific infections (e.g., malaria), donors are asked about recent travel to areas where some infections are more common.

Examples of parasitic diseases that can be transmitted by blood transfusion are listed below.

Babesiosis

Babesiosis is caused by microscopic parasites that infect red blood cells and are spread by certain ticks. In the United States, tick-borne transmission is most common in particular regions and seasons; it mainly occurs in parts of the Northeast and upper Midwest and usually peaks during the warm months.

Chagas Disease

Chagas disease is caused by the parasite *Trypanosoma cruzi*, which is transmitted to animals and people by insects. *Trypanosoma cruzi* is found only in the Americas, and transmission of the parasite occurs mainly in rural areas of Latin America where poverty is widespread. Since 2007, first time blood donors have been screened for antibodies to *T. cruzi* in the United States, making the risk of transfusion-transmitted *Trypanosoma cruzi* extremely rare.

Leishmaniasis

Leishmaniasis includes 2 major diseases, cutaneous leishmaniasis and visceral leishmaniasis, caused by more than 20 different leishmanial species. Leishmaniasis is transmitted by the bite of small insects called "sand flies." The distribution of leishmaniasis is worldwide. Several transfusion-transmitted cases of visceral form of the Leishmania have been reported.

Malaria

Malaria is a serious and sometimes fatal disease caused by a parasite that commonly infects a certain type of mosquito which feeds on humans. People who get malaria are typically very sick with high fevers, shaking chills, and flu-like illness. About 1,700 cases of malaria are diagnosed in the United States each year. The vast majority of cases in the United States are in travelers and immigrants returning from countries where malaria transmission occurs, many from sub-Saharan Africa and South Asia.

Viral Diseases

As with bacteria and parasites, viruses that are bloodborne can be transmitted by blood transfusion. Donors are asked questions about their social behavior and health history to help minimize the risk of transfusion-transmitted viral diseases.

Examples of viral diseases that can be transmitted through transfusion are listed below.

Chikungunya Virus

Chikungunya virus (CHIKV) is an arbovirus spread to humans from mosquitos. CHIKV outbreaks have occurred in Africa, Asia, Europe, the Indian and Pacific Oceans, and the Caribbean. No CHIKV outbreaks have been reported in the United States. Symptoms include fever and joint pain, and there is no vaccine or medicine to prevent or treat CHIKV.

Dengue Fever

Dengue fever (DF) is caused by any 1 of 4 related viruses transmitted by mosquitoes. With more than one-third of the world's population living in areas at risk for transmission, dengue infection is a leading cause of illness and death in the tropics and subtropics. As many as 100 million people are infected yearly.

Hepatitis A Virus

Hepatitis A is a contagious liver disease that results from infection with the Hepatitis A virus (HAV). Hepatitis A is spread primarily by the fecal-oral route, but transfusion-transmitted HAV infection has been reported. Hepatitis A can range in severity from a mild illness lasting a few weeks to a severe illness lasting several months and, in rare occasions, can cause death.

Hepatitis B Virus

Hepatitis B is a contagious liver disease caused by the Hepatitis B virus (HBV). 1.2 million Americans are living with chronic Hepatitis B, and most are unaware of their infection. Over time, approximately 15 to 25 percent of people with chronic Hepatitis B develop serious liver problems, including liver damage, cirrhosis, liver failure, and liver cancer. Every year, approximately 3,000 people in the United States and more than 600,000 people worldwide die from Hepatitis B-related liver disease. Since 1972, the blood supply has been screened for Hepatitis B in the United States, making the risk of transfusion-transmitted HBV extremely rare.

Hepatitis C Virus

Hepatitis C is a contagious liver disease caused by the Hepatitis C virus (HCV). Hepatitis C is the most common chronic bloodborne infection in the United States. 3.2 million Americans are living with chronic Hepatitis C, and most are unaware of their infection. Chronic Hepatitis C is a serious disease that can result in long-term health problems, including liver damage, cirrhosis, liver failure, and liver cancer. Since 1992, the blood supply has been screened for Hepatitis C in the United States, making the risk of transfusion-transmitted HCV extremely rare.

Hepatitis E Virus

Hepatitis E is a contagious liver disease caused by the Hepatitis E Virus (HEV). HEV is transmitted via the fecal-oral route, generally through contaminated water in areas with poor sanitation. Though HEV is rare in the United States, it is more common in other countries. Hepatitis E-related lived disease is self-limiting and does not lead to chronic infection.

Human Immunodeficiency Virus

Human immunodeficiency virus is the cause of AIDS. The Centers for Disease Control and Prevention (CDC) estimates that about 38,500 people in the United States contracted HIV in 2015. This risk of transfusion-transmitted HIV is extremely remote due to the rigorous testing of the U.S. blood supply.

Human T-Cell Lymphotropic Virus

Human T-cell lymphotropic virus (HTLV) is a viral infection prevalent in Japan, sub-Saharan Africa, the Caribbean Islands, and South America. HTLV can be spread mother to child, through sexual contact, or via infected blood products. Though many infected remain asymptomatic, HTLV can lead to neoplastic diseases, inflammatory syndromes, and opportunistic infections.

West Nile Virus

West Nile virus (WNV) is a potentially serious illness. Experts believe WNV is established as a seasonal epidemic in North America that flares up in the summer and continues into the fall. Symptoms of the illness include fever, headache, tiredness, aches, and sometimes rash. Although WNV is most often transmitted by the bite of infected mosquitoes, the virus can also be transmitted through contact with infected animals, their blood, or other tissues.

Zika Virus

Zika virus (ZIKV) is a mosquito-borne arbovirus spread by the *Aedes aegypti* mosquito. ZIKV can be passed from a pregnant woman to her fetus, and infection during pregnancy can lead to serious birth defects. Symptoms of Zika include fever, rash, headache, joint pain, red eyes, and muscle pain. Transfusion-transmitted cases of ZIKV have been reported.

Prion Diseases

Prion diseases, or transmissible spongiform encephalopathies (TSEs), are a family of rare, progressive neurodegenerative disorders that affect both humans and animals. The causative agent of TSEs is believed to be a prion. A prion is an abnormal, transmissible agent that is able to induce abnormal folding of normal cellular prion proteins in the brain, leading to brain damage and the characteristics signs and symptoms of the disease. Prion diseases are usually rapidly progressive and always fatal. As with viruses, bacteria, and parasites, prions are bloodborne and may be transmitted by blood transfusion.

Variant Creutzfeldt-Jakob Disease

Variant Creutzfeldt-Jakob disease (vCJD) is a rare, rapidly progressing neurological disease that causes dementia and death. In 1996, cases of vCJD were first reported in the United Kingdom.

Transmission of vCJD in the United Kingdom has been thought to be related to transfusions received years earlier with nonleukoreduced red blood cells from healthy donors who became ill with vCJD months to less than four years after the donations. Recipients of blood components from other donors later diagnosed with vCJD remain under surveillance in the United Kingdom and France. The magnitude of the risk of acquiring vCJD from transfusion is uncertain.

Section 4.4

Contagious Disease Transmission on Airplanes and Cruise Ships

This section contains text excerpted from the following sources: Text under the heading "Air Travel and Transmission of Communicable Diseases" is excerpted from "Air Travel," Centers for Disease Control and Prevention (CDC), June 12, 2017; Text under the heading "Protecting Travelers' Health from Airport to Community" is excerpted from "Protecting Travelers' Health from Airport to Community: Investigating Contagious Diseases on Flights," Centers for Disease Control and Prevention (CDC), April 3, 2019; Text under the heading "Cruise Ship Travel and Transmission of Communicable Diseases" is excerpted from "Cruise Ship Travel," Centers for Disease Control and Prevention (CDC), June 12, 2017.

Air Travel and Transmission of Communicable Diseases

Worldwide, more than 2.8 billion people travel by commercial aircraft every year, and this number continues to rise. Travelers often have concerns about the health risks of flying in airplanes. Those with underlying illness need to be aware that the entire point-to-point travel experience, including buses, trains, taxis, public waiting areas, and even movement within the airport, can pose challenges. Although illness may occur as a direct result of air travel, it is uncommon; the main concerns are:

- Exacerbations of chronic medical problems due to changes in air pressure and humidity

- Relative immobility during flights (risk of thromboembolic disease)

- Close proximity to other passengers with certain communicable diseases

In-Flight Transmission of Communicable Diseases

Communicable diseases may be transmitted to other travelers during air travel; therefore, people who are acutely ill, or still within the infectious period for a specific disease, should delay their travel until they are no longer contagious. For example, otherwise healthy adults can transmit influenza to others for 5 to 7 days. Travelers should be up-to-date on routine vaccinations and receive destination-specific vaccinations before travel. Travelers should be reminded to wash their hands frequently and thoroughly (or use an alcohol-based hand sanitizer containing more than 60 percent alcohol), especially after using the toilet and before preparing or eating food, and to cover their noses and mouths when coughing or sneezing.

Aircraft contact investigations may be conducted for certain serious communicable diseases. If a passenger with a serious communicable disease was infectious during a flight, passengers who may have been exposed may be contacted by public health authorities for possible screening or prophylaxis. When necessary, public health authorities will obtain contact information from the airline for potentially exposed travelers so they may be contacted and offered an intervention.

To request a consultation, public health authorities may contact the Centers for Disease Control and Prevention (CDC) quarantine station of jurisdiction or the CDC Emergency Operations Center (EOC) by calling 770-488-7100.

Tuberculosis (Mycobacterium tuberculosis)

Tuberculosis (TB) is transmitted from person-to-person via airborne respiratory droplet nuclei. Although the risk of transmission onboard aircraft is low, the CDC recommends conducting passenger contact investigations for flights longer than eight hours if the person with TB has sputum that is smear-positive for acid-fast bacilli and cavitation on chest radiograph or has multidrug-resistant TB. People known to have active TB disease should not travel by commercial air (or any other commercial means) until they are determined to be noninfectious. State health department TB controllers are valuable resources for advice to determine when a person can be considered noninfectious.

Meningococcal Disease (Neisseria meningitidis)

Meningococcal disease caused by *N. meningitidis* is transmitted by direct contact with respiratory droplets and secretions, and it can be rapidly fatal. Therefore, close contacts of ill travelers need to be quickly identified and provided with prophylactic antimicrobial agents. Antimicrobial prophylaxis should be considered for any of the following:

- Household members traveling with the ill traveler
- Travel companions with prolonged close contact

- Travelers seated directly next to the ill traveler on flights longer than 8 hours (gate to gate) or who have had direct contact with respiratory secretions or vomit.

Measles (Rubeola)

Measles is a viral illness transmitted by respiratory droplets, direct contact, or airborne routes. Most measles cases diagnosed in the United States are imported from countries where measles is endemic. An ill traveler is considered infectious during a flight of any duration if she or he traveled during the 4 days before rash onset through 4 days after rash onset. Flight-related contact investigations are initiated as quickly as possible, so postexposure prophylaxis may be provided to susceptible travelers. If indicated, the measles, mumps, and rubella (MMR) vaccine given within 72 hours of exposure or immune globulin, given within 6 days of exposure, may prevent measles or decrease its severity in people who are not immune.

Disinsection

To reduce the accidental spread of mosquitoes and other vectors via airline cabins and luggage compartments, a number of countries require disinsection of all inbound flights or flights from certain areas. Although disinsection, when done appropriately, was declared safe by the World Health Organization (WHO) in 1995, there is still much debate about the safety of the agents and the effectiveness of disinsection as a public health measure to prevent the spread of vector-borne diseases. Although the CDC reserves the right to require disinsection to control importation and spread of vector-borne infectious diseases, it is not currently required for aircraft arriving at the U.S. airports. The WHO information on aircraft disinsection, including available procedures, can be found on their website. An updated list of countries that require disinsection, and the types of methods used, is available at the Department of Transportation's website.

Protecting Travelers' Health from Airport to Community

What if a passenger was sick on your flight? What if that person was later diagnosed with a serious infectious disease and was contagious during your flight? Are you at risk? If you were exposed, how do you protect yourself?

Although the risk of getting a contagious disease on an airplane is low, public health officers sometimes need to find and alert travelers who may have been exposed to a sick passenger on a flight. The search for these travelers is known as a "contact investigation." A contact investigation is one of the ways the CDC works with partners in the United States and other countries to protect the health of people exposed to an illness during travel and to protect their communities from contagious diseases that are just a flight away.

Answering the Call

A contact investigation often starts with a phone call to a CDC Quarantine Station located at a U.S. international airport. The caller is a public health official who informs the CDC about a recent air traveler diagnosed with a specific contagious disease. Sometimes, the CDC is notified about a sick traveler while the plane is still in the air or shortly after the plane has landed. However, in most cases, the CDC is notified when a sick traveler seeks treatment at a medical facility. These notifications can be made days, weeks, or even months after the travel. This sick traveler is now referred to as the "index patient."

The caller notifies the CDC because other passengers on the arriving international flight or connecting domestic flights may have been exposed and need to be notified. Or an international partner calls the CDC about exposed U.S. passengers on overseas flights. The passengers exposed to the index patient are called "contacts."

The CDC is responsible for coordinating contact investigations of illness exposures on arriving international flights or flights between states. A single infected traveler can trigger more than one contact investigation if the traveler takes connecting flights to reach a U.S. destination.

A person can be contagious without showing any symptoms while the disease is developing (incubating) in the body. Quarantine public health officers must determine whether the index patient was contagious during a flight. Their decision is based on the disease, history of symptoms, and the date of the flight.

Starting the Contact Investigation

If the index patient was contagious during the flight, passengers seated nearby may have been exposed to the disease. The CDC will start a contact investigation to find these passengers.

The CDC requests the flight manifest for passengers seated near the index patient. The flight manifest is a document that contains passengers' names, seat numbers, and contact information. The CDC guards the privacy of passengers by keeping this information secure.

This is a good reminder to make sure you give the correct contact information to the airlines when you book your flight. Also, remember to update your frequent flyer program contact information.

Diseases of Concern during Air Travel

Most flight contact investigations are performed for infectious tuberculosis (TB), measles, rubella (German measles), pertussis (whooping cough), and meningococcal disease (meningitis).

The CDC has developed instructions (protocols) for investigating contagious diseases. The CDC uses these protocols to identify passengers who may have been exposed during a flight. Identifying contacts is based on the disease, how it spreads, and where a passenger was seated in relation to the index patient.

Two types of passengers will be considered contacts regardless of where they sat:

1. All traveling companions of the index patient who were on the same flight

2. For measles and rubella, all children younger than two years of age sitting anywhere on the plane. These children may be too young to have been vaccinated and would be at high risk for getting the disease.

Did You Provide Accurate Information?

Contact information from the flight manifest is often incomplete.

The CDC relies on the U.S. Customs and Border Protection (CBP) for help with contact investigations involving international flights. The CBP can often provide more information that fills in the gaps.

Remember to provide a current telephone number when making your flight reservations. Otherwise, how will you know if you were exposed if no one can reach you?

The CDC staff then combine the information from the CBP and the airline's flight manifest for locating exposed passengers (contacts). At every step, the CDC protects the privacy of this information.

Protecting the Health of Passengers

The CDC provides the exposed passengers' contact information to state and local health departments or ministries of health in the countries where the passengers live. These agencies then try to locate these passengers and inform them about their exposure and what to do.

Exposed passengers may be asked whether they are protected against (immune to) the specific disease. They can be immune if they had the disease in the past or have received a vaccine.

Public health officers will educate contacts about how to watch for and report symptoms of the illness being investigated. Contacts who are not immune (for example, because they have not been vaccinated for the disease) may need to receive preventive drugs or a vaccine to protect them from the disease. Any recommendations will be based on the disease, availability of preventive drugs or vaccines, and amount of time passed since exposure.

The contact investigation process is how federal agencies and airlines work together to help state and local health departments find exposed passengers. If you are considered a contact of an index patient on an airplane, they will call you. So make sure you leave a number where they can reach you.

Cruise Ship Travel and Transmission of Communicable Diseases

Cruise ship travel presents a unique combination of health concerns. Travelers from diverse regions brought together in often crowded, semi-enclosed environments onboard ships can facilitate the spread of person-to-person, foodborne, or waterborne diseases. Outbreaks on ships can be sustained for multiple voyages by transmission among crew members who remain onboard or by persistent environmental contamination. Port visits can expose travelers to local vector-borne diseases. The remote location of the travelers at sea means that they may need to rely on the medical capabilities and supplies available onboard the ship for extended periods of time, and cruise travelers and their physicians should be aware of ships' medical limitations and prepare accordingly. Certain groups, such as pregnant women, the elderly, or those with chronic health conditions or who are immunocompromised, require special consideration when considering cruise travel.

Illnesses and Injury Aboard Cruise Ships

Cruise ship medical clinics deal with a wide variety of illnesses and injuries. Approximately 3 to 11 percent of conditions reported to cruise ship infirmaries are urgent or an emergency. Approximately 95 percent of illnesses are treated or managed onboard, and 5 percent require evacuation and shoreside consultation for medical, surgical, or dental problems. Roughly half of the passengers who seek medical care are older than 65 years of age. Most infirmary visits are due to acute illnesses, of which respiratory illnesses (19 to 29%); seasickness (10 to 25%); injuries from slips, trips, or falls (12 to 18%); and gastrointestinal (GI) illness (9 to 10%) are the most frequently reported diagnoses. Death rates for cruise ship passengers, most often from cardiovascular events, range from 0.6 to 9.8 deaths per million passenger-nights.

The most frequently reported cruise ship outbreaks involve respiratory infections; GI infections (norovirus); and vaccine-preventable diseases other than influenza, such as varicella (chickenpox). To reduce the risk of onboard introduction of communicable diseases by embarking passengers, ships may conduct medical screening during embarkation to identify ill passengers, preventing them from boarding or requiring isolation if they are allowed to board.

The following measures should be encouraged to limit the introduction and spread of communicable diseases on cruise ships:

- Passengers and their clinicians should consult the CDC's Travelers' Health website (www.cdc.gov/travel) before travel for updates on outbreaks and travel health notices.

- Passengers ill with communicable diseases before a voyage should delay travel until they are no longer contagious.

- Passengers who become ill during the voyage should seek care in the ship's infirmary to receive clinical management, facilitate infection control measures, and maximize reporting of potential public health events.

Specific Health Risks
Gastrointestinal Illness

From 2008 through 2014, rates of GI illness among passengers on voyages lasting 3 to 21 days decreased from 27.2 to 22.3 cases per

100,000 travel days. Despite this decrease, GI illness outbreaks continue to occur. Updates on these outbreaks involving ships with the U.S. ports of call can be found at www.cdc.gov/nceh/vsp/surv/gilist.htm.

More than 90 percent of GI outbreaks with a confirmed cause are due to norovirus. Characteristics of norovirus that facilitate outbreaks are a low infective dose, easy person-to-person transmissibility, prolonged viral shedding, no long-term immunity, and the organism's ability to survive routine cleaning procedures. From 2010 through 2015, 8 to 16 outbreaks of norovirus infections occurred on cruise ships each year. GI outbreaks on cruise ships from food and water sources have also been associated with *Salmonella spp., enterotoxigenic Escherichia coli, Shigella spp., Vibrio spp., Staphylococcus aureus, Clostridium perfringens, Cyclospora cayetanensis*, and hepatitis A and E viruses.

To protect themselves from infections and reduce the spread of GI illnesses on cruise ships, passengers should be counseled on the following:

- Passengers should wash their hands with soap and water often, especially before eating and after using the restroom.

- Passengers who develop a GI illness, even if symptoms are mild, should promptly call the ship's medical center (or the ship's master, if no medical center exists) and follow cruise ship guidance regarding isolation and other infection control measures.

- Additional information on cruise ship outbreaks is available at www.cdc.gov/nceh/vsp.

Respiratory Illness
Influenza

Respiratory illnesses are the most common medical complaint, and influenza is the most commonly reported vaccine-preventable illness on cruise ships. Since passengers and crew originate from all regions of the world, shipboard outbreaks of influenza A and B can occur year-round, and travelers on cruise ships can be exposed to strains circulating in different parts of the world. Using 2008 to 2011 surveillance data, the CDC found a mean rate of influenza-like illness (defined as having a temperature higher than 100°F along with a cough or sore throat) of 0.065 cases per 1,000 person-nights, without a detectable seasonal pattern.

Given the cruise ship environment, population, and variable medical capabilities, the following measures are recommended year round to protect travelers from influenza:

- Clinicians should provide cruise travelers, particularly those at high risk for influenza complications, with the current seasonal influenza vaccine (if available) at least two weeks before travel.

- Passengers at high risk for influenza complications should discuss antiviral treatment and chemoprophylaxis with their healthcare provider before travel.

- Passengers should practice good respiratory hygiene and cough etiquette.

- Passengers should report their respiratory illness to the infirmary promptly and follow isolation recommendations, if indicated.

Legionnaires' Disease

Although it is not a common cause of respiratory illness on cruise ships, Legionnaires' disease is a treatable infection that can result in severe pneumonia, leading to death. More than 20 percent of all Legionnaires' disease cases reported to the CDC are travel-associated. Clusters of Legionnaires' disease associated with hotel or cruise ship travel are difficult to identify because travelers often disperse from the source of infection before symptoms begin. A total of 83 ship-associated cases of Legionnaires' disease were reported in the literature from 1977 through 2012. The cases involved outbreaks on 8 ships, with a median of 4 cases per outbreak (range, 2 to 50 cases); 6 cases resulted in death.

In general, Legionnaires' disease is not transmitted person-to-person but is contracted by inhaling or aspirating warm, aerosolized water contaminated with Legionella organisms. Person-to-person transmission may be possible in rare cases. Contaminated ships' hot tubs are the most commonly implicated sources of shipboard Legionella outbreaks; potable water supply systems have also been implicated. Improvements in ship design and the standardization of water disinfection have reduced the risk of Legionella growth and colonization.

Most cruise ships have healthcare personnel who can perform Legionella urine antigen testing. People with suspected Legionnaires' disease require prompt antibiotic treatment.

In evaluating cruise travelers for Legionnaires' disease, clinicians should do the following:

- Obtain a thorough travel history of all destinations from 10 days before symptom onset (to assist in the identification of potential source of exposure).

- Collect urine for antigen testing.

- Culture lower respiratory secretions on selective media, which is essential to identify the species or serogroup.

- Inform the CDC of any travel-associated Legionnaires' disease cases by sending an email to travellegionella@cdc.gov. Cases of Legionnaires' disease should be quickly reported to public health officials in order to determine if there are links to previously reported clusters and to stop potential clusters and new outbreaks.

Vaccine-Preventable Diseases

Although most cruise ship passengers are from countries with routine vaccination programs (such as the United States and Canada), many crew members originate from developing countries with low immunization rates. Outbreaks of measles, rubella, meningococcal disease and, most commonly, varicella have been reported on cruise ships. Preventive measures to reduce the spread of vaccine-preventable diseases (VPDs) onboard cruise ships should be followed:

- Crew members should have documented proof of immunity to VPDs

- Passengers, especially older passengers (older than 65 years of age) and immunocompromised people, should be up-to-date with routine vaccinations before travel, as well as any required or recommended vaccinations specific for their destinations.

- Women of childbearing age should be immune to varicella and rubella before cruise ship travel.

Vector-Borne Diseases

Cruise ship port visits may include countries where vector-borne diseases, such as malaria, dengue, yellow fever, Japanese encephalitis, and Zika, are endemic. New diseases might surface in unexpected locations. For example, chikungunya was reported in late 2013 for the first time in the Caribbean (with subsequent spread throughout the Caribbean and numerous North, Central, and South American countries and territories). Zika virus was first reported in Brazil in 2015 and subsequently spread across the Caribbean and Latin America.

Passengers should follow recommendations for avoiding mosquito bites and vector-borne infections:

- Use an effective insect repellent.

- Treat clothing and gear with permethrin, or purchase permethrin-treated items.

- While indoors, remain in well-screened or air-conditioned areas.

- When outdoors, wear long-sleeved shirts, long pants, boots, and hats.

- Obtain yellow fever vaccination if recommended or required.

- Take antimalarial chemoprophylaxis if needed

Other Health Concerns

Stresses of cruise ship travel include varying weather and environmental conditions, as well as unaccustomed changes in diet and physical activity. Foreign travel may increase the likelihood of risk-taking behaviors, such as alcohol misuse, drug use, and unsafe sex. In spite of modern stabilizer systems, seasickness is a common complaint (affecting up to one-fourth of travelers). Cruise lines may not allow women to board after the 24th week of pregnancy, and pregnant women should contact the cruise line for specific policies and recommendations before booking.

Chapter 5

Screening Internationally Adopted Children for Contagious Diseases

In the past 15 years, more than 250,000 children have come to the United States to join their families through international adoption. Families traveling to unite with their adopted child, siblings who wait at home for the child's arrival, extended family members, and child care providers are all at risk for acquiring infectious diseases secondary to travel or resulting from contact with the newly arrived child. International adoptees may be underimmunized and are at an increased risk for infections—such as measles, hepatitis A, and hepatitis B—because of crowded living conditions, malnutrition, lack of clean water, lack of immunizations, and exposure to endemic diseases that are not commonly seen in the United States. Challenges in providing care to internationally adopted children include the absence of a complete medical history, lack of availability of a biological family history, questionable reliability of immunization records, variation in preadoption living standards, varying disease epidemiology in the countries of origin, the presence of previously unidentified medical problems, and the increased risk for developmental delays and psychological issues in these children.

This chapter includes text excerpted from "International Adoption," Centers for Disease Control and Prevention (CDC), June 12, 2017.

Travel Preparation for Adoptive Parents and Their Families

A pretravel clinic visit is strongly recommended for prospective adoptive parents. In preparation, the travel health provider must know the disease risks in the adopted child's country of origin and the medical and social histories of the adoptee (if available), as well as which family members will be traveling, their immunization and medical histories, the season of travel, the length of stay in the country, and the itinerary while in country. Family members who remain at home, including extended family, should be current on their routine immunizations. Protection against measles, varicella, tetanus, diphtheria, pertussis, hepatitis A, hepatitis B, and polio must be ensured for everyone who will be in the household or in close contact by providing care for the adopted child. Measles immunity or 2 doses of measles-mumps-rubella (MMR) vaccine separated by more than 28 days should be documented for all people born in or after 1957. Varicella vaccine should be given to those without a history of varicella disease or documentation of 2 doses of varicella vaccine more than 3 months apart. Adults who have not received tetanus-diphtheria-acellular pertussis (Tdap) vaccine, including adults older than 65 years of age, should receive a single dose of Tdap to protect against *Bordetella pertussis* in addition to tetanus and diphtheria. Unprotected family members and close contacts of the adopted child should be immunized against hepatitis A virus (HAV) before the child's arrival. Most adult family members and caretakers will need to be immunized with hepatitis B vaccine, since it has only been routinely given since 1990.

If the adopted child is from a polio-endemic area, family members and caretakers should ensure that they have completed the recommended age-appropriate polio vaccine series. A one-time inactivated polio booster for adults who have completed the primary series in the past is recommended if they are traveling to these areas and can be considered for adults who remain at home but who will be in close contact caring for the child. Additional polio vaccination requirements for long-term travelers (those staying longer than 4 weeks) and residents departing from countries with polio transmission may affect travel.

Prospective adoptive parents and any children traveling with them should receive advice on travel safety, food safety, immunization, malaria chemoprophylaxis, diarrhea prevention and treatment, and other travel-related health issues. Instructions on car seats, injury prevention, food safety, and air travel apply equally to the adoptive child, so the travel health provider should also be familiar with and provide information on these child-specific issues.

Follow-Up Medical Examination after Arrival in the United States

The adopted child should have a medical examination within two weeks of arrival in the United States or earlier if the child has fever, anorexia, diarrhea, vomiting, or other medical concerns. Items to consider during medical examination of an adopted child include the following:

- **Temperature** (fever requires further investigation)

- **General appearance:** alert, interactive

- **Anthropometric measurements:** weight/age, height/age, weight/height, head circumference/age, body mass index (BMI)

- **Facial features:** length of palpebral fissures, philtrum, upper lip (fetal alcohol syndrome: short palpebral fissures, thin upper lip, indistinct philtrum), other facial features suggestive of a genetic syndrome

- **Hair:** texture, color, areas of alopecia with dry patches (tinea capitis)

- **Eyes:** jaundice, pallor, strabismus, visual acuity screen

- **Ears:** hearing screen, otitis media

- **Mouth:** palate, thrush, presence of a uvula, teeth (number and condition)

- **Neck:** thyroid (enlargement secondary to hypothyroidism, iodine deficiency), lymph nodes

- **Heart:** murmurs

- **Chest:** symmetry, Tanner stage breasts

- **Abdomen:** liver or spleen enlargement

- **Skin:** Mongolian spots, scars, bacillus Calmette-Guérin (BCG) scar, birthmarks, molluscum contagiosum, tinea capitis, tinea corporis

- **Lymph nodes:** enlargement suggestive of TB or other infections

- **Back:** scoliosis, sacral dimple

- **Genitalia:** Tanner stage, presence of both testicles, findings of sexual abuse

- **Extremities:** presence of bowing (rickets) or deformities

- **Neurologic:** presence and quality of reflexes

In addition, all children should receive a developmental screening by a clinician with experience in child development to determine if immediate referrals should be made for a more detailed neurodevelopmental examination and therapies. Further evaluation will depend on the country of origin, the age of the child, previous living conditions, nutritional status, developmental status, and the adoptive family's specific questions. Concerns raised during the preadoption medical review may dictate further investigation.

Screening for Infectious Diseases

The current panel of tests for infectious diseases recommended by the American Academy of Pediatrics (AAP) for screening internationally adopted children is as follows:

- Hepatitis A virus (HAV) serologic testing (IgG and IgM)

- Hepatitis B virus (HBV) serologic testing (repeat at 6 months if initial testing is negative)

- Hepatitis C antibody (repeat at 6 months if initial testing is negative)

- Syphilis serologic testing (treponemal and nontreponemal testing)

- Human immunodeficiency virus (HIV) 1 and 2 serologic testing (antigen/antibody)

- Complete blood cell count with differential and red blood cell indices

- Stool examination for ova and parasites (3 specimens)

- Stool examination for Giardia intestinalis and *Cryptosporidium* antigen (1 specimen)

- Tuberculin skin test (TST) (all ages) or interferon-γ release assay (IGRA) (for children older than 5 years of age) (repeat at 6 months if initial test is negative)

Additional screening tests may be useful, depending on the child's country of origin or specific risk factors. These screens may include Chagas disease serologic tests, malaria smears, or serologic testing for schistosomiasis, strongyloidiasis, and filariasis.

Immunizations

The U.S. Immigration and Nationality Act requires that any person seeking an immigrant visa for permanent residency must show proof of having received the Advisory Committee on Immunization Practices (ACIP)-recommended vaccines before immigration. This requirement applies to all immigrant infants and children entering the United States, but internationally adopted children younger than 10 years of age are exempt from the overseas immunization requirements. Adoptive parents are required to sign a waiver indicating their intention to comply with the immunization requirements within 30 days of the child's arrival in the United States.

Most children throughout the developing world receive bacillus Calmette-Guérin, oral polio, measles, diphtheria, tetanus, and pertussis vaccines per the original immunization schedule of the United Nations Expanded Programme of Immunizations (begun in 1974). In many developing countries, HBV, *Haemophilus influenzae type b* (Hib), and rotavirus vaccines have become more widely available. Upon arrival in the United States, more than 90 percent of newly arrived internationally adopted children need catch-up immunizations to meet ACIP guidelines. Hepatitis A, Hib, human papillomavirus, mumps, pneumococcal conjugate, rotavirus, rubella, and varicella vaccines are often not available in developing countries. Reliability of vaccine records appears to differ by, and even within, country of origin. Some children may have an immunization record with documentation of the vaccines and dates they were given, and others may have incomplete documentation or no record at all. In addition, some children may be immune to vaccine-preventable diseases such as hepatitis A, measles, mumps, rubella, or varicella. A clinical diagnosis of any of these diseases should not be accepted as evidence of immunity.

Providers can choose one of two approaches for vaccination of internationally adopted children. The first is to re-immunize, regardless of immunization record. The second, applicable to children aged older than six months of age, is to test antibody titers to the vaccines reportedly administered and re-immunize only for those diseases to which the child has no protective titers. Immunity to *B. pertussis* is an exception; antibody titers do not correlate with immune status to

B. pertussis. However, protective antibody levels to diphtheria and tetanus imply protective antibody levels to *B. pertussis*. For children older than 6 months of age, testing can be done for diphtheria (IgG), tetanus (IgG), polio (neutralizing antibody to each serotype), hepatitis B (surface antibody), and Hib. Reimmunization for pneumococcus is recommended, given that there are 13 serotypes in the vaccine. Most experts recommend serologic testing for infants and children older than 6 months of age. For children older than 12 months of age, testing can be done for measles, mumps, rubella, hepatitis A, and varicella. The MMR vaccine is not given in most countries of origin; the measles vaccine is often administered as a single antigen.

Immunizations should be given according to the current ACIP schedule for catch-up vaccination. If the infant is younger than 6 months of age and there is uncertainty regarding immunization status or validity of the immunization record, the child should be re-immunized according to the ACIP schedule.

Chapter 6

Bioterrorism: Disease Used as a Weapon

Chapter Contents

Section 6.1—Bioterrorism Overview.. 72

Section 6.2—Strategic National Stockpile of Medicine............... 74

Section 6.3—U.S. Preparedness for Health
　　　　　　　Emergencies from Bioterrorism (Anthrax)............ 79

Section 6.1

Bioterrorism Overview

This section includes text excerpted from "Bioterrorism," Centers for Disease Control and Prevention (CDC), September 15, 2017.

What Is the Problem?

The word "bioterrorism" refers to biological agents (microbes or toxins) used as weapons to further personal or political agendas. Acts of bioterrorism range from a single exposure directed at an individual by another individual to government-sponsored biological warfare resulting in mass casualties. Bioterrorism differs from other methods of terrorism in that the materials needed to make an effective biological agent are readily available, require little specialized knowledge, and are inexpensive to produce. Until the aftermath of 9/11, few instances of bioterrorism were documented in the United States.

A bioterrorist attack could be caused by virtually any pathogenic microorganism. The agents of greatest concern are anthrax (a bacterium) and smallpox (a virus). Both can be lethal. Anthrax is not communicable, while smallpox is readily transmitted from person to person. In humans, the three forms of anthrax are inhalational, cutaneous, and intestinal. Symptoms vary depending upon how the person was exposed but generally occur within 7 days of the exposure. Initial symptoms of inhalational anthrax may resemble the flu. If untreated, symptoms will progress to breathing difficulties and eventual shock. The incubation period for smallpox is 7 to 17 days following exposure. Symptoms include high fever, fatigue, and head and back pain. A characteristic rash follows in 2 to 3 days.

Who Is at Risk?

In the United States, the risk of contracting anthrax is extremely low. The intentional release of anthrax following the events of 9/11 resulted in only 22 recognized cases of cutaneous and inhalational anthrax. Any risk for inhalational anthrax due to cross-contaminated mail is also very low, even for postal workers. The possibility does exist, however, that if anthrax was dispersed in a public place, a large number of people could be affected. Smallpox has not occurred in the U.S. since 1949. If the virus was intentionally released, the number of people affected could run to the tens of thousands.

Can It Be Prevented?

Bioterrorism differs from other methods of terrorism in that the effects are not always immediately apparent. An attack may be difficult to distinguish from a naturally occurring infectious disease outbreak. The first evidence of an attack will be in hospital emergency rooms, where the proper diagnosis will be essential in treating and preventing the spread of the disease. In the event of intentional anthrax distribution, people at risk should take a 60-day course of prophylactic antibiotics, either doxycycline or ciprofloxacin. Vaccination against smallpox is not recommended to prevent the disease in the general public. In people exposed to smallpox, however, the vaccine can lessen the severity of, or even prevent, illness if given within 4 days of exposure. The U.S. has a supply of vaccine for emergency use.

The Bottom Line

A story about bioterrorism carries inherent drama but also certain responsibilities. A story can raise concerns and heighten the public's awareness of the topic, or it could cause alarm and panic. And because biological materials are inexpensive and readily available, some thought should be given to whether or not the show will give ideas to potential terrorists. If a person thinks that they have been exposed to a biological incident or they suspect a biological threat is planned, they should contact their local health department and/or their local police department. Either of these agencies will promptly notify the Federal Bureau of Investigation (FBI), which is responsible for coordinating the interagency investigation of bioterrorism. The symptoms for early inhalational anthrax resemble those of the common cold or flu. Anthrax is diagnosed by isolating B. anthracis from the infected person or through other diagnostic tests. The fatality rate for cutaneous anthrax is about 20 percent; for inhalational anthrax, the rate is closer to 75 percent. Smallpox is spread from person to person via airborne saliva droplets. The majority of people infected with smallpox do recover. There is a fatality rate of approximately 30 percent.

Section 6.2

Strategic National Stockpile of Medicine

This section includes text excerpted from "Strategic National
Stockpile," Office of the Assistant Secretary for Preparedness and
Response (ASPR), U.S. Department of Health and
Human Services (HHS), December 12, 2018.

About the Strategic National Stockpile

The Strategic National Stockpile (SNS) is the nation's largest supply of potentially life-saving pharmaceuticals and medical supplies for use in a public health emergency severe enough to cause local supplies to run out.

When state, local, tribal, and territorial responders request federal assistance to support their response efforts, the stockpile ensures that the right medicines and supplies get to those who need them most during an emergency. Organized for scalable response to a variety of public health threats, this repository contains enough supplies to respond to multiple large-scale emergencies simultaneously.

With approximately 200 federal and contract employees, the SNS is organized to support any public health threat. Stockpile staff represents a variety of specialties, and all work together to ensure that the right resources are ready and can get to the right place at the right time.

Stockpile Products
Inventory

The majority of stockpile assets are held in storage and kept as managed inventory. Maintaining a supply of medications and medical supplies for specific health threats allows the stockpile to respond with the right product when a specific disease or agent is known.

Products in the stockpile may require an Emergency Use Authorization, which is granted by the U.S. Food and Drug Administration (FDA). The authorization allows for the emergency use of an unapproved medical product (e.g., drugs, vaccines, and devices) or unapproved use of an approved medical product to diagnose, treat, or prevent serious or life-threatening diseases or conditions for which no adequate, FDA-approved alternative is available.

If a community experiences a large-scale public health incident in which the disease or agent is unknown, the first line of support from the stockpile is to send a broad range of pharmaceuticals and medical supplies. Contents are pre-packed and configured in transport-ready containers for rapid delivery anywhere in the United States within 12 hours of the federal decision to deploy. Each package contains 50 tons of emergency medical resources.

The stockpile has medicines and supplies stored in strategically located warehouses throughout the country, ready for deployment. Immediately shipping a variety of items to the affected state allows authorities to begin or sustain response efforts. All states have plans to receive and distribute these medical countermeasures quickly to local jurisdictions.

CHEMPACK

CHEMPACKs are containers of nerve agent antidotes placed in secure locations in local jurisdictions around the country to allow rapid response to a chemical incident. These medications treat the symptoms of nerve agent exposure and can be used even when the actual agent is unknown.

Because these antidotes must be administered quickly, the CHEMPACK team maintains 1,960 containers strategically placed in more than 1,340 locations in the United States. More than 90 percent of the U.S. population is within 1 hour of a CHEMPACK location. Most are located in hospitals or fire stations selected by local authorities to support a rapid hazmat response and can be accessed quickly if hospitals or first responders need them.

Federal Medical Stations

Somewhere between a temporary shelter and temporary hospital, a Federal Medical Station is a nonemergency medical center set up during a natural disaster to care for displaced persons with special health needs—including those with chronic health conditions, limited mobility, or common mental-health issues—that cannot be met in a shelter for the general population during an incident.

The modular and rapidly deployable reserve of beds, supplies, and medicines provides equipment to care for 50 to 250 people for 3 days before resupply is needed. Flexible and scalable, it can be tailored to meet the requirements of each incident and has the ability to increase local healthcare capabilities in mass casualty events or in response to potential public health threats.

Federal Medical Stations operate through the cooperation of federal, state, and local authorities and require pre-planning and pre-identification of potential locations based on specific selection criteria. Prior to an emergency event, state, local, tribal, and territorial agencies collaborate with the U.S. Department of Health and Human Services (HHS) Regional Emergency Coordinators to survey sites and identify any gaps that may need addressing during a response.

The stockpile also deploys the Federal Medical Station Strike Team, which is a group of technical specialists with specific, in-depth knowledge of the stockpile and supply operations. This specialized team can assist federal and state responders, clinicians, and public health staff with identifying a suitable facility, receiving and staging equipment, and on-the-spot training to volunteers who will assemble the equipment (e.g., beds and nurses stations). The strike team can also request additional material as needed.

Sustaining the Stockpile

Sustaining the Strategic National Stockpile involves managing the entire life cycle of stockpile assets, as well as acquiring, storing, and transporting supplies.

Strategic National Stockpile management includes:

- Overseeing the shelf life of medicines to ensure the stock is rotated and kept within the FDA potency shelf-life limits
- Conducting routine quality assurance on all products
- Performing annual inventory of all products
- Inspecting environmental conditions, security, and package maintenance
- Ensuring SNS holdings are based on the latest scientific data and threat levels
- Ensuring the ability to transport items during a public health emergency

Shelf Life Extension Program

The SNS participates in the Federal Shelf Life Extension Program (for federal stockpiles), which is managed by the Department of Defense and the FDA. Once the FDA conducts stability testing and determines that products are stable and safe for continued use, the program will extend the use-by dates of pharmaceuticals beyond their original expiration dates. Testing typically provides an added 12 to 24 months of extended shelf life. More testing can lead to even longer extensions. Products that fail FDA testing are removed from stockpile inventory.

Participation in the Shelf Life Extension Program requires:

- Tracking the expiration date and manufacturer lot numbers of eligible products

- Coordinating the shipment of products to the FDA for stability testing

- Receiving and tracking the FDA testing results for each lot of product

- Disposing of and replacing product lots that have failed FDA testing

Inventory Management and Tracking System

In a large-scale public health crisis, state and local public health agencies will have to manage large quantities of medical countermeasures (MCMs) to help prevent or treat diseases. Responders need an effective software tool to manage the large and rapidly moving MCM inventory they may receive from the SNS.

The Inventory Management and Tracking System (IMATS) was created by the SNS to help state and local public health agencies manage these MCMs during a crisis. IMATS allows responders to track MCM inventory down to local levels; monitor reorder thresholds; and support warehouse operations. This tool can also be used in regular day-to-day operations.

Global Responders
What Is the Global Health Security Agenda?

The Global Health Security Agenda (GHSA) is a partnership between U.S. government sister agencies, other nations, international organizations, and public and private stakeholders. The program seeks to accelerate progress toward a world safe and secure from infectious disease threats and to promote global health security as an international security priority, to prevent, detect, and respond to public health threats within their borders.

Stockpile Support

The stockpile supports GHSA's Medical Countermeasures and Personnel Deployment Action Package. This five-year goal is to create a national framework for sending and receiving medical countermeasures (medicines and supplies) and public health and medical personnel among international partners during public health emergencies.

Stockpile experts work with health and emergency management authorities in other countries to improve the supply chain that gets critical medicines and supplies (medical countermeasures) where they are needed most during a public health emergency, such as an influenza pandemic or Ebola outbreak. This effort helps protect the United States by slowing down or stopping health threats early and close to the source.

Medical Countermeasures Workshop

In 2018, the stockpile deployed experts to host medical countermeasure workshops in developing countries including Liberia, Guinea, and Sierra Leone. These workshops enhanced their ability to detect and respond to public health threats within their borders and manage medicines and supplies in a large-scale public health emergency. Stockpile experts also validated two national medical supply chain plans for Uganda and Cameroon. The workshop includes lessons on medical supply chain operations and addresses planning issues, modern supply chain functions, supply chain information requirements, stockpiling operations, logistics operations, planning, and more.

Stockpile experts also provided two three-day medical countermeasure training events for the CDC's Public Health Emergency Management (PHEM) fellows during their time at the CDC. The PHEM Fellowship is designed to build capacity among members of the international community who work in preparedness and response. Students travel to Atlanta from as far away as Japan, South Korea, Pakistan, Uganda, Ethiopia, Burkina Faso, Malaysia, Kazakhstan, Bangladesh, Cameroon, and Senegal for a four-month fellowship to gain an understanding of public health emergency management principles and the functions that support an emergency operations center.

Section 6.3

U.S. Preparedness for Health Emergencies from Bioterrorism (Anthrax)

This section includes text excerpted from "Anthrax—Preparedness," Centers for Disease Control and Prevention (CDC), September 1, 2015. Reviewed July 2019.

Hopefully, an attack involving anthrax will never happen in the United States. However, there are steps that you and your family can take to help prepare if an anthrax emergency ever did happen. If such an emergency were to occur in the United States, the Centers for Disease Control and Prevention (CDC) and other federal agencies would be ready to respond.

What You Can Do to Prepare
Get a Kit, Make a Plan, Stay Informed

For details about how to put together an emergency kit, how to develop a family disaster plan, and how to stay informed about all types of emergencies, go to the CDC's Emergency Preparedness and You website. These basic preparedness steps would be essential during an anthrax emergency.

People in areas where anthrax is released would also need to know how to get antibiotics, how to create a family medical history, and how to recognize the symptoms of anthrax.

Know How You Would Get Antibiotics during an Anthrax Crisis

If an anthrax emergency happened in your area, your community might need to receive large amounts of antibiotics and medical supplies from the federal government. The supplies would be sent to sites that are usually called "points of dispensing" (PODs). PODs would be located in your community in safe, familiar places, such as schools or convention centers.

In an anthrax emergency, you would be able to find out where the nearest POD is located and what to bring to the POD by listening to news updates on television and the radio, visiting your health department's website, and staying alert for messages from community leaders.

PODs are designed to provide medicine to a large number of people in a short period of time, so you should expect to stand in line. While at the POD, you would be asked to fill out a form that includes some basic information about your medical history. Once you complete your form, a POD staff member would review it and determine which antibiotic is best for you.

Keep a Family Medical History

In some cases, you may be able to pick up antibiotics for others in your household. If you live with family members, it is important to keep a medical history for each person in your family, including:

- Medical conditions
- Allergies
- Any medicines they are taking
- Each child's weight

During an emergency, you may be asked to bring this information to a POD to make sure you get the right antibiotics for everyone in your family.

In an anthrax emergency, many lives would be saved if people started taking antibiotics right away. It is very important to start taking antibiotics as soon as you get them, take them as directed, and keep taking them as for as long as you are told to.

We hope there is never an anthrax emergency that requires PODs to open, but if there is, be assured the process is in place to get antibiotics to you and your family as quickly as possible.

Be Aware of the Symptoms of Anthrax

During an anthrax emergency, you would need to be able to recognize the symptoms of anthrax, especially inhalation anthrax, and be prepared to get medical care if you are experiencing any symptoms.

What the Centers for Disease Control and Prevention Is Doing to Prepare

The CDC is working with other federal agencies and health departments across the country to prepare for an anthrax attack. Activities include:

- Providing funds and guidance to help health departments strengthen their ability to respond to all types of public health incidents and build more resilient communities

- Providing training in emergency response for the public health workforce and healthcare providers, as well as leaders in the public and private sector

- Coordinating response activities and providing resources to health departments through the CDC Emergency Operations Center

- Regulating the possession, use, and transfer of biological agents and toxins that could pose a severe threat to public health and safety through the CDC Select Agent Program

- Promoting science and practices to strengthen preparedness and response activities

- Ensuring that the United States has enough laboratories that can quickly conduct tests when anthrax is suspected

- Working with hospitals, laboratories, emergency response teams, and healthcare providers to make sure they have the medicine and supplies they would need if an anthrax attack occurred

- Developing guidance to protect the health and safety of workers who would be responding during an anthrax emergency

Part Two

Viral Contagious Diseases

Chapter 7

Adenovirus

Adenoviruses are common viruses that cause a range of illness. They can cause cold-like symptoms, a sore throat, bronchitis, pneumonia, diarrhea, and pink eye (conjunctivitis). You can get an adenovirus infection at any age. People with weakened immune systems or existing respiratory or cardiac disease are more likely than others to get very sick from an adenovirus infection.

Symptoms of Adenovirus

Adenoviruses can cause a wide range of illnesses, such as:

- The common cold
- A sore throat
- Bronchitis (a condition that occurs when the airways in the lungs become filled with mucus and may spasm, which causes a person to cough and have shortness of breath)
- Pneumonia (infection of the lungs)
- Diarrhea
- Pink eye
- Fever

This chapter includes text excerpted from "Adenoviruses," Centers for Disease Control and Prevention (CDC), April 26, 2018.

- Bladder inflammation or infection

- Inflammation of the stomach and intestines

- Neurologic disease (conditions that affect the brain and spinal cord)

Adenoviruses can cause mild to severe illness, though serious illness is less common. People with weakened immune systems, or existing respiratory or cardiac disease, are at a higher risk of developing severe illness from an adenovirus infection.

Transmission of Adenovirus

Adenoviruses are usually spread from an infected person to others through:

- Close personal contact, such as touching or shaking hands

- The air, by coughing and sneezing

- Touching an object or surface with adenoviruses on it, then touching your mouth, nose, or eyes before washing your hands

Some adenoviruses can spread through an infected person's stool, for example, during diaper changing. Adenovirus can also spread through the water, such as swimming pools, but this is less common.

Sometimes, the virus can be shed (released from the body) for a long time after a person recovers from an adenovirus infection, especially among people who have weakened immune systems.

This "virus shedding" usually occurs without any symptoms, even though the person can still spread adenovirus to other people.

Treatment of Adenovirus

There is no specific treatment for people with adenovirus infection. Most adenovirus infections are mild and may require only care to help relieve symptoms.

Prevention of Adenovirus
The Adenovirus Vaccine Is for U.S. Military Only

There is currently no adenovirus vaccine available to the general public.

A vaccine specific for adenovirus types 4 and 7 was approved by the U.S. Food and Drug Administration (FDA) in March 2011 for use only in U.S. military personnel who may be at a higher risk for infection from these two adenovirus types.

Follow Simple Steps to Protect Yourself and Others

You can protect yourself and others from adenoviruses and other respiratory illnesses by following a few simple steps:

- Wash your hands often with soap and water.
- Avoid touching your eyes, nose, or mouth with unwashed hands.
- Avoid close contact with people who are sick.

If you are sick, you can help protect others by following a few simple steps:

- Stay home when you are sick.
- Cover your mouth and nose when coughing or sneezing.
- Avoid sharing cups and eating utensils with others.
- Refrain from kissing others.
- Wash your hands often with soap and water, especially after using the bathroom.

Frequent handwashing is especially important in child care settings and healthcare facilities.

Maintain Proper Chlorine Levels to Prevent Outbreaks

Adenoviruses are resistant to many common disinfectant products and can remain infectious for long periods on surfaces and objects. It is important to keep adequate levels of chlorine in swimming pools to prevent outbreaks of conjunctivitis caused by adenoviruses.

Chapter 8

Avian Flu

Although avian influenza A viruses usually do not infect people, rare cases of human infection with these viruses have been reported. Infected birds shed avian influenza virus in their saliva, mucus, and feces. Human infections with bird flu viruses can happen when enough virus gets into a person's eyes, nose, or mouth, or enough is inhaled. This can happen when the virus is in the air (in droplets or possibly dust) and a person breathes it in, or when a person touches something that has the virus on it then touches their mouth, eyes, or nose. Rare human infections with some avian viruses have occurred most often after unprotected contact with infected birds or surfaces contaminated with avian influenza viruses. However, some infections have been identified where direct contact was not known to have occurred. Illness in people has ranged from mild to severe.

The spread of avian influenza A viruses from one ill person to another has been reported very rarely, and when it has been reported, it has been limited, inefficient, and not sustained. However, because of the possibility that avian influenza A viruses could change and gain the ability to spread easily between people, monitoring for human infection and person-to-person spread is extremely important for public health.

This chapter includes text excerpted from "Avian Influenza A Virus Infections in Humans," Centers for Disease Control and Prevention (CDC), April 18, 2017.

Signs and Symptoms of Avian Influenza A Virus Infections in Humans

The reported signs and symptoms of avian influenza A virus infections in humans have ranged from mild to severe and include conjunctivitis; influenza-like illness (e.g., fever, cough, sore throat, muscle aches), sometimes accompanied by nausea, abdominal pain, diarrhea, and vomiting; severe respiratory illness (e.g., shortness of breath, difficulty breathing, pneumonia, acute respiratory distress, viral pneumonia, respiratory failure); neurologic changes (altered mental status, seizures); and the involvement of other organ systems.

Asian lineage H7N9 and HPAI Asian lineage H5N1 viruses have been responsible for most human illness worldwide to date, including most serious illnesses and highest mortality.

Detecting Avian Influenza A Virus Infection in Humans

Avian influenza A virus infection in people cannot be diagnosed by clinical signs and symptoms alone; laboratory testing is needed. Avian influenza A virus infection is usually diagnosed by collecting a swab from the upper respiratory tract (nose or throat) of the sick person. (Testing is more accurate when the swab is collected during the first few days of illness.) This specimen is sent to a laboratory; the laboratory looks for avian influenza A virus either by using a molecular test, by trying to grow the virus, or both. (Growing avian influenza A viruses should only be done in laboratories with high levels of biosafety.)

For critically ill patients, the collection and testing of lower respiratory tract specimens also may lead to the diagnosis of avian influenza virus infection. However, for some patients who are no longer very sick or who have fully recovered, it may be difficult to detect avian influenza A virus in the specimen. Sometimes, it may still be possible to diagnose avian influenza A virus infection by looking for evidence of antibodies the body has produced in response to the virus. This is not always an option because it requires two blood specimens (one taken during the first week of illness and another taken three to four weeks later). Also, it can take several weeks to verify the results, and testing must be performed in a special laboratory, such as at the Centers for Disease Control and Prevention (CDC).

The CDC has posted guidance for clinicians and public health professionals in the United States on appropriate testing, specimen collection, and processing of samples from patients who may be infected with avian influenza A viruses.

Treating Avian Influenza A Virus Infections in Humans

The CDC currently recommends a neuraminidase inhibitor for the treatment of human infection with avian influenza A viruses. The CDC has posted avian influenza guidance for healthcare professionals and laboratorians, including guidance on the use of antiviral medications for the treatment of human infections with novel influenza viruses associated with severe disease. Analyses of available avian influenza viruses circulating worldwide suggest that most viruses are susceptible to oseltamivir, peramivir, and zanamivir. However, some evidence of antiviral resistance has been reported in Asian H5N1 and Asian H7N9 viruses isolated from some human cases. Monitoring for antiviral resistance among avian influenza A viruses is crucial and ongoing.

Preventing Human Infection with Avian Influenza A Viruses

The best way to prevent infection with avian influenza A virus is to avoid sources of exposure. Most human infections with avian influenza A viruses have occurred following direct or close contact with infected poultry.

People who have had contact with infected birds may be given influenza antiviral drugs preventatively. While antiviral drugs are most often used to treat influenza, they also can be used to prevent infection in someone who has been exposed to influenza viruses. When used to prevent seasonal influenza, antiviral drugs are 70 to 90 percent effective. The CDC has posted interim guidance for clinicians and public health professionals in the United States regarding the follow-up and influenza antiviral chemoprophylaxis of persons exposed to birds infected with avian influenza A viruses.

The seasonal influenza vaccination will not prevent infection with avian influenza A viruses, but it can reduce the risk of co-infection with human and avian influenza A viruses. It is also possible to make a vaccine that can protect people against avian influenza viruses. For example, the United States government maintains a stockpile of vaccines to protect against some Asian avian influenza A H5N1 viruses.

The stockpiled vaccine could be used if similar H5N1 viruses were to begin transmitting easily from person to person. Since influenza viruses change, the CDC continues to make new candidate vaccine viruses as needed. Creating a candidate vaccine virus is the first step in producing a vaccine.

Chapter 9

Chickenpox (Varicella) and Shingles

About Chickenpox

Chickenpox is a highly contagious disease caused by the varicella-zoster virus (VZV). It can cause an itchy, blister-like rash. The rash first appears on the chest, back, and face, and then spreads over the entire body, causing between 250 and 500 itchy blisters. Chickenpox can be serious, especially in babies, adolescents, adults, pregnant women, and people with a weakened immune system. The best way to prevent chickenpox is to get the chickenpox vaccine.

Chickenpox used to be very common in the United States. In the early 1990s, an average of 4 million people got chickenpox, 10,500 to 13,000 were hospitalized, and 100 to 150 died each year.

The chickenpox vaccine became available in the United States in 1995. Each year, more than 3.5 million cases of chickenpox, 9,000 hospitalizations, and 100 deaths are prevented by chickenpox vaccination in the United States.

This chapter contains text excerpted from the following sources: Text under the heading "About Chickenpox" is excerpted from "About Chickenpox," Centers for Disease Control and Prevention (CDC), December 31, 2018; Text under the heading "About Shingles" is excerpted from "Shingles," National Institute on Aging (NIA), National Institutes of Health (NIH), October 29, 2018.

Signs and Symptoms of Chickenpox

Anyone who has not had chickenpox or gotten the chickenpox vaccine can get the disease. Chickenpox illness usually lasts about four to seven days.

The classic symptom of chickenpox is a rash that turns into itchy, fluid-filled blisters that eventually turn into scabs. The rash may first show up on the chest, back, and face, and then spread over the entire body, including inside the mouth, eyelids, or genital area. It usually takes about one week for all of the blisters to become scabs.

Other typical symptoms that may begin to appear one to two days before rash include:

- Fever

- Tiredness

- Loss of appetite

- Headache

Children usually miss five to six days of school or child care due to chickenpox

Chickenpox in Vaccinated People

Some people who have been vaccinated against chickenpox can still get the disease. However, the symptoms are usually milder, with fewer or no blisters (or just red spots), mild or no fever, and a shorter duration of illness. But some vaccinated people who get chickenpox may have a disease similar to unvaccinated people.

People at Risk for Severe Chickenpox

Some people who get chickenpox may have more severe symptoms and may be at a higher risk for complications.

Complications of Chickenpox

Complications from chickenpox can occur, but they are not common in healthy people who get the disease. People who may get a serious case of chickenpox and may be at high risk for complications include:

- Infants

- Adolescents

- Adults
- Pregnant women
- People with weakened immune systems because of illness or medications, such as:
  - People with human immunodeficiency virus/acquired immunodeficiency syndrome (HIV/AIDS) or cancer
  - Patients who have had transplants
  - People on chemotherapy, immunosuppressive medications, or long-term use of steroids

Serious complications from chickenpox include:

- Bacterial infections of the skin and soft tissues in children, including Group A streptococcal infections
- Infection of the lungs (pneumonia)
- Infection or inflammation of the brain (encephalitis, cerebellar ataxia)
- Bleeding problems (hemorrhagic complications)
- Bloodstream infections (sepsis)
- Dehydration
- Some people with serious complications from chickenpox can become so sick that they need to be hospitalized. Chickenpox can also cause death.

Deaths are very rare now due to the vaccine program. However, some deaths from chickenpox continue to occur in healthy, unvaccinated children and adults. In the past, many of the healthy adults who died from chickenpox contracted the disease from their unvaccinated children.

Transmission of Chickenpox

Chickenpox is a highly contagious disease caused by the VZV. The virus spreads easily from people with chickenpox to others who have never had the disease or never been vaccinated. The virus spreads mainly through close contact with someone who has chickenpox.

The VZV also causes shingles. Chickenpox can be spread from people with shingles to others who have never had chickenpox or received the chickenpox vaccine. This can happen through close contact with someone who has shingles.

A person with chickenpox is contagious, beginning 1 to 2 days before rash onset until all the chickenpox lesions have crusted (scabbed). Vaccinated people who get chickenpox may develop lesions that do not crust. These people are considered contagious until no new lesions have appeared for 24 hours.

It takes about 2 weeks (from 10 to 21 days) after exposure to a person with chickenpox or shingles for someone to develop chickenpox. If a vaccinated person gets the disease, they can still spread it to others. For most people, getting chickenpox once provides immunity for life. However, for a few people, it is possible to get chickenpox more than once; although, this is not common.

Treatment of Chickenpox
Treatments at Home for People with Chickenpox

There are several things that you can do at home to help relieve chickenpox symptoms and prevent skin infections. Calamine lotion and a cool bath with added baking soda, uncooked oatmeal, or colloidal oatmeal may help relieve some of the itching. Try to minimize scratching to prevent the virus from spreading to others and potential bacterial infection from occurring. Keeping fingernails trimmed short may help prevent skin infections caused by scratching blisters.

Over-the-Counter Medications

Do not use aspirin or aspirin-containing products to relieve fever from chickenpox. The use of aspirin in children with chickenpox has been associated with Reye syndrome, a severe disease that affects the liver and brain and can cause death. Instead, use nonaspirin medications, such as acetaminophen, to relieve fever from chickenpox. The American Academy of Pediatrics (AAP) recommends avoiding treatment with ibuprofen if possible because it has been associated with life-threatening bacterial skin infections.

When to Call a Healthcare Provider

For people exposed to chickenpox, call a healthcare provider if the person:

- Has never had chickenpox and is not vaccinated with the chickenpox vaccine

- Is pregnant
- Has a weakened immune system caused by disease or medication; for example:
  - A person with HIV/AIDS or cancer
  - A person who has had a transplant
  - A person on chemotherapy, immunosuppressive medications, or long-term use of steroids

Call a healthcare provider if:

- The person is at risk of serious complications because she or he:
  - Is less than 1 year of age
  - Is older than 12 years of age
- Has a weakened immune system
- Is pregnant
- The person develops any of the following symptoms:
  - Fever that lasts longer than 4 days
  - Fever that rises above 102°F (38.9°C)
- Any areas of the rash or any part of the body becomes very red, warm, or tender, or begins leaking pus (thick, discolored fluid), as these symptoms may indicate a bacterial infection
- Difficulty waking up or confused behavior
- Difficulty walking
- Stiff neck
- Frequent vomiting
- Difficulty breathing
- Severe cough
- Severe abdominal pain
- Rash with bleeding or bruising (hemorrhagic rash)

Treatments Prescribed by Your Doctor for People with Chickenpox

Your healthcare provider can advise you on treatment options. Antiviral medications are recommended for people with chickenpox that are more likely to develop serious illness, including:

- Otherwise healthy people older than 12 years of age

- People with chronic skin or lung disease

- People receiving long-term salicylate therapy or steroid therapy

- Pregnant women

- People with a weakened immune system

There are antiviral medications licensed for the treatment of chickenpox. The medication works best if it is given as early as possible, preferably within the first 24 hours after the rash starts.

Prevention of Chickenpox

The best way to prevent chickenpox is to get the chickenpox vaccine. Everyone—including children, adolescents, and adults—should get two doses of the chickenpox vaccine if they have never had chickenpox or were never vaccinated.

The chickenpox vaccine is very safe and effective at preventing the disease. Most people who get the vaccine will not get chickenpox. If a vaccinated person does get chickenpox, the symptoms are usually milder with fewer or no blisters (they may have just red spots) and mild or no fever.

The chickenpox vaccine prevents almost all cases of severe illness. Since the varicella vaccination program began in the United States, there has been over 90 percent decrease in chickenpox cases, hospitalizations, and deaths.

About Shingles

Shingles is a disease that affects your nerves. It can cause burning, shooting pain, tingling, and/or itching, as well as a rash and blisters. You may recall having chickenpox as a child. Shingles is caused by the same virus, the VZV. After you recover from chickenpox, the virus continues to live in some of your nerve cells. It is usually inactive, so you do not even know it is there. In fact, most adults live with VZV in their bodies and never get shingles. But, for about one in three adults, the virus will become active again. Instead of causing another case of chickenpox, it produces shingles. It is not totally understood what makes the virus go from inactive to active. Having shingles does not mean you have any other underlying disease.

How Do You Get Shingles?

Everyone who has had chickenpox has VZV in their body and is at risk for getting shingles. Right now, there is no way of knowing who will get the disease. But, some things make it more likely:

Advanced age. The risk of getting shingles increases as you age. People may have a harder time fighting off infections as they get older. About half of all shingles cases are in adults 60 years of age or older. The chance of getting shingles becomes much greater by the age of 70.

Trouble fighting infections. Your immune system is the part of your body that responds to infections. Age can affect your immune system, as can an HIV infection, cancer, cancer treatments, too much sun, or organ transplant drugs. Even stress or a cold can weaken your immune system for a short time. These all can put you at risk for shingles.

Can You Catch Shingles?

Shingles is not contagious. You cannot catch it from someone. But, you can catch chickenpox from someone with shingles. So, if you have never had chickenpox, try to stay away from anyone who has shingles.

If you have shingles, try to stay away from anyone who has not had chickenpox or who might have a weak immune system.

What Are the Symptoms of Shingles?

Usually, shingles develop only on one side of the body or face and in a small area rather than all over. The most common place for shingles is a band that goes around one side of your waistline.

Most people have some of the following shingles symptoms:

- Burning, tingling, or numbness of the skin
- Feeling sick—chills, fever, upset stomach, or headache
- Fluid-filled blisters
- Skin that is sensitive to touch
- Mild itching to strong pain

Depending on where shingles develop, it could also cause symptoms, such as hiccups or even loss of vision.

For some people, the symptoms of shingles are mild. They might just have some itching. For others, shingles can cause intense pain that can be felt from the gentlest touch or breeze.

How Long Does Shingles Last?

Most cases of shingles last three to five weeks. Shingles follow a pattern:

- The first sign is often burning or tingling pain; sometimes, it includes numbness or itching on one side of the body.

- Somewhere between one and five days after the tingling or burning feeling on the skin, a red rash will appear.

- A few days later, the rash will turn into fluid-filled blisters.

- About a week to 10 days after that, the blisters dry up and crust over.

- A couple of weeks later, the scabs clear up.

Most people get shingles only one time. But, it is possible to have it more than once.

Long-Term Pain and Other Lasting Problems

After the shingles rash goes away, some people may be left with ongoing pain called "postherpetic neuralgia" (PHN). The pain is felt in the area where the rash had been. For some people, PHN is the longest lasting and worst part of shingles. The older you are when you get shingles, the greater your chance of developing PHN.

Postherpetic neuralgia pain can cause depression, anxiety, sleeplessness, and weight loss. Some people with PHN find it hard to go about their daily activities, such as dressing, cooking, and eating. Talk to your doctor if you have any of these problems.

There are medicines that may help with PHN. Steroids may lessen the pain and shorten the time you are sick. Analgesics, antidepressants, and anticonvulsants may also reduce pain. Usually, PHN will get better over time.

Some people have other problems that last after shingles has cleared up. For example, the blisters caused by shingles can become infected. They may also leave a scar. It is important to keep the area clean and try not to scratch the blisters. Your doctor can prescribe an antibiotic treatment if needed.

See your doctor right away if you notice blisters on your face—this is an urgent problem. Blisters near or in the eye can cause lasting eye damage or blindness. Hearing loss, a brief paralysis of the face, or, very rarely, swelling of the brain (encephalitis) can also occur.

Do You Have a Rash?

If you think you might have shingles, talk to your doctor as soon as possible. It is important to see your doctor no later than three days after the rash starts. The doctor will confirm whether or not you have shingles and can make a treatment plan. Although there is no cure for shingles, early treatment with drugs that fight the virus can help the blisters dry up faster and limit severe pain. Shingles can often be treated at home. People with shingles rarely need to stay in a hospital.

Should You Get the Shingles Vaccine?

The shingles vaccine is safe and easy, and it may keep you from getting shingles and PHN. Healthy adults 50 years of age and older should get vaccinated with a shingles vaccine called "Shingrix." It is given in 2 doses, 2 to 6 months apart. Shingrix is preferred over Zostavax, an older shingles vaccine. Zostavax may still be used to prevent shingles in healthy adults 60 years of age and older. For example, you could use Zostavax if a person is allergic to Shingrix, prefers Zostavax, or requests immediate vaccination and Shingrix is not available.

You should try to get the second dose of Shingrix between two and six months after you got the first dose. If your doctor or pharmacist is out of Shingrix, you can use the Vaccine Finder (www.vaccinefinder. org) to help find other providers who have Shingrix. You can also contact pharmacies in your area and ask to be put on a waiting list for Shingrix. If it is been more than six months since you got the first dose, you should get the second dose as soon as possible. You do not need to get a first dose again.

You should get Shingrix even if you have already had shingles, received Zostavax, or do not remember having had chickenpox. However, you should not get Shingrix if you have a fever or illness, have a weakened immune system, or have had an allergic reaction to Shingrix. Check with your doctor if you are not sure what to do.

You can get the shingles vaccine at your doctor's office and at some pharmacies. All Medicare Part D plans and most private health insurance plans will cover the cost.

What Can You Do about Shingles?

If you have shingles, here are some tips that might help you feel better:

• Get plenty of rest, and eat well-balanced meals.

101

- Try simple exercises, such as stretching or walking. Check with your doctor before starting a new exercise routine.

- Apply a cool washcloth to your blisters to ease the pain and help dry the blisters.

- Do things that take your mind off your pain. For example, watch television, read, talk with friends, listen to relaxing music, or work on a hobby you like.

- Avoid stress. It can make the pain worse.

- Wear loose-fitting, natural-fiber clothing.

- Take an oatmeal bath, or use calamine lotion to see if it soothes your skin.

- Share your feelings about your pain with family and friends. Ask for their understanding.

Also, you can limit spreading the virus by:

- Keeping the rash covered

- Not touching or scratching the rash

- Washing your hands often

Chapter 10

Common Colds

A sore throat and runny nose are usually the first signs of a cold, followed by coughing and sneezing. Most people recover in about 7 to 10 days. You can help reduce your risk of getting a cold by washing your hands often, avoiding close contact with sick people, and not touching your face with unwashed hands.

Common colds are the main reason that children miss school and adults miss work. Each year in the United States, there are millions of cases of the common cold. Adults have an average of two to three colds per year, and children have even more.

Most people get colds in the winter and spring, but it is possible to get a cold any time of the year. Symptoms usually include:

- A sore throat
- Runny nose
- Coughing
- Sneezing
- Headaches
- Body aches

This chapter includes text excerpted from "Common Colds: Protect Yourself and Others," Centers for Disease Control and Prevention (CDC), February 11, 2019.

Most people recover within about 7 to 10 days. However, people with weakened immune systems, asthma, or respiratory conditions may develop a serious illness, such as bronchitis or pneumonia.

How to Protect Yourself

Viruses that cause colds can spread from infected people to others through the air and close personal contact. You can also get infected through contact with stool or respiratory secretions from an infected person. This can happen when you shake hands with someone who has a cold or when you touch a surface, such as a doorknob, that has respiratory viruses on it, then touch your eyes, mouth, or nose.

You can help reduce your risk of getting a cold by:

- Washing your hands often with soap and water. Wash them for 20 seconds, and help young children do the same. If soap and water are not available, use an alcohol-based hand sanitizer. Viruses that cause colds can live on your hands, and regular handwashing can help protect you from getting sick.

- Avoid touching your eyes, nose, and mouth with unwashed hands. Viruses that cause colds can enter your body this way and make you sick

- Stay away from people who are sick. Sick people can spread viruses that cause the common cold through close contact with others.

How to Protect Others

If you have a cold, you should follow these tips to help prevent spreading it to other people:

- Stay at home while you are sick, and keep children out of school or day care while they are sick.

- Avoid close contact with others, such as hugging, kissing, or shaking hands.

- Move away from people before coughing or sneezing.

- Cough and sneeze into a tissue then throw it away, or cough and sneeze into your upper shirt sleeve, completely covering your mouth and nose.

- Wash your hands after coughing, sneezing, or blowing your nose.

- Disinfect frequently touched surfaces and objects, such as toys and doorknobs.

There is no vaccine to protect you against the common cold.

How to Feel Better

There is no cure for a cold. To feel better, you should get lots of rest and drink plenty of fluids. Over-the-counter (OTC) medicines may help ease symptoms but will not make your cold go away any faster. Always read the label, and use medications as directed. Talk to your doctor before giving your child nonprescription cold medicines because some medicines contain ingredients that are not recommended for children.

Antibiotics will not help you recover from a cold caused by a respiratory virus. They do not work against viruses, and they may make it harder for your body to fight future bacterial infections if you take them unnecessarily.

When to See a Doctor

You should call your doctor if you or your child has one or more of these conditions:

- Symptoms that last more than 10 days

- Symptoms that are severe or unusual

- If your child is younger than three months of age and has a fever or is lethargic

You should also call your doctor right away if you are at high risk for serious flu complications and experience flu symptoms such as fever, chills, and muscle or body aches. People at high risk for flu complications include young children (younger than 5 years of age); adults 65 years of age and older; pregnant women; and people with certain medical conditions, such as asthma, diabetes, and heart disease.

Your doctor can determine if you or your child has a cold or the flu, and they can recommend treatment to help with symptoms.

Causes of the Common Cold

Many different respiratory viruses can cause the common cold, but rhinoviruses are the most common. Rhinoviruses can also trigger asthma attacks and have been linked to sinus and ear infections. Other viruses that can cause colds include respiratory syncytial virus, human parainfluenza viruses, adenovirus, human coronaviruses, and human metapneumovirus.

Know the Difference between Common Cold and Flu

The flu, which is caused by influenza viruses, also spreads and causes illness around the same time as the common cold. Because these two illnesses have similar symptoms, it can be difficult (or even impossible) to tell the difference between them based on symptoms alone. In general, flu symptoms are worse than the common cold and can include fever or feeling feverish/chills, cough, a sore throat, a runny or stuffy nose, muscle or body aches, headaches and fatigue (tiredness). Flu can also have very serious complications. The Centers for Disease Control and Prevention (CDC) recommends yearly flu vaccination as the first and best way to prevent the flu. If you get the flu, antiviral drugs may be a treatment option.

Chapter 11

Conjunctivitis

People often call conjunctivitis "pink eye" because it can cause the white of the eye to take on a pink or red color. Symptoms of pink eye can vary but typically include redness or swelling of the white of the eye.

Causes of Conjunctivitis

The most common causes of conjunctivitis (pink eye) are:

- Viruses
- Bacteria
- Allergens

Other causes include:

- Chemicals
- Contact lens wear
- Foreign bodies in the eye (such as a loose eyelash)
- Indoor and outdoor air pollution caused, for example, by smoke, dust, fumes, or chemical vapors
- Fungi
- Ameba and parasites

This chapter includes text excerpted from "Conjunctivitis (Pink Eye)," Centers for Disease Control and Prevention (CDC), January 4, 2019.

It can be difficult to determine the exact cause of conjunctivitis because some symptoms may be the same no matter the cause.

Viral Conjunctivitis

- Infection of the eye caused by a virus

- Can be caused by a number of different viruses, such as adenoviruses

- Very contagious

- Sometimes can result in large outbreaks depending on the virus

Bacterial Conjunctivitis

- Infection of the eye caused by certain bacteria

- Can be caused by *Staphylococcus aureus*, *Streptococcus pneumoniae*, *Haemophilus influenzae*, *Moraxella catarrhalis*, or, less commonly, *Chlamydia trachomatis* and *Neisseria gonorrhoeae*

- Can be spread easily, especially with certain bacteria and in certain settings

- Children with conjunctivitis without fever or behavioral changes can usually continue going to school.

- More common in kids than adults

- Observed more frequently December through April

Allergic Conjunctivitis

- The result of the body's reaction to allergens, such as pollen from trees, plants, grasses, and weeds; dust mites; molds; dander from pets; medicines; or cosmetics

- Not contagious

- Occurs more frequently among people with other allergic conditions, such as hay fever, asthma, and eczema

- Can occur seasonally when allergens, such as pollen counts, are high

- Can also occur year-round due to indoor allergens, such as dust mites and animal dander

Conjunctivitis Caused by Irritants

- Caused by irritation from a foreign body in the eye or contact with smoke, dust, fumes, or chemicals
- Not contagious
- Can occur when contact lenses are worn longer than recommended or not cleaned properly

Symptoms of Conjunctivitis

Symptoms of conjunctivitis (pink eye) can include:

- The pink or red color in the white of the eye(s)
- Swelling of the conjunctiva (the thin layer that lines the white part of the eye and the inside of the eyelid) and/or eyelids
- Increased tear production
- Feeling such as a foreign body is in the eye(s) or an urge to rub the eye(s)
- Itching, irritation, and/or burning
- Discharge (pus or mucus)
- Crusting of eyelids or lashes, especially in the morning
- Contact lenses that feel uncomfortable and/or do not stay in place on the eye

Depending on the cause, other symptoms may occur.

Viral Conjunctivitis

- Can occur with symptoms of a cold, flu, or other respiratory infection
- Usually begins in one eye and may spread to the other eye within days
- Discharge from the eye is usually watery rather than thick

Bacterial Conjunctivitis

- More commonly associated with discharge (pus), which can lead to eyelids sticking together
- Sometimes occurs with an ear infection

Allergic Conjunctivitis

• Usually occurs in both eyes

• Can produce intense itching, tearing, and swelling in the eyes

• May occur with symptoms of allergies, such as an itchy nose, sneezing, a scratchy throat, or asthma

Conjunctivitis Caused by Irritants

• Can produce watery eyes and mucus discharge

Transmission of Conjunctivitis
How It Spreads

Several viruses and bacteria can cause conjunctivitis, some of which are very contagious. Each of these types of germs can spread from person to person in different ways. They usually spread from an infected person to others through:

• Close personal contact, such as touching or shaking hands

• The air by coughing and sneezing

• Touching an object or surface with germs on it, then touching your eyes before washing your hands

When to Go Back to Work or School

If you have conjunctivitis but do not have a fever or other symptoms, you may be allowed to remain at work or school with your doctor's approval. However, if you still have symptoms, and your activities at work or school include close contact with other people, you should not attend.

Diagnosis of Conjunctivitis

A doctor can often determine whether a virus, bacterium, or allergen is causing conjunctivitis based on patient history, symptoms, and an examination of the eye. Conjunctivitis always involves eye redness or swelling, but it also has other symptoms that can vary depending on the cause. These symptoms can help a healthcare professional diagnose the cause of conjunctivitis. However, it can sometimes be difficult to make a firm diagnosis because some symptoms are the same no matter the cause.

It can also sometimes be difficult to determine the cause without doing laboratory testing. Although not routinely done, your healthcare provider may collect a sample of eye discharge from the infected eye and send it to the laboratory to help them determine which form of infection you have and how best to treat it.

Viral Conjunctivitis

The cause is likely a virus if:

- Conjunctivitis accompanies a common cold or respiratory tract infection
- Discharge from the eye is watery rather than thick

Bacterial Conjunctivitis

The cause may be bacterial if:

- Conjunctivitis occurs at the same time as an ear infection
- Occurs shortly after birth
- Discharge from the eye is thick rather than watery

Allergic Conjunctivitis

The cause is likely allergic if:

- Conjunctivitis occurs seasonally when pollen counts are high
- The patient's eyes itch intensely
- It occurs with other signs of allergic diseases, such as hay fever, asthma, or eczema

Treatment of Conjunctivitis

There are times when it is important to seek medical care for conjunctivitis. However, this is not always necessary. To help relieve some of the inflammation and dryness caused by conjunctivitis, you can use cold compresses and artificial tears, which you can purchase over-the-counter (OTC) without a prescription. You should also stop wearing contact lenses until your eye doctor says it is okay to start wearing them again. If you did not need to see a doctor, do not wear your contacts until you no longer have symptoms of pink eye.

111

When to Seek Medical Care

You should see a healthcare provider if you have conjunctivitis along with any of the following:

- Pain in the eye(s)

- Sensitivity to light or blurred vision that does not improve when discharge is wiped from the eye(s)

- Intense redness in the eye(s)

- Symptoms that get worse or do not improve, including pink eye thought to be caused by bacteria that does not improve after 24 hours of antibiotic use

- A weakened immune system, for example from human immunodeficiency virus (HIV) infection, cancer treatment, or other medical conditions or treatments

Newborns with symptoms of conjunctivitis should see a doctor right away.

Viral Conjunctivitis

Most cases of viral conjunctivitis are mild. The infection will usually clear up in 7 to 14 days without treatment and without any long-term consequences. However, in some cases, viral conjunctivitis can take 2 to 3 weeks or more to clear up.

A doctor can prescribe antiviral medication to treat more serious forms of conjunctivitis. For example, conjunctivitis caused by herpes simplex virus (HSV) or varicella-zoster virus (VZV). Antibiotics will not improve viral conjunctivitis; these drugs are not effective against viruses.

Bacterial Conjunctivitis

Your doctor may prescribe an antibiotic, usually given topically as eye drops or ointment, for bacterial conjunctivitis. Antibiotics may help shorten the length of infection, reduce complications, and reduce the spread to others. Antibiotics may be necessary in the following cases:

- With discharge (pus)

- When conjunctivitis occurs in people whose immune system is compromised

- When certain bacteria are suspected

Mild bacterial conjunctivitis may get better without antibiotic treatment and without causing any complications. It often improves in two to five days without treatment but can take two weeks to go away completely.

Talk with your doctor about the best treatment options for your infection.

Allergic Conjunctivitis

Conjunctivitis caused by an allergen (such as pollen or animal dander) usually improves by removing the allergen from the person's environment. Allergy medications and certain eye drops (topical antihistamine and vasoconstrictors), including some prescription eye drops, can also provide relief from allergic conjunctivitis. In some cases, your doctor may recommend a combination of drugs to improve symptoms. Your doctor can help if you have conjunctivitis caused by an allergy.

Prevention of Conjunctivitis
Preventing the Spread of Conjunctivitis

Viral and bacterial conjunctivitis are very contagious. They can spread easily from person to person. You can greatly reduce the risk of getting conjunctivitis or spreading it to someone else by following some simple steps for good hygiene.

If You Have Conjunctivitis

If you have conjunctivitis, you can help limit its spread to other people by following these steps:

- Wash your hands often with soap and warm water for at least 20 seconds. Wash them especially well before and after cleaning, or applying eye drops or ointment to your infected eye. If soap and water are not available, use an alcohol-based hand sanitizer that contains at least 60 percent alcohol to clean your hands.

- Avoid touching or rubbing your eyes. This can worsen the condition or spread it to your other eye.

- With clean hands, wash any discharge from around your eye(s) several times a day using a clean, wet washcloth or fresh cotton ball. Throw away cotton balls after use, and wash used washcloths with hot water and detergent, then wash your hands again with soap and warm water.

- Do not use the same eye drop dispenser/bottle for your infected and noninfected eyes.

- Wash pillowcases, sheets, washcloths, and towels often in hot water and detergent; wash your hands after handling such items.

- Stop wearing contact lenses until your eye doctor says it is okay to start wearing them again.

- Clean eyeglasses, being careful not to contaminate items (such as hand towels) that might be shared by other people.

- Clean, store, and replace your contact lenses as instructed by your eye doctor.

- Do not share personal items, such as pillows, washcloths, towels, eye drops, eye or face makeup, makeup brushes, contact lenses, contact lens storage cases, or eyeglasses.

- Do not use swimming pools.

If You Are around Someone with Conjunctivitis

If you are around someone with conjunctivitis, you can reduce your risk of infection by following these steps:

- Wash your hands often with soap and warm water for at least 20 seconds. If soap and warm water are not available, use an alcohol-based hand sanitizer that contains at least 60 percent alcohol to clean your hands.

- Wash your hands after contact with an infected person or items she or he uses; for example, wash your hands after applying eye drops or ointment to an infected person's eye(s) or after putting their bed linens in the washing machine.

- Avoid touching your eyes with unwashed hands.

- Do not share items used by an infected person; for example, do not share pillows, washcloths, towels, eye drops, eye or face makeup, makeup brushes, contact lenses, contact lens storage cases, or eyeglasses.

Avoid Getting Sick Again

In addition, if you have conjunctivitis, there are steps you can take to avoid reinfection once the infection goes away:

- Throw away and replace any eye or face makeup or makeup brushes you used while infected.

- Throw away disposable contact lenses and cases that you used while your eyes were infected.

- Throw away contact lens solutions that you used while your eyes were infected.

- Clean extended wear lenses as directed.

- Clean eyeglasses and cases that you used while infected.

Vaccines Can Prevent Some Infections Associated with Conjunctivitis

There is no vaccine that prevents all types of conjunctivitis. However, there are vaccines to protect against some viral and bacterial diseases that are associated with conjunctivitis:

- Rubella

- Measles

- Chickenpox

- Shingles

- Pneumococcal

- *Haemophilus influenzae type b* (Hib)

Conjunctivitis caused by allergens or irritants is not contagious unless a secondary viral or bacterial infection develops.

Chapter 12

Ebola Virus Disease

What Is Ebola Virus Disease?

Ebola virus disease (EVD) is a rare and deadly disease most commonly affecting people and nonhuman primates (monkeys, gorillas, and chimpanzees). It is caused by an infection with a group of viruses within the genus *Ebolavirus*:

- Ebola virus (species *Zaire ebolavirus*)

- Sudan virus (species *Sudan ebolavirus*)

- Taï Forest virus (species *Taï Forest ebolavirus*, formerly *Côte d'Ivoire ebolavirus*)

- Bundibugyo virus (species *Bundibugyo ebolavirus*)

- Reston virus (species *Reston ebolavirus*)

- Bombali virus (species *Bombali ebolavirus*)

Of these, only four (Ebola, Sudan, Taï Forest, and Bundibugyo viruses) are known to cause disease in people. Reston virus is known to cause disease in nonhuman primates and pigs, but it does not affect people. It is unknown if the Bombali virus, which was identified in bats, causes disease in either animals or people.

This chapter includes text excerpted from "What Is Ebola Virus Disease?" Centers for Disease Control and Prevention (CDC), May 20, 2017.

Ebola virus was first discovered in 1976 near the Ebola River in what is now the Democratic Republic of Congo. Since then, the virus has been infecting people from time to time, leading to outbreaks in several African countries. Scientists do not know where the Ebola virus comes from. However, based on the nature of similar viruses, they believe that the virus is animal-borne, with bats being the most likely source. The bats carrying the virus can transmit it to other animals, such as apes, monkeys, duikers, and humans.

Ebola virus spreads to people through direct contact with bodily fluids of a person who is sick with or has died from EVD. This can occur when a person touches the infected bodily fluids (or objects that are contaminated with them), and the virus gets in through broken skin or mucous membranes in the eyes, nose, or mouth. The virus can also spread to people through direct contact with the blood, bodily fluids, and tissues of infected fruit bats or primates. People can get the virus through sexual contact as well.

Ebola survivors may experience difficult side effects after their recovery, such as tiredness, muscle aches, eye and vision problems, and stomach pain. Survivors may also experience stigma as they reenter their communities.

Transmission of Ebola Virus Disease

Scientists think that people are initially infected with Ebola virus through contact with an infected animal, such as a fruit bat or a nonhuman primate. This is called a "spillover event." After that, the virus spreads from person to person, potentially affecting a large number of people.

The virus spreads through direct contact (such as through broken skin or mucous membranes in the eyes, nose, or mouth) with:

- Blood or bodily fluids (urine, saliva, sweat, feces, vomit, breast milk, and semen) of a person who is sick with or has died from EVD

- Objects (such as needles and syringes) contaminated with bodily fluids from a person sick with EVD or the body of a person who died from EVD

- Infected fruit bats or nonhuman primates (such as apes and monkeys)

- Semen from a human who recovered from EVD (through oral, vaginal, or anal sex). The virus can remain in certain bodily fluids (including semen) of a patient who has recovered from EVD, even if they no longer have symptoms of severe illness

When someone gets infected with Ebola, they will not show signs or symptoms of illness right away. The Ebola virus cannot spread to others until a person develops signs or symptoms of EVD. After a person infected with Ebola develops symptoms of illness, they can spread Ebola to others.

Additionally, the Ebola virus usually is not transmitted by food. However, in certain parts of the world, Ebola virus may spread through the handling and consumption of bushmeat (wild animals hunted for food). There is also no evidence that mosquitoes or other insects can transmit Ebola virus.

Persistence of the Virus

There is no known risk of becoming infected with Ebola virus through casual contact with a survivor. However, the virus can remain in certain bodily fluids and continue to spread to others after a person has recovered from the infection. The virus can persist in semen, breast milk, ocular (eye) fluid, and spinal column fluid. Areas of the body that contain these fluids are known as "immunologically privileged sites." These are the sites of the body where viruses and pathogens, such as Ebola virus, can remain undetected even after the immune system has cleared the virus from other sites of the body. Scientists are now studying how long the virus stays in these bodily fluids among Ebola survivors.

During an Ebola outbreak, the virus can spread quickly within healthcare settings (such as clinics or hospitals). Clinicians and other healthcare personnel providing care should use dedicated medical equipment, preferably disposable. Proper cleaning and disposal of instruments, such as needles and syringes, are important. If instruments are not disposable, they must be sterilized before additional use.

Ebola virus is killed using a U.S. Environmental Protection Agency (EPA)-registered hospital disinfectant with a label claim for a nonenveloped virus. On dry surfaces, such as doorknobs and countertops, the virus can survive for several hours. However, in bodily fluids, such as blood, the virus can survive up to several days at room temperature.

Pets and Livestock

Serologic studies show that Ebola virus has been detected in dogs and cats found in Ebola-affected areas, but there are no reports of dogs or cats becoming sick with EVD or spreading the Ebola virus to people or other animals.

Certain exotic or unusual pets (monkeys, apes, or pigs) have been known to be infected with the Ebola virus. Pigs are the only species of livestock known to be at risk of infection by an Ebola virus. In the Philippines and China, pigs are naturally infected with Ebola Reston virus (*Reston ebolavirus*), which does not cause illness in people. In a laboratory setting, pigs have developed illness when infected with an extremely high dose of *Zaire ebolavirus*, but they are not known to be involved in the spread of this virus strain to humans.

Signs and Symptoms of Ebola Virus Disease

Symptoms of EVD include:

- Fever
- Severe headache
- Muscle pain
- Weakness
- Fatigue
- Diarrhea
- Vomiting
- Abdominal (stomach) pain
- Unexplained hemorrhage (bleeding or bruising)

Symptoms may appear anywhere from 2 to 21 days after contact with the virus, with an average of 8 to 10 days. Many common illnesses can have these same symptoms, including influenza (flu) or malaria.

Ebola virus disease is a rare but severe and often deadly disease. Recovery from EVD depends on good supportive clinical care and the patient's immune response. Studies show that survivors of Ebola virus infection have antibodies (molecules that are made by the immune system to label invading pathogens for destruction) that can be detected in the blood up to 10 years after recovery.

Diagnosis of Ebola Virus Disease

Diagnosing EVD shortly after infection can be difficult. Early symptoms of EVD, such as fever, headache, and weakness, are not specific to Ebola virus infection and often are seen in patients with other more common diseases, such as malaria and typhoid fever.

To determine whether Ebola virus infection is a possible diagnosis, there must be a combination of symptoms suggestive of EVD and possible exposure to EVD within 21 days before the onset of symptoms. Exposure may include contact with:

- Blood or bodily fluids from a person sick with or who died from EVD

- Objects contaminated with blood or bodily fluids of a person sick with or who died from EVD

- Infected fruit bats and primates (apes or monkeys)

- Semen from a human who has recovered from EVD

If a person shows early signs of EVD and has had a possible exposure, she or he should be isolated (separated from other people) and public health authorities notified. Blood samples from the patient should be collected and tested to confirm infection. Ebola virus can be detected in blood after the onset of symptoms, most notably fever. It may take up to three days after symptoms start for the virus to reach detectable levels. A positive laboratory test means that Ebola infection is confirmed. Public health authorities will conduct a public health investigation, including tracing of all possibly exposed contacts.

Treatment of Ebola Virus Disease

Symptoms of EVD are treated as they appear. When used early, basic interventions can significantly improve the chances of survival. These include:

- Providing fluids and electrolytes (body salts) through infusion into a vein (intravenously)

- Offering oxygen therapy to maintain oxygen status

- Using medication to support blood pressure, reduce vomiting and diarrhea, and to manage fever and pain

- Treating other infections, if they occur

Recovery from EVD depends on good supportive care and the patient's immune response. Those who do recover develop antibodies that can last 10 years, possibly longer. It is not known if people who recover are immune for life or if they can later become infected with a different species of Ebola virus. Some survivors may have long-term complications, such as joint and vision problems.

Antiviral Drugs

There is no antiviral drug licensed by the Food and Drug Administration (FDA) to treat EVD in people. Drugs that are being developed to treat EVD work by stopping the virus from making copies of itself.

Blood transfusions from survivors and mechanical filtering of blood from patients are also being explored as possible treatments for EVD.

Prevention of Ebola Virus Disease

In the United States, EVD is a very rare disease that has only occurred because of cases that were acquired in other countries, eventually followed by human-to-human transmission. The reservoir of the virus does not exist in the United States. EVD is more common in some parts of sub-Saharan Africa, with occasional outbreaks occurring in people. In these areas, the Ebola virus is believed to circulate at low rates in certain animal populations (enzootic). Occasionally, people become sick with Ebola after coming into contact with these infected animals, which can then lead to Ebola outbreaks where the virus spreads between people.

When living in or traveling to a region where Ebola virus is present, there are a number of ways to protect yourself and prevent the spread of EVD.

While in an area affected by Ebola, it is important to avoid the following:

- Contact with blood and bodily fluids (such as urine, feces, saliva, sweat, vomit, breast milk, semen, and vaginal fluids)

- Items that may have come in contact with an infected person's blood or bodily fluids (such as clothes, bedding, needles, and medical equipment)

- Funeral or burial rituals that require handling the body of someone who died from EVD

- Contact with bats and nonhuman primates or blood, fluids, and raw meat prepared from these animals (bushmeat) or meat from an unknown source

- Contact with semen from a human who had EVD until you know the virus is gone from the semen

These same prevention methods apply when living in or traveling to an area affected by an Ebola outbreak. After returning from an area affected by Ebola, monitor your health for 21 days and seek medical care immediately if you develop symptoms of EVD.

Is There Any Vaccine for Ebola Virus Disease?

There is no vaccine licensed by the FDA to protect people from the Ebola virus.

An experimental vaccine called "rVSV-ZEBOV" was found to be highly protective against the virus in a trial conducted by the World Health Organization (WHO) and other international partners in Guinea in 2015. The FDA licensure for the vaccine is expected in 2019. In the meantime, 300,000 doses have been committed for an emergency use stockpile under the appropriate regulatory mechanism (Investigational New Drug application (IND) or Emergency Use Authorization (EUA)) in the event an outbreak occurs before the FDA approval is received. Scientists continue to study the safety of this vaccine in populations such as children and people with human immunodeficiency virus (HIV).

Another Ebola vaccine candidate, the recombinant adenovirus type-5 Ebola vaccine, was evaluated in a phase 2 trial in Sierra Leone in 2015. An immune response was stimulated by this vaccine within 28 days of vaccination, the response decreased over 6 months after injection. Research on this vaccine is ongoing.

Chapter 13

Epstein-Barr Virus and Infectious Mononucleosis

About Epstein-Barr Virus

Epstein-Barr virus (EBV), is one of the most common human viruses in the world. It spreads primarily through saliva. EBV can cause infectious mononucleosis, also called "mono," and other illnesses. Most people will get infected with EBV in their lifetime and will not have any symptoms. Mono caused by EBV is most common among teens and adults.

Epstein-Barr virus, also known as "human herpesvirus 4," is a member of the herpes virus family. It is one of the most common human viruses. EBV spreads most commonly through bodily fluids, primarily saliva. EBV can cause infectious mononucleosis and other illnesses.

Symptoms of Epstein-Barr Virus

Symptoms of EBV infection can include:

- Fatigue

- Fever

This chapter includes text excerpted from "Epstein-Barr Virus and Infectious Mononucleosis," Centers for Disease Control and Prevention (CDC), May 8, 2018.

- Inflamed throat

- Swollen lymph nodes in the neck

- Enlarged spleen

- Swollen liver

- Rash

Many people become infected with EBV in their childhood. EBV infections in children usually do not cause symptoms, or the symptoms are not distinguishable from other mild, brief childhood illnesses. People who get symptoms from EBV infection, usually teenagers or adults, get better in two to four weeks. However, some people may feel fatigued for several weeks or even months.

After you get an EBV infection, the virus becomes latent (inactive) in your body. In some cases, the virus may reactivate. This does not always cause symptoms, but people with weakened immune systems are more likely to develop symptoms if EBV reactivates.

Transmission of Epstein-Barr Virus

Epstein-Barr virus spreads most commonly through bodily fluids, especially saliva. However, EBV can also spread through blood and semen during sexual contact, blood transfusions, and organ transplantations.

Epstein-Barr virus can be spread by using objects, such as a toothbrush or drinking glass, that an infected person recently used. The virus probably survives on an object at least as long as the object remains moist.

The first time you get infected with EBV (primary EBV infection) you can spread the virus for weeks and even before you have symptoms. Once the virus is in your body, it stays there in a latent state. If the virus reactivates, you can potentially spread EBV to others no matter how much time has passed since the initial infection.

Diagnosis of Epstein-Barr Virus

Diagnosing EBV infection can be challenging because the symptoms are similar to other illnesses. EBV infection can be confirmed with a blood test that detects antibodies. About 9 out of 10 of adults have antibodies that show that they have a current or past EBV infection.

Prevention and Treatment of Epstein-Barr Virus

There is no vaccine to protect against EBV infection. You can help protect yourself by not kissing or sharing drinks; food; or personal items, such as toothbrushes, with people who have EBV infection.

There is no specific treatment for EBV. However, some things can be done to help relieve symptoms, including:

- Drinking fluids to stay hydrated

- Getting plenty of rest

- Taking over-the-counter (OTC) medications for pain and fever

About Infectious Mononucleosis

Infectious mononucleosis, also called "mono," is a contagious disease. EBV is the most common cause of infectious mononucleosis, but other viruses can also cause this disease. It is common among teenagers and young adults, especially college students. At least one out of four teenagers and young adults who get infected with EBV will develop infectious mononucleosis.

Symptoms of Infectious Mononucleosis

Typical symptoms of infectious mononucleosis usually appear four to six weeks after you get infected with EBV. Symptoms may develop slowly and may not all occur at the same time.

These symptoms include:

- Extreme fatigue

- Fever

- Sore throat

- Head and body aches

- Swollen lymph nodes in the neck and armpits

- Swollen liver or spleen or both

- Rash

An enlarged spleen and a swollen liver are less common symptoms. For some people, their liver or spleen or both may remain enlarged even after their fatigue ends.

Most people get better in two to four weeks; however, some people may feel fatigued for several more weeks. Occasionally, the symptoms of infectious mononucleosis can last for six months or longer.

Diagnosing Infectious Mononucleosis

Healthcare providers typically diagnose infectious mononucleosis-based on symptoms.

Laboratory tests are not usually needed to diagnose infectious mononucleosis. However, specific laboratory tests may be needed to identify the cause of illness in people who do not have a typical case of infectious mononucleosis.

The blood work of patients who have infectious mononucleosis due to EBV infection may show:

- More white blood cells (lymphocytes) than normal

- Unusual looking white blood cells (atypical lymphocytes)

- Fewer than normal neutrophils or platelets

- Abnormal liver function

Transmission of Infectious Mononucleosis

Epstein-Barr virus is the most common cause of infectious mononucleosis, but other viruses can cause this disease. Typically, these viruses spread most commonly through bodily fluids, especially saliva.

However, these viruses can also spread through blood and semen during sexual contact, blood transfusions, and organ transplantations.

Prevention and Treatment

There is no vaccine to protect against infectious mononucleosis. You can help protect yourself by not kissing or sharing drinks; food; or personal items, such as toothbrushes, with people who have infectious mononucleosis.

You can help relieve symptoms of infectious mononucleosis by:

- Drinking fluids to stay hydrated

- Getting plenty of rest

- Taking OTC medications for pain and fever

If you have infectious mononucleosis, you should not take penicillin antibiotics, such as ampicillin or amoxicillin. Based on the severity of the symptoms, a healthcare provider may recommend treatment of specific organ systems affected by infectious mononucleosis.

Because your spleen may become enlarged as a result of infectious mononucleosis, you should avoid contact sports until you fully recover. Participating in contact sports can be strenuous and may cause the spleen to rupture.

Chapter 14

Fifth Disease (Parvovirus B19)

Fifth disease is a mild rash illness caused by *Parvovirus B19*. It is more common in children than in adults. A person usually gets sick with the fifth disease within 4 to 14 days after getting infected with *Parvovirus B19*. This disease, also called "erythema infectiosum," got its name because it was fifth in a list of historical classifications of common skin rash illnesses in children.

Signs and Symptoms of Fifth Disease

The symptoms of fifth disease are usually mild and may include:

- Fever
- Runny nose
- Headache
- Rash

This chapter includes text excerpted from "*Parvovirus B19* and Fifth Disease— Fifth Disease," Centers for Disease Control and Prevention (CDC), November 2, 2015. Reviewed July 2019.

You Can Get a Rash on Your Face and Body

You may get a red rash on your face called "slapped cheek" rash. This rash is the most recognized feature of fifth disease. It is more common in children than adults.

Some people may get a second rash a few days later on their chest, back, buttocks, or arms and legs. The rash may be itchy, especially on the soles of the feet. It can vary in intensity and usually goes away in 7 to 10 days, but it can come and go for several weeks. As it starts to go away, it may look lacy.

You May Also Have Painful or Swollen Joints

People with fifth disease can also develop pain and swelling in their joints. This is called "polyarthropathy syndrome." It is more common in adults, especially women. Some adults with fifth disease may only have painful joints, usually in the hands, feet, or knees, and no other symptoms. The joint pain usually lasts one to three weeks, but it can last for months or longer. It usually goes away without any long-term problems.

Complications of Fifth Disease

Fifth disease is usually mild for children and adults who are otherwise healthy. But for some people, fifth disease can cause serious health complications, such as chronic anemia that requires medical treatment.

You may be at risk for serious complications from fifth disease if you have a weakened immune system caused by leukemia, cancer, organ transplants, or human immunodeficiency virus (HIV) infection.

Transmission of Parvovirus B19

Parvovirus B19—which causes fifth disease—spreads through respiratory secretions, such as saliva, sputum, or nasal mucus, when an infected person coughs or sneezes. You are most contagious when it seems like you have "just a fever and/or cold" and before you get the rash or joint pain and swelling. After you get the rash, you are not likely to be contagious, so then it is usually safe for you or your child to go back to work or school.

People with fifth disease who have weakened immune systems may be contagious for a longer amount of time.

Parvovirus B19 can also spread through blood or blood products. A pregnant woman who is infected with *Parvovirus B19* can pass the virus to the fetus.

Once you recover from fifth disease, you develop immunity that generally protects you from *Parvovirus B19* infection in the future.

Diagnosis of Fifth Disease

Healthcare providers can often diagnose fifth disease just by seeing "slapped cheek" rash on a patient's face. They can also do a blood test to determine if you are susceptible or immune to *Parvovirus B19* infection or if you were recently infected. This is not a routine test, but it can be performed in special circumstances. Talk to your healthcare provider. The blood test may be particularly helpful for pregnant women who may have been exposed to *Parvovirus B19* and are suspected to have fifth disease.

Treatment of Fifth Disease

Fifth disease is usually mild and will go away on its own. Children and adults who are otherwise healthy usually recover completely. Treatment usually involves relieving symptoms, such as fever, itching, and joint pain and swelling.

People who have complications from fifth disease should see their healthcare provider for medical treatment.

Prevention of Parvovirus B19 Infection

There is no vaccine or medicine that can prevent *Parvovirus B19* infection. You can reduce your chance of being infected or infecting others by:

- Washing your hands often with soap and water

- Covering your mouth and nose when you cough or sneeze

- Not touching your eyes, nose, or mouth

- Avoiding close contact with people who are sick

- Staying home when you are sick

Once you get the rash, you are probably not contagious. So, it is usually then safe for you to go back to work or for your child to return to school or a child care center.

Infected persons who are pregnant should know about potential risks to the fetus and discuss this with their doctor.

All healthcare providers and patients should follow strict infection control practices to prevent *Parvovirus B19* from spreading.

Chapter 15

Genital Herpes

What Is Genital Herpes?

Genital herpes is a sexually transmitted disease (STD) caused by the herpes simplex virus type 1 (HSV-1) or type 2 (HSV-2).

How Common Is Genital Herpes?

Genital herpes infection is common in the United States. The Centers for Disease Control and Prevention (CDC) estimates that, annually, 776,000 people in the United States get new genital herpes infections. Nationwide, 11.9 percent of persons between 14 and 49 years of age have HSV-2 infection (12.1% when adjusted for age). However, the prevalence of genital herpes infection is higher than that, because an increasing number of genital herpes infections are caused by HSV-1. Oral HSV-1 infection is typically acquired in childhood; because the prevalence of oral HSV-1 infection has declined in recent decades, people may have become more susceptible to contracting a genital herpes infection from HSV-1.

HSV-2 infection is more common among women than among men; the percentages of those infected during 2015 to 2016 were 15.9 percent versus 8.2 percent, respectively, among persons between 14 and 49 years of age. This is possible because genital infection is more easily transmitted from men to women than from women to men

This chapter includes text excerpted from "Genital Herpes—CDC Fact Sheet (Detailed)," Centers for Disease Control and Prevention (CDC), January 31, 2017.

during penile-vaginal sex. HSV-2 infection is more common among non-Hispanic Blacks (34.6%) than among non-Hispanic Whites (8.1%). A previous analysis found that these disparities exist even among persons with similar numbers of lifetime sexual partners. Most infected persons may be unaware of their infection; in the United States, an estimated 87.4 percent of 14 to 49 year olds infected with HSV-2 have never received a clinical diagnosis.

The age-adjusted percentage of persons in the United States infected with HSV-2 decreased from 18.0 percent in 1999 to 2000 to 12.1 percent in 2015 to 2016.

How Do People Get Genital Herpes?

Infections are transmitted through contact with HSV in herpes lesions, mucosal surfaces, genital secretions, or oral secretions. HSV-1 and HSV-2 can be shed from normal-appearing oral or genital mucosa or skin. Generally, a person can only get HSV-2 infection during genital contact with someone who has a genital HSV-2 infection. However, receiving oral sex from a person with an oral HSV-1 infection can result in getting a genital HSV-1 infection. Transmission commonly occurs from contact with an infected partner who does not have visible lesions and who may not know that she or he is infected. In persons with asymptomatic HSV-2 infections, genital HSV shedding occurs on 10.2 percent of days, compared to 20.1 percent of days among those with symptomatic infections.

What Are the Symptoms of Genital Herpes?

Most individuals infected with HSV are asymptomatic, or they have very mild symptoms that go unnoticed or are mistaken for another skin condition. When symptoms do occur, herpes lesions typically appear as one or more vesicles, or small blisters, on or around the genitals, rectum or mouth. The average incubation period for initial herpes infection is 4 days (ranging from 2 to 12) after exposure. The vesicles break and leave painful ulcers that may take 2 to 4 weeks to heal after the initial herpes infection. Experiencing these symptoms is referred to as having the first herpes "outbreak" or "episode."

Clinical manifestations of genital herpes differ between the first and recurrent (i.e., subsequent) outbreaks. The first outbreak of herpes is often associated with a longer duration of herpetic lesions; increased viral shedding (making HSV transmission more likely); and systemic symptoms, including fever, body aches, swollen lymph nodes, or headache. Recurrent outbreaks of genital herpes are common, and many patients who recognize recurrences have prodromal symptoms, either localized genital pain, or tingling or shooting pains in the legs, hips, or buttocks, which occurs hours to days before the eruption of herpetic lesions. Symptoms of recurrent outbreaks are typically shorter in duration and less severe than the first outbreak of genital herpes. Long-term studies have indicated that the number of symptomatic recurrent outbreaks may decrease over time. Recurrences and subclinical shedding are much less frequent for genital HSV-1 infection than for genital HSV-2 infection.

What Are the Complications of Genital Herpes?

Genital herpes may cause painful genital ulcers that can be severe and persistent in persons with suppressed immune systems, such as human immunodeficiency virus (HIV)-infected persons. Both HSV-1 and HSV-2 can also cause rare but serious complications, such as aseptic meningitis (inflammation of the linings of the brain). Development of extragenital lesions (e.g., buttocks, groin, thigh, finger, or eye) may occur during the course of infection.

Some persons who contract genital herpes have concerns about how it will impact their overall health, sex life, and relationships. There can be a considerable embarrassment, shame, and stigma associated with a herpes diagnosis that can substantially interfere with a patient's relationships. Clinicians can address these concerns by encouraging patients to recognize that while herpes is not curable, it is a manageable condition. Three important steps that providers can take for their newly-diagnosed patients are giving information, providing support and resources, and helping define treatment and prevention options. Patients can be counseled that risk of genital herpes transmission can be reduced, but not eliminated, by disclosure of infection to sexual partners, avoiding sex during a recurrent outbreak, use of suppressive antiviral therapy, and consistent condom use. Since a diagnosis of genital herpes may affect perceptions about existing or future sexual relationships, it is important for patients to understand how to talk to sexual partners about STDs.

There are also potential complications for a pregnant woman and her newborn child.

What Is the Link between Genital Herpes and Human Immunodeficiency Virus?

Genital ulcerative disease caused by herpes makes it easier to transmit and acquire HIV infection sexually. There is an estimated two- to four-fold increased risk of acquiring HIV if individuals with genital herpes infection are genitally exposed to HIV. Ulcers or breaks in the skin or mucous membranes (lining of the mouth, vagina, and rectum) from a herpes infection may compromise the protection normally provided by the skin and mucous membranes against infections, including HIV. In addition, having genital herpes increases the number of CD4 cells (the target cell for HIV entry) in the genital mucosa. In persons with both HIV and genital herpes, local activation of HIV replication at the site of genital herpes infection can increase the risk that HIV will be transmitted during contact with the mouth, vagina, or rectum of an HIV-uninfected sex partner.

How Does Genital Herpes Affect a Pregnant Woman and Her Baby?

Neonatal herpes is one of the most serious complications of genital herpes. Healthcare providers should ask all pregnant women if they have a history of genital herpes. Herpes infection can be passed from mother to child during pregnancy or childbirth, or babies may be infected shortly after birth, resulting in a potentially fatal neonatal herpes infection. Infants born to women who acquire genital herpes close to the time of delivery and are shedding virus at delivery are at a much higher risk for developing neonatal herpes, compared with women who have recurrent genital herpes. Thus, it is important that women avoid contracting herpes during pregnancy. Women should be counseled to abstain from intercourse during the third-trimester with partners known to have, or suspected of having, genital herpes.

While women with genital herpes may be offered antiviral medication late in pregnancy through delivery to reduce the risk of a recurrent herpes outbreak, third-trimester antiviral prophylaxis has not been shown to decrease the risk of herpes transmission to the neonate. Routine serologic HSV screening of pregnant women is not recommended. However, at onset of labor, all women should undergo careful examination and questioning to evaluate for the presence of prodromal symptoms or herpetic lesions. If herpes symptoms are present, a cesarean delivery is recommended to prevent HSV transmission to the infant. There are detailed guidelines for how to manage asymptomatic infants born to women with active genital herpes lesions.

How Is Genital Herpes Diagnosed?

The preferred HSV tests for patients with active genital ulcers are detection of HSV DNA by nucleic acid amplification tests, such as polymerase chain reaction (PCR), or isolation by viral culture. HSV culture requires collection of a sample from the lesion, and once viral growth is seen, specific cell staining to differentiate between HSV-1 and HSV-2. However, culture sensitivity is low, especially for recurrent lesions, and declines as lesions heal. PCR is more sensitive, allows for more rapid and accurate results, and is increasingly being used. Because viral shedding is intermittent, failure to detect HSV by culture or PCR does not indicate an absence of HSV infection. Tzanck preparations are insensitive and nonspecific and should not be used.

Herpes serologic tests are blood tests that detect antibodies to the herpes virus. Providers should only request type-specific glycoprotein G (gG)-based serologic assays when serology is performed for their patients. Several ELISA-based serologic tests are approved by the U.S. Food and Drug Administration (FDA) and are available commercially. While the presence of HSV-2 antibody can be presumed to reflect genital infection, patients should be counseled that the presence of HSV-1 antibody may represent either oral or genital infection. The sensitivities of glycoprotein G type-specific serologic tests for HSV-2 vary from 80 to 98 percent; false-negative results might be more frequent at early stages of infection. The most commonly used test, HerpeSelect HSV-2 Elisa might be falsely positive at low index values.

Such low values should be confirmed with another test, such as Biokit or the Western Blot. Negative HSV-1 results should be interpreted with caution because some ELISA-based serologic tests are insensitive for detection of HSV-1 antibody, HSV-2 infection is more common among women than among men; the percentages of those infected during 2015 to 2016 were 15.9 percent versus 8.2 percent, respectively, among 14 to 49 year-olds. This is possible because the genital infection is more easily transmitted from men to women than from women to men during penile-vaginal sex. HSV-2 infection is more common among non-Hispanic Blacks (34.6%) than among non-Hispanic Whites (8.1%). A previous analysis found that these disparities exist even among persons with similar numbers of lifetime sexual partners. Most infected persons may be unaware of their infection; in the United States, an estimated 87.4 percent of individuals between 14 and 49 years of age infected with HSV-2 have never received a clinical diagnosis.

The age-adjusted percentage of persons in the United States infected with HSV-2 decreased from 18.0 percent in 1999 to 2000 to 12.1 percent in 2015-y. Immunoglobulin M (IgM) testing for HSV-1 or HSV-2 is not useful, because IgM tests are not type-specific and might be positive during recurrent genital or oral episodes of herpes.

For the symptomatic patient, testing with both virologic and serologic assays can determine whether it is a new infection or a newly-recognized old infection. A primary infection would be supported by a positive virologic test and a negative serologic test, while the diagnosis of recurrent disease would be supported by positive virologic and serologic test results.

The CDC does not recommend screening for HSV-1 or HSV-2 in the general population. Several scenarios where type-specific serologic HSV tests may be useful include:

- Patients with recurrent genital symptoms or atypical symptoms and negative HSV PCR or culture

- Patients with a clinical diagnosis of genital herpes but no laboratory confirmation

- Patients who report having a partner with genital herpes

- Patients presenting for an STD evaluation (especially those with multiple sex partners)

- Persons with HIV infection

- Methylsulfonylmethane (MSM) at an increased risk for HIV acquisition

Please note that while type-specific herpes testing can determine if a person is infected with HSV-1 or HSV-2 (or both), there is no commercially available test to determine if a herpes infection in one individual was acquired from another specific person. The CDC encourages patients to discuss any herpes questions and concerns with their healthcare provider or seek counsel at an STD clinic.

Is There a Cure or Treatment for Herpes?

There is no cure for herpes. Antiviral medications can, however, prevent or shorten outbreaks during the period of time the person takes the medication. In addition, daily suppressive therapy (i.e., daily use of antiviral medication) for herpes can reduce the likelihood of transmission to partners.

There is currently no commercially available vaccine that is protective against genital herpes infection. Candidate vaccines are in clinical trials.

How Can Herpes Be Prevented?

Correct and consistent use of latex condoms can reduce, but not eliminate, the risk of transmitting or acquiring genital herpes because herpes virus shedding can occur in areas that are not covered by a condom.

The surest way to avoid transmission of STDs, including genital herpes, is to abstain from sexual contact or to be in a long-term mutually monogamous relationship with a partner who has been tested for STDs and is known to be uninfected.

Persons with herpes should abstain from sexual activity with partners when herpes lesions or other symptoms of herpes are present. It is important to know that even if a person does not have any symptoms, she or he can still infect sex partners. Sex partners of infected persons should be advised that they may become infected, and they should use condoms to reduce the risk. Sex partners can seek testing to determine if they are infected with HSV.

Daily treatment with valacyclovir decreases the rate of HSV-2 transmission in discordant, heterosexual couples in which the source partner has a history of genital HSV-2 infection. Such couples should be encouraged to consider suppressive antiviral therapy as part of a strategy to prevent transmission, in addition to consistent condom use and avoidance of sexual activity during recurrences.

Chapter 16

Gonorrhea

What Is Gonorrhea?

Gonorrhea is a sexually transmitted disease (STD) caused by infection with the *Neisseria gonorrhoeae* bacterium. *N. gonorrhoeae* infects the mucous membranes of the reproductive tract, including the cervix, uterus, and fallopian tubes in women, and the urethra in women and men. *N. gonorrhoeae* can also infect the mucous membranes of the mouth, throat, eyes, and rectum.

How Common Is Gonorrhea?

Gonorrhea is a very common infectious disease. The Centers for Disease Control and Prevention (CDC) estimates that approximately 820,000 new gonococcal infections occur in the United States each year, and more than half of these infections are detected and reported to the CDC. The CDC estimates that 570,000 of them were among young people between 15 and 24 years of age. In 2017, 555,608 cases of gonorrhea were reported to the CDC.

This chapter includes text excerpted from "Gonorrhea—CDC Fact Sheet (Detailed Version)," Centers for Disease Control and Prevention (CDC), October 25, 2016.

How Do People Get Gonorrhea?

Gonorrhea is transmitted through sexual contact with the penis, vagina, mouth, or anus of an infected partner. Ejaculation does not have to occur for gonorrhea to be transmitted or acquired. Gonorrhea can also be spread perinatally from mother to baby during childbirth.

People who have had gonorrhea and received treatment may be reinfected if they have sexual contact with a person infected with gonorrhea.

Who Is at Risk for Gonorrhea?

Any sexually active person can be infected with gonorrhea. In the United States, the highest reported rates of infection are among sexually active teenagers, young adults, and African Americans.

What Are the Signs and Symptoms of Gonorrhea?

Many men with gonorrhea are asymptomatic. When present, signs and symptoms of urethral infection in men include dysuria or a white, yellow, or green urethral discharge that usually appears 1 to 14 days after infection. In cases where the urethral infection is complicated by epididymitis, men with gonorrhea may also complain of testicular or scrotal pain.

Most women with gonorrhea are asymptomatic. Even when a woman has symptoms, they are often so mild and nonspecific that they are mistaken for a bladder or vaginal infection. The initial symptoms and signs in women include dysuria, increased vaginal discharge, or vaginal bleeding between periods. Women with gonorrhea are at risk of developing serious complications from the infection, regardless of the presence or severity of symptoms.

Symptoms of rectal infection in both men and women may include discharge, anal itching, soreness, bleeding, or painful bowel movements. Rectal infection also may be asymptomatic. Pharyngeal infection may cause a sore throat but usually is asymptomatic.

What Are the Complications of Gonorrhea?

Untreated gonorrhea can cause serious and permanent health problems in both women and men.

In women, gonorrhea can spread into the uterus or fallopian tubes and cause pelvic inflammatory disease (PID). The symptoms may be quite mild or can be very severe and can include abdominal pain and fever. PID can lead to internal abscesses and chronic pelvic pain. PID can also damage the fallopian tubes enough to cause infertility or increase the risk of ectopic pregnancy.

In men, gonorrhea may be complicated by epididymitis. In rare cases, this may lead to infertility.

If left untreated, gonorrhea can also spread to the blood and cause disseminated gonococcal infection (DGI). DGI is usually characterized by arthritis, tenosynovitis, and/or dermatitis. This condition can be life-threatening.

What about Gonorrhea and Human Immunodeficiency Virus?

Untreated gonorrhea can increase a person's risk of acquiring or transmitting the human immunodeficiency virus (HIV), the virus that causes acquired immunodeficiency syndrome (AIDS).

How Does Gonorrhea Affect a Pregnant Woman and Her Baby?

If a pregnant woman has gonorrhea, she may give the infection to her baby as the baby passes through the birth canal during delivery. This can cause blindness, joint infection, or a life-threatening blood infection in the baby. Treatment of gonorrhea as soon as it is detected in pregnant women will reduce the risk of these complications. Pregnant women should consult a healthcare provider for appropriate examination, testing, and treatment as necessary.

Who Should Be Tested for Gonorrhea?

Any sexually active person can be infected with gonorrhea. Anyone with genital symptoms, such as discharge, burning during urination, unusual sores, or rash, should stop having sex and see a healthcare provider immediately.

Also, anyone with an oral, anal, or vaginal sex partner who has been recently diagnosed with an STD should see a healthcare provider for evaluation.

Some people should be tested (screened) for gonorrhea even if they do not have symptoms or know of a sex partner who has gonorrhea. Anyone who is sexually active should discuss her or his risk factors with a healthcare provider and ask whether she or he should be tested for gonorrhea or other STDs.

145

The CDC recommends yearly gonorrhea screening for all sexually active women younger than 25 years of age, as well as older women with risk factors, such as new or multiple sex partners or a sex partner who has a sexually transmitted infection (STI).

People who have gonorrhea should also be tested for other STDs.

How Is Gonorrhea Diagnosed?

Urogenital gonorrhea can be diagnosed by testing urine, urethral (for men), or endocervical or vaginal (for women) specimens using nucleic acid amplification testing (NAAT). It can also be diagnosed using gonorrhea culture, which requires endocervical or urethral swab specimens.

If a person has had oral and/or anal sex, pharyngeal and/or rectal swab specimens should be collected either for culture or for NAAT (if the local laboratory has validated the use of NAAT for extra-genital specimens).

What Is the Treatment for Gonorrhea?

Gonorrhea can be cured with the right treatment. The CDC now recommends dual therapy (i.e., using two drugs) for the treatment of gonorrhea. It is important to take all of the medication prescribed to cure gonorrhea. Medication for gonorrhea should not be shared with anyone. Although medication will stop the infection, it will not repair any permanent damage done by the disease. Antimicrobial resistance in gonorrhea is of increasing concern, and successful treatment of gonorrhea is becoming more difficult. If a person's symptoms continue for more than a few days after receiving treatment, she or he should return to a healthcare provider to be reevaluated.

What about Partners

If a person has been diagnosed and treated for gonorrhea, she or he should tell all recent anal, vaginal, or oral sex partners (all sex partners within 60 days before the onset of symptoms or diagnosis) so they can see a health provider and be treated. This will reduce the risk that the sex partners will develop serious complications from gonorrhea and will also reduce the person's risk of becoming reinfected. A person with gonorrhea and all of her or his sex partners must avoid having sex until they have completed their treatment for gonorrhea and until they no longer have symptoms.

How Can Gonorrhea Be Prevented?

Latex condoms, when used consistently and correctly, can reduce the risk of transmission of gonorrhea. The surest way to avoid transmission of gonorrhea or other STDs is to abstain from vaginal, anal, and oral sex, or to be in a long-term mutually monogamous relationship with a partner who has been tested and is known to be uninfected.

Chapter 17

Hand, Foot, and Mouth Disease

Hand, foot, and mouth disease (HFMD) is a common viral illness that usually affects infants and children younger than five years of age. However, it can sometimes occur in older children and adults.

Signs and Symptoms of Hand, Foot, and Mouth Disease

Typical symptoms of hand, foot, and mouth disease include:

- Fever
- Reduced appetite
- Sore throat
- A feeling of being unwell (malaise)

One or two days after the fever starts, painful sores can develop in the mouth (herpangina). They usually begin as small red spots, often in the back of the mouth, that blister and can become painful.

A skin rash on the palms of the hands and soles of the feet may also develop over one or two days as flat, red spots, sometimes with blisters. It may also appear on the knees, elbows, buttocks or genital area.

This chapter includes text excerpted from "Hand, Foot, and Mouth Disease (HFMD)," Centers for Disease Control and Prevention (CDC), February 22, 2019.

Some people, especially young children, may get dehydrated if they are not able to swallow enough liquids because of painful mouth sores. You should seek medical care in these cases.

Not everyone will get all of these symptoms. Some people, especially adults, may become infected and show no symptoms at all, but they can still pass the virus to others.

Most people who get hand, foot, and mouth disease will have mild illness or no symptoms at all. But a small proportion of cases can be more severe.

Complications of Hand, Foot, and Mouth Disease

Health complications from hand, foot, and mouth disease are not common:

- Viral or "aseptic" meningitis can occur with hand, foot, and mouth disease, but it is rare. It causes fever, headache, stiff neck, or back pain and may require the infected person to be hospitalized for a few days.

- Encephalitis (inflammation of the brain) or polio-like paralysis can occur, but this is even rarer.

- Fingernail and toenail loss have been reported, occurring mostly in children within a few weeks after having the hand, foot, and mouth disease. At this time, it is not known whether nail loss was a result of the disease in reported cases. However, in the reports reviewed, the nail loss was temporary, and the nail grew back without medical treatment.

Causes of Hand, Foot, and Mouth Disease

Hand, foot, and mouth disease is caused by viruses that belong to the Enterovirus genus (group), which includes polioviruses, coxsackieviruses, echoviruses, and other enteroviruses.

- Coxsackievirus A16 is typically the most common cause of hand, foot, and mouth disease in the United States, but other coxsackieviruses can also cause the illness.

- Enterovirus 71 has also been associated with cases and outbreaks of hand, foot, and mouth disease, mostly in children in East and Southeast Asia. Less often, enterovirus 71 has been associated with severe disease, such as encephalitis.

- Several types of enteroviruses may be identified in outbreaks of hand, foot and mouth disease, but most of the time, only one or two enteroviruses are identified.

Transmission of Hand, Foot, and Mouth Disease

The viruses that cause hand, foot, and mouth disease can be found in an infected person's:

- Nose and throat secretions (such as saliva, sputum, or nasal mucus)

- Blister fluid

- Feces

You can get exposed to the viruses that cause hand, foot, and mouth disease through:

- Close personal contact, such as hugging an infected person

- The air when an infected person coughs or sneezes

- Contact with feces, such as changing diapers of an infected person, then touching your eyes, nose, or mouth before washing your hands

- Contact with contaminated objects and surfaces, such as touching a doorknob that has viruses on it, then touching your eyes, mouth, or nose before washing your hands

It is also possible to get infected with the viruses that cause hand, foot, and mouth disease if you swallow recreational water, such as water in swimming pools. However, this is not very common. This can happen if the water is not properly treated with chlorine and becomes contaminated with feces from a person who has the hand, foot, and mouth disease.

Generally, a person with hand, foot, and mouth disease is most contagious during the first week of illness. People can sometimes be contagious for days or weeks after symptoms go away. Some people, especially adults, may become infected and not develop any symptoms, but they can still spread the virus to others. This is why people should always try to maintain good hygiene, such as frequent handwashing, so they can minimize their chance of spreading or getting infections.

You should stay home while you are sick with hand, foot, and mouth disease. Talk with your healthcare provider if you are not sure when you should return to work or school. The same applies to children returning to day care.

Hand, foot, and mouth disease is not transmitted to or from pets or other animals.

Diagnosis of Hand, Foot, and Mouth Disease

Hand, foot, and mouth disease is one of the many infections that causes mouth sores. Healthcare providers can usually identify mouth sores caused by hand, foot, and mouth disease by considering:

- How old the patient is
- What symptoms the patient has
- How the rash and mouth sores look

A healthcare professional may sometimes collect samples from the patient's throat or feces then send them to a laboratory to test for the virus.

Treatment of Hand, Foot, and Mouth Disease

There is no specific treatment for hand, foot, and mouth disease. However, you can do some things to relieve symptoms:

- Take over-the-counter (OTC) medications to relieve pain and fever. (Caution: Aspirin should not be given to children.)
- Use mouthwashes or sprays that numb mouth pain.

If a person has mouth sores, it might be painful for them to swallow. However, it is important for people with hand, foot, and mouth disease to drink enough liquids to prevent dehydration (loss of body fluids). If a person cannot swallow enough liquids to avoid dehydration, they may need to receive them through an intravenous (IV) line in their vein.

If you are concerned about your or your child's symptoms you should contact your healthcare provider.

Prevention of Hand, Foot, and Mouth Disease

There is currently no vaccine in the United States to protect against the viruses that cause hand, foot, and mouth disease. But, researchers are working to develop vaccines to help prevent hand, foot, and mouth disease in the future.

You can lower your risk of being infected by doing the following:

- Wash your hands often with soap and water for at least 20 seconds, especially after changing diapers and using the toilet.

- Clean and disinfect frequently touched surfaces and soiled items, including toys.

- Avoid close contact, such as kissing, hugging, or sharing eating utensils or cups, with people with hand, foot, and mouth disease.

Chapter 18

Hepatitis: A through E and Beyond

What Is Viral Hepatitis?

Viral hepatitis is inflammation of the liver caused by a virus. Several different viruses, named hepatitis A, B, C, D, and E viruses, cause viral hepatitis.

All of these viruses cause acute or short-term viral hepatitis. Hepatitis B, C, and D viruses can also cause chronic hepatitis, in which the infection is prolonged, sometimes lifelong. Chronic hepatitis can lead to cirrhosis, liver failure, and liver cancer.

Researchers are looking for other viruses that may cause hepatitis, but none have been identified with certainty. Other viruses that less often affect the liver include cytomegalovirus (CMV); Epstein-Barr virus (EBV), also called "infectious mononucleosis"; herpesvirus; Parvovirus; and adenovirus.

What Are the Symptoms of Viral Hepatitis?

Symptoms include:

- Jaundice, which causes a yellowing of the skin and eyes

This chapter includes text excerpted from "Viral Hepatitis: A through E and Beyond," National Institute of Diabetes and Digestive and Kidney Diseases (NIDDK), February 2008. Reviewed July 2019.

- Fatigue
- Abdominal pain
- Loss of appetite
- Nausea
- Vomiting
- Diarrhea
- Low-grade fever
- Headache

However, some people do not have symptoms.

Hepatitis A
How Is Hepatitis A Spread?

Hepatitis A is spread primarily through food or water contaminated by feces from an infected person. Rarely, it spreads through contact with infected blood.

Who Is at Risk for Hepatitis A?

People most likely to get hepatitis A are:

- International travelers, particularly those traveling to developing countries
- People who live with or have sex with an infected person
- People living in areas where children are not routinely vaccinated against hepatitis A, where outbreaks are more likely
- Day care children and employees, during outbreaks
- Men who have sex with men (MSM)
- Users of illicit drugs

How Can Hepatitis A Be Prevented?

The hepatitis A vaccine offers immunity to adults and children older than the age of 1. The Centers for Disease Control and Prevention (CDC) recommends routine hepatitis A vaccination for children between 12 and 23 months of age and for adults who are at high risk for infection. Treatment with immune globulin can provide short-term immunity to hepatitis A when given before exposure or within 2 weeks of exposure to the virus. Avoiding tap water when traveling internationally and practicing good hygiene and sanitation also help prevent hepatitis A.

What Is the Treatment for Hepatitis A?

Hepatitis A usually resolves on its own over several weeks.

Hepatitis B
How Is Hepatitis B Spread?

Hepatitis B is spread through contact with infected blood; through sex with an infected person; and from mother to child during childbirth, whether the delivery is vaginal or via cesarean section.

Who Is at Risk for Hepatitis B?

People most likely to get hepatitis B are:

- People who live with or have sexual contact with an infected person
- Men who have sex with men
- People who have multiple sex partners
- Injection drug users
- Immigrants and children of immigrants from areas with high rates of hepatitis b
- Infants born to infected mothers
- Healthcare workers
- Hemodialysis patients
- People who received a transfusion of blood or blood products before 1987, when better tests to screen blood donors were developed
- International travelers

How Can Hepatitis B Be Prevented?

The hepatitis B vaccine offers the best protection. All infants and unvaccinated children, adolescents, and at-risk adults should be vaccinated. For people who have not been vaccinated, reducing exposure to the virus can help prevent hepatitis B. Reducing exposure means using latex condoms, which may lower the risk of transmission; not sharing drug needles; and not sharing personal items, such as toothbrushes, razors, and nail clippers, with an infected person.

What Is the Treatment for Hepatitis B?

Drugs approved for the treatment of chronic hepatitis B include alpha interferon and peginterferon, which slow the replication of the virus in the body and also boost the immune system, and the antiviral drugs lamivudine, adefovir dipivoxil, entecavir, and telbivudine. Other drugs are also being evaluated. Infants born to infected mothers should receive hepatitis B immune globulin and the hepatitis B vaccine within 12 hours of birth to help prevent infection.

People who develop acute hepatitis B are generally not treated with antiviral drugs because, depending on their age at infection, the disease often resolves on its own. Infected newborns are most likely to progress to chronic hepatitis B, but by young adulthood, most people with acute infection recover spontaneously. Severe acute hepatitis B can be treated with an antiviral drug, such as lamivudine.

Hepatitis C
How Is Hepatitis C Spread?

Hepatitis C is spread primarily through contact with infected blood. Less commonly, it can spread through sexual contact and childbirth.

Who Is at Risk for Hepatitis C?

People most likely to be exposed to the hepatitis C virus are:

- Injection drug users
- People who have sex with an infected person
- People who have multiple sex partners
- Healthcare workers
- Infants born to infected women
- Hemodialysis patients
- People who received a transfusion of blood or blood products before July 1992, when sensitive tests to screen blood donors for hepatitis C were introduced

- People who received clotting factors made before 1987, when methods to manufacture these products were improved

How Can Hepatitis C Be Prevented?

There is no vaccine for hepatitis C. The only way to prevent the disease is to reduce the risk of exposure to the virus. Reducing exposure means avoiding behaviors like sharing drug needles or personal items, such as toothbrushes, razors, and nail clippers, with an infected person.

What Is the Treatment for Hepatitis C?

Chronic hepatitis C is treated with peginterferon together with the antiviral drug ribavirin. If acute hepatitis C does not resolve on its own within two to three months, drug treatment is recommended.

Hepatitis D
How Is Hepatitis D Spread?

Hepatitis D is spread through contact with infected blood. This disease only occurs at the same time as infection with hepatitis B or in people who are already infected with hepatitis B.

Who Is at Risk for Hepatitis D?

Anyone infected with hepatitis B is at risk for hepatitis D. Injection drug users have the highest risk. Others at risk include:

- People who live with or have sex with a person infected with hepatitis D

- People who received a transfusion of blood or blood products before 1987

How Can Hepatitis D Be Prevented?

People not already infected with hepatitis B should receive the hepatitis B vaccine. Other preventive measures include avoiding exposure to infected blood; contaminated needles; and an infected person's personal items, such as toothbrushes, razors, and nail clippers.

What Is the Treatment for Hepatitis D?

Chronic hepatitis D is usually treated with pegylated interferon; although, other potential treatments are under study.

Hepatitis E

How Is Hepatitis E Spread?

Hepatitis E is spread through food or water contaminated by feces from an infected person. This disease is uncommon in the United States.

Who Is at Risk for Hepatitis E?

People most likely to be exposed to the hepatitis E virus are:

- International travelers, particularly those traveling to developing countries

- People living in areas where hepatitis E outbreaks are common

- People who live with or have sex with an infected person

How Can Hepatitis E Be Prevented?

There is no U.S. Food and Drug Administration (FDA)-approved vaccine for hepatitis E. The only way to prevent the disease is to reduce the risk of exposure to the virus. Reducing the risk of exposure means avoiding tap water when traveling internationally and practicing good hygiene and sanitation.

What Is the Treatment for Hepatitis E?

Hepatitis E usually resolves on its own over several weeks to months.

What Else Causes Viral Hepatitis

Some cases of viral hepatitis cannot be attributed to hepatitis A, B, C, D, or E viruses, or even the less common viruses that can infect the liver, such as cytomegalovirus, EBV, herpesvirus, Parvovirus, and adenovirus. These cases are called "non-A–E hepatitis." Scientists continue to study the causes of non-A–E hepatitis.

Chapter 19

Human Immunodeficiency Virus and Acquired Immunodeficiency Syndrome

What Is Human Immunodeficiency Virus?

Human immunodeficiency virus (HIV) is a virus that attacks cells that help the body fight infection, making a person more vulnerable to other infections and diseases. It is spread by contact with certain bodily fluids of a person with HIV, most commonly during unprotected sex (sex without a condom or HIV medicine to prevent or treat HIV), or through sharing injection drug equipment.

If left untreated, HIV can lead to the disease acquired immunodeficiency syndrome (AIDS).

The human body cannot get rid of HIV and no effective HIV cure exists. So, once you have HIV, you have it for life.

However, by taking HIV medicine (called "antiretroviral therapy" or ART), people with HIV can live long and healthy lives and prevent transmitting HIV to their sexual partners. In addition, there are effective methods to prevent getting HIV through sex or drug use, including pre-exposure prophylaxis (PrEP) and post-exposure prophylaxis (PEP).

This chapter includes text excerpted from "What Are HIV and AIDS?" HIV. gov, U.S. Department of Health and Human Services (HHS), June 17, 2019.

First identified in 1981, HIV is the cause of one of humanity's deadliest and most persistent epidemics.

What Is Acquired Immunodeficiency Syndrome?

Acquired immunodeficiency syndrome is the late stage of human immunodeficiency virus (HIV) infection that occurs when the body's immune system is badly damaged because of the virus.

In the United States, most people with HIV do not develop AIDS because taking HIV medicine every day as prescribed stops the progression of the disease.

A person with HIV is considered to have progressed to AIDS when:

- The number of their CD4 cells falls below 200 cells per cubic millimeter of blood (200 cells/mm3). (In someone with a healthy immune system, CD4 counts are between 500 and 1,600 cells/mm3.)

  or

- They develop one or more opportunistic infections regardless of their CD4 count.

Without HIV medicine, people with AIDS typically survive about three years. Once someone has a dangerous opportunistic illness, life expectancy without treatment falls to about one year. HIV medicine can still help people at this stage of HIV infection, and it can even be lifesaving. But people who start ART soon after they get HIV experience more benefits—that's why HIV testing is so important.

How Do You Know If You Have Human Immunodeficiency Virus?

The only way to know for sure if you have HIV is to get tested. Testing is relatively simple. You can ask your healthcare provider for an HIV test. Many medical clinics, substance abuse programs, community health centers, and hospitals offer them too. You can also buy a home testing kit at a pharmacy or online.

How Is Human Immunodeficiency Virus Transmitted?

You can get or transmit HIV only through specific activities. Most commonly, people get or transmit HIV through sexual behaviors and needle or syringe use.

Only certain body fluids—blood, semen, preseminal fluid, rectal fluids, vaginal fluids, and breast milk—from a person who has HIV can transmit HIV. These fluids must come in contact with a mucous membrane or damaged tissue or be directly injected into the bloodstream (from a needle or syringe) for transmission to occur. Mucous membranes are found inside the rectum, vagina, penis, and mouth.

In the United States, HIV is spread mainly by:

- Having anal or vaginal sex with someone who has HIV without using a condom or taking medicines to prevent or treat HIV.

  - For the HIV-negative partner, receptive anal sex (bottoming) is the highest-risk sexual behavior, but you can also get HIV from insertive anal sex (topping).

  - Either partner can get HIV through vaginal sex, though it is less risky for getting HIV than receptive anal sex.

- Sharing needles or syringes, rinse water, or other equipment (works) used to prepare drugs for injection with someone who has HIV. HIV can live in a used needle up to 42 days depending on temperature and other factors.

Less commonly, HIV may be spread:

- From mother to child during pregnancy, birth, or breastfeeding. Although the risk can be high if a mother is living with HIV and not taking medicine, recommendations to test all pregnant women for HIV and start HIV treatment immediately have lowered the number of babies who are born with HIV.

- By being stuck with an HIV-contaminated needle or other sharp object. This is a risk mainly for healthcare workers.

In extremely rare cases, HIV has been transmitted by:

- Oral sex—putting the mouth on the penis (fellatio), vagina (cunnilingus), or anus (rimming). In general, there's little to no risk of getting HIV from oral sex. But transmission of HIV, though extremely rare, is theoretically possible if an HIV-positive man ejaculates in his partner's mouth during oral sex.

- Receiving blood transfusions, blood products, or organ/tissue transplants that are contaminated with HIV. This was more common in the early years of HIV, but now the risk is extremely small because of rigorous testing of the U.S. blood supply and donated organs and tissues.

- Eating food that has been prechewed by an HIV-infected person. The contamination occurs when infected blood from a caregiver's mouth mixes with food while chewing. The only known cases are among infants.

- Being bitten by a person with HIV. Each of the very small number of documented cases has involved severe trauma with extensive tissue damage and the presence of blood. There is no risk of transmission if the skin is not broken.

- Contact between broken skin, wounds, or mucous membranes and HIV-infected blood or blood-contaminated body fluids.

- Deep, open-mouth kissing if both partners have sores or bleeding gums and blood from the HIV-positive partner gets into the bloodstream of the HIV-negative partner. HIV is not spread through saliva.

Can You Get Human Immunodeficiency Virus from Casual Contact, Using a Public Space, or from a Mosquito Bite?

No. HIV is NOT transmitted:

- By hugging, shaking hands, sharing toilets, sharing dishes, or closed-mouth or "social" kissing with someone who is HIV-positive

- Through saliva, tears, or sweat that is not mixed with the blood of an HIV-positive person

- By mosquitoes, ticks or other blood-sucking insects

- Through the air

As noted above, only certain body fluids—blood, semen, preseminal fluid, rectal fluids, vaginal fluids, and breast milk—from an HIV-infected person can transmit HIV. Most commonly, people get or transmit HIV through sexual behaviors and needle or syringe use. Babies can also get HIV from an HIV-positive mother during pregnancy, birth, or breastfeeding.

Who Is at Risk for Human Immunodeficiency Virus?

HIV can affect anyone regardless of sexual orientation, race, ethnicity, gender or age. However, certain groups are at higher risk for HIV and merit special consideration because of particular risk factors.

Is the Risk of Human Immunodeficiency Virus Different for Different People?

Some groups of people in the United States are more likely to get HIV than others because of many factors, including the status of their sex partners, their risk behaviors, and where they live.

When you live in a community where many people have HIV infection, the chances of having sex or sharing needles or other injection equipment with someone who has HIV are higher. You can use the Centers for Disease Control and Prevention's (CDC) HIV, STD, hepatitis, and tuberculosis Atlas Plus to see the percentage of people with HIV ("prevalence") in different U.S. communities. Within any community, the prevalence of HIV can vary among different populations.

Gay and bisexual men have the largest number of new diagnoses in the United States. Blacks/African Americans and Hispanics/Latinos are disproportionately affected by HIV compared to other racial and ethnic groups. Also, transgender women who have sex with men are among the groups at highest risk for HIV infection, and injection drug users remain at significant risk for getting HIV.

Risky behaviors, such as having anal or vaginal sex without using a condom or taking medicines to prevent or treat HIV, and sharing needles or syringes play a big role in HIV transmission. Anal sex is the highest-risk sexual behavior. If you do not have HIV, being a receptive partner (or bottom) for anal sex is the highest-risk sexual activity for getting HIV. If you do have HIV, being the insertive partner (or top) for anal sex is the highest-risk sexual activity for transmitting HIV.

But there are more tools available to prevent HIV than ever before. Choosing less risky sexual behaviors, taking medicines to prevent and treat HIV, and using condoms with lubricants are all highly effective ways to reduce the risk of getting or transmitting HIV.

How Can You Tell If You Have Human Immunodeficiency Virus?

The only way to know for sure if you have HIV is to get tested. You cannot rely on symptoms to tell whether you have HIV.

Knowing your HIV status gives you powerful information so you can take steps to keep yourself and your partner(s) healthy:

- If you test positive, you can take medicine to treat HIV. People with HIV who take HIV medicine daily as prescribed can live a long and healthy life and prevent transmission to others. Without HIV medicine (ART), the virus replicates in the body and damages the immune system. This is why people need to start treatment as soon as possible after testing positive.

- If you test negative, there are several ways to prevent getting HIV.

- If you are pregnant, you should be tested for HIV so that you can begin treatment if you are HIV-positive. If an HIV-positive woman is treated for HIV early in her pregnancy, the risk of transmitting HIV to her baby can be very low.

Use the HIV Services Locator to find an HIV testing site near you.

What Are the Symptoms of Human Immunodeficiency Virus?

There are several symptoms of HIV. Not everyone will have the same symptoms. It depends on the person and what stage of the disease they are in.

Below are the three stages of HIV and some of the symptoms people may experience.

Stage 1: Acute Human Immunodeficiency Virus Infection

Within two to four weeks after infection with HIV, about two-thirds of people will have a flu-like illness. This is the body's natural response to HIV infection.

Flu-like symptoms can include:

- Fever

- Chills

- Rash

- Night sweats

- Muscle aches

- Sore throat

- Fatigue

- Swollen lymph nodes

- Mouth ulcers

These symptoms can last anywhere from a few days to several weeks. But some people do not have any symptoms at all during this early stage of HIV.

Do not assume you have HIV just because you have any of these symptoms—they can be similar to those caused by other illnesses. But if you think you may have been exposed to HIV, get an HIV test.

- Request an HIV test for recent infection—Most HIV tests detect antibodies (proteins your body makes as a reaction to HIV), not HIV itself. But it can take a few weeks after you are infected for your body to produce them. There are other types of tests that can detect HIV infection sooner. Tell your doctor or clinic if you think you were recently exposed to HIV, and ask if their tests can detect early infection.

- Know your status—After you get tested, be sure to learn your test results. If you are HIV-positive, see a doctor as soon as possible so you can start treatment with HIV medicine. And be aware: when you are in the early stage of infection, you are at very high risk of transmitting HIV to others. It is important to take steps to reduce your risk of transmission. If you are HIV-negative, there are prevention options like PrEP that can help you stay negative.

Stage 2: Clinical Latency

In this stage, the virus still multiplies, but at very low levels. People in this stage may not feel sick or have any symptoms. This stage is also called "chronic HIV infection."

Without HIV treatment, people can stay in this stage for 10 or 15 years, but some move through this stage faster.

If you take HIV treatment every day, exactly as prescribed and get and keep an undetectable viral load, you can protect your health and prevent transmission to others. But if your viral load is detectable, you can transmit HIV during this stage, even when you have no symptoms. It is important to see your healthcare provider regularly to get your level checked.

Stage 3: Acquired Immunodeficiency Syndrome

If you have HIV and you are not on HIV treatment, eventually the virus will weaken your body's immune system and you will progress to AIDS. This is the late stage of HIV infection.

Symptoms of AIDS can include:

- Rapid weight loss

- Recurring fever or profuse night sweats

- Extreme and unexplained tiredness

- Prolonged swelling of the lymph glands in the armpits, groin, or neck

- Diarrhea that lasts for more than a week

- Sores of the mouth, anus, or genitals

- Pneumonia

- Red, brown, pink, or purplish blotches on or under the skin or inside the mouth, nose, or eyelids

- Memory loss, depression, and other neurologic disorders

Each of these symptoms can also be related to other illnesses. The only way to know for sure if you have HIV is to get tested.

Many of the severe symptoms and illnesses of HIV disease come from the opportunistic infections that occur because your body's immune system has been damaged. See your healthcare provider if you are experiencing any of these symptoms.

Chapter 20

Human Papillomavirus

Human papillomavirus (HPV) is the most common sexually transmitted infection (STI) in the United States. Some health effects caused by HPV can be prevented by the HPV vaccines.

What Is Human Papillomavirus?

Human papillomavirus is a different virus than human immunodeficiency virus (HIV) and herpes simplex virus (HSV). 79 million Americans, most in their late teens and early twenties, are infected with HPV. There are many different types of HPV. Some types can cause health problems, including genital warts and cancers. But, there are vaccines that can stop these health problems from happening.

How Is Human Papillomavirus Spread?

You can get HPV by having vaginal, anal, or oral sex with someone who has the virus. It is most commonly spread during vaginal or anal sex. HPV can be passed even when an infected person has no signs or symptoms.

Anyone who is sexually active can get HPV, even if you have had sex with only one person. You also can develop symptoms years after you have sex with someone who is infected. This makes it hard to know when you first became infected.

This chapter includes text excerpted from "Genital HPV Infection—Fact Sheet," Centers for Disease Control and Prevention (CDC), November 16, 2017.

Does Human Papillomavirus Cause Health Problems?

In most cases, HPV goes away on its own and does not cause any health problems. But when HPV does not go away, it can cause health problems, such as genital warts and cancer.

Genital warts usually appear as a small bump or group of bumps in the genital area. They can be small or large, raised or flat, or shaped like a cauliflower. A healthcare provider can usually diagnose warts by looking at the genital area.

Does Human Papillomavirus Cause Cancer?

Human papillomavirus can cause cervical and other cancers, including cancer of the vulva, vagina, penis, or anus. It can also cause cancer in the back of the throat, including the base of the tongue and tonsils (called "oropharyngeal cancer").

Cancer often takes years, even decades, to develop after a person gets HPV. The types of HPV that can cause genital warts are not the same as the types of HPV that can cause cancers.

There is no way to know which people who have HPV will develop cancer or other health problems. People with weak immune systems (including those with HIV/AIDS (acquired immunodeficiency syndrome)) may be less able to fight off HPV. They may also be more likely to develop health problems from HPV.

How Can I Avoid Human Papillomavirus and the Health Problems It Can Cause?

You can do several things to lower your chances of getting HPV.

Get vaccinated. The HPV vaccine is safe and effective. It can protect against diseases (including cancers) caused by HPV when given in the recommended age groups. The Centers for Disease Control and Prevention (CDC) recommends 11 to 12 year olds get 2 doses of the HPV vaccine to protect against cancers caused by HPV.

Get screened for cervical cancer. Routine screening for women between the ages of 21 and 65 can prevent cervical cancer.

If you are sexually active:

- Use latex condoms the right way every time you have sex. This can lower your chances of getting HPV. But, HPV can infect areas not covered by a condom—so condoms may not fully protect against getting HPV.

170

- Be in a mutually monogamous relationship or have sex only with someone who only has sex with you.

Who Should Get Vaccinated?

All boys and girls 11 or 12 years of age should get vaccinated.

Catch-up vaccines are recommended for boys and men through the age of 21 and for girls and women through the age of 26 if they did not get vaccinated when they were younger.

The HPV vaccine is also recommended for the following people if they did not get vaccinated when they were younger:

- Young men who have sex with men, including young men who identify as gay or bisexual or who intend to have sex with men through the age of 26

- Young adults who are transgender through the age of 26

- Young adults with certain immunocompromising conditions (including HIV) through the age of 26

How Do I Know If I Have Human Papillomavirus?

There is no test to find out a person's "HPV status." Also, there is no approved HPV test to find HPV in the mouth or throat.

There are HPV tests that can be used to screen for cervical cancer. These tests are only recommended for screening in women 30 years of age and older. HPV tests are not recommended to screen men, adolescents, or women under 30 years of age.

Most people with HPV do not know that they are infected, and they never develop symptoms or health problems from it. Some people find out they have HPV when they get genital warts. Women may find out they have HPV when they get an abnormal Papanicolaou test (Pap test) result (during cervical cancer screening). Others may only find out once they have developed more serious problems from HPV, such as cancers.

How Common Is Human Papillomavirus and the Health Problems Caused by Human Papillomavirus?

Human papillomavirus: About 79 million Americans are currently infected with HPV. About 14 million people become newly infected each year. HPV is so common that almost every person who is sexually active will get HPV at some time in their life if they do not get the HPV vaccine.

Health problems related to HPV include genital warts and cervical cancer.

Genital warts: Before HPV vaccines were introduced, roughly 340,000 to 360,000 women and men were affected by genital warts caused by HPV every year.* Also, about 1 in 100 sexually active adults in the United States has genital warts at any given time.

Cervical cancer: Every year, nearly 12,000 women living in the United States will be diagnosed with cervical cancer, and more than 4,000 women die from cervical cancer—even with screening and treatment.

There are other conditions and cancers caused by HPV that occur in people living in the United States. Every year, approximately 19,400 women and 12,100 men are affected by cancers caused by HPV.

* These figures only look at the number of people who sought care for genital warts. This could be an underestimate of the actual number of people who get genital warts.

I Am Pregnant. Will Having Human Papillomavirus Affect My Pregnancy?

If you are pregnant and have HPV, you can get genital warts or develop abnormal cell changes on your cervix. Abnormal cell changes can be found with routine cervical cancer screening. You should get routine cervical cancer screening even when you are pregnant.

Can I Be Treated for Human Papillomavirus or Health Problems Caused by Human Papillomavirus?

There is no treatment for the virus itself. However, there are treatments for the health problems that HPV can cause:

- Genital warts can be treated by your healthcare provider or with prescription medication. If left untreated, genital warts may go away, stay the same, or grow in size or number.

- Cervical precancer can be treated. Women who get routine Pap tests and follow up as needed can identify problems before cancer develops. Prevention is always better than treatment.

- Other HPV-related cancers are also more treatable when diagnosed and treated early.

Chapter 21

Influenza

Chapter Contents

Section 21.1—Seasonal Flu 176

Section 21.2—Pandemic Flu... 182

Section 21.3—H1N1 Flu 187

Section 21.1

Seasonal Flu

This section includes text excerpted from "About Flu,"
Centers for Disease Control and Prevention (CDC), August 23, 2018.

What Is Influenza?

Influenza, also referred to as "flu," is a contagious respiratory illness caused by influenza viruses. It can cause mild to severe illness. Serious outcomes of flu infection can result in hospitalization or death. Some people, such as older people, young children, and people with certain health conditions, are at a high risk of serious flu complications. There are two main types of influenza (flu) virus: types A and B. The influenza A and B viruses that routinely spread in people (human influenza viruses) are responsible for seasonal flu epidemics each year.

The best way to prevent flu is by getting vaccinated each year.

Flu Symptoms

Flu is different from a cold, as it usually comes on suddenly. People who are sick with flu often feel some or all of these symptoms:

- Fever* or feeling feverish/chills
- Cough
- Sore throat
- Runny or stuffy nose
- Muscle or body aches
- Headaches
- Fatigue (tiredness)
- Some people may experience vomiting and diarrhea, though this is more common in children than adults.

* It is important to note that not everyone with flu will have a fever.

How Flu Spreads

Most experts believe that flu viruses spread mainly by tiny droplets made when people with flu cough, sneeze, or talk. These droplets can land in the mouths or noses of people who are nearby. Less often, a person might get flu by touching a surface or object that has flu virus on it and then touching their own mouth, nose, or yes.

How Many People Get Sick with Flu Every Year?

A 2018 Centers for Disease Control and Prevention (CDC) study published in *Clinical Infectious Diseases* (CID) looked at the percentage of the U.S. population who were sickened by flu using 2 different methods and compared the findings. Both methods had similar findings, which suggested that, on average, about 8 percent of the U.S. population gets sick from flu each season, with a range of between 3 and 11 percent depending on the season.

Why Is the 3 to 11 Percent Estimate Different from the Previously Cited 5 to 20 Percent Range?

The commonly cited 5 to 20 percent estimate was based on a study that examined both symptomatic and asymptomatic influenza illness, which means it also looked at people who may have had the flu but never knew it because they did not have any symptoms. The 3 to 11 percent range is an estimate of the proportion of people who have symptomatic flu illness.

Who Is Most Likely to Be Infected with Influenza?

The same CID study found that children are most likely to get sick from flu and that people 65 and older are least likely to get sick from influenza. Median incidence values (or attack rate) by age group were 9.3 percent for children between 0 and 17 years of age, 8.8 percent for adults between 18 and 64 years of age, and 3.9 percent for adults 65 years of age and older. This means that children younger than 18 years of age are more than twice as likely to develop a symptomatic flu infection than adults 65 years of age and older.

How Is the Seasonal Incidence of Influenza Estimated?

Influenza virus infection is so common that the number of people infected each season can only be estimated. These statistical estimations are based on the CDC-measured flu hospitalization rates that are adjusted to produce an estimate of the total number of influenza infections in the United States for a given flu season.

The estimates for the number of infections are then divided by the census population to estimate the seasonal incidence (or attack rate) of influenza.

Does Seasonal Incidence of Influenza Change Based on the Severity of Flu Season?

Yes. The proportion of people who get sick from the flu varies. A paper published in CID found that between 3 and 11 percent of the U.S. population gets infected and develops flu symptoms each year. The 3 percent estimate is from the 2011 to 2012 season, which was an H1N1-predominant season classified as being of low severity. The estimated incidence of flu illness during 2 seasons was around 11 percent; 2012 to 2013 was an H3N2-predominant season classified as being of moderate severity, while 2014 to 2015 was an H3N2 predominant season classified as being of high severity.

Period of Contagiousness

You may be able to pass on flu to someone else before you know you are sick, as well as while you are sick.

- People with flu are most contagious in the first three to four days after their illness begins.

- Some otherwise healthy adults may be able to infect others beginning one day before symptoms develop and up to five to seven days after becoming sick.

- Some people, especially young children and people with weakened immune systems, might be able to infect others with flu viruses for an even longer time.

Onset of Symptoms

The time from when a person is exposed and infected with flu to when symptoms begin is about two days, but it can range from about one to four days.

Table 21.1. Estimates of the Incidence of Symptomatic Influenza by Season and Age-Group, United States, 2010–2016

Season	Predominant Virus(es)	Season Severity	Incidence, %, by Age Group						
			0–4 Years	5–17 Years	18–49 Years	50–64 Years	≥65 Years	All Ages
2010–11	A/H3N2, A/H1N1pdm09	Moderate	14.1	8.4	5.3	8.1	4.3	6.8
2011–12	A/H3N2	Low	4.8	3.6	2.5	3.1	2.3	3
2012–13	A/H3N2	Moderate	18.6	12.7	8.9	14.3	9.9	11.3
2013–14	A/H1N1pdm09	Moderate	12.4	7.2	9.2	13	3.4	9
2014–15	A/H3N2	High	150	12.7	7.8	12.9	12.4	10.8
2015–16	A/H1N1pdm09	Moderate	11.1	7.4	7.1	11	3.5	7.6
Median			13.2	7.9	7.4	12	3.9	8.3

Complications of Flu

Complications of flu can include bacterial pneumonia, ear infections, sinus infections and worsening of chronic medical conditions, such as congestive heart failure, asthma, or diabetes.

People at High Risk from Flu

Anyone can get flu (even healthy people), and serious problems related to flu can happen at any age; but, some people are at a high risk of developing serious flu-related complications if they get sick. This includes people 65 years of age and older, people of any age with certain chronic medical conditions (such as asthma, diabetes, or heart disease), pregnant women, and children younger than 5 years of age.

Preventing Seasonal Flu

The first and most important step in preventing flu is to get a flu vaccine each year. The flu vaccine has been shown to reduce flu-related illnesses and the risk of serious flu complications that can result in hospitalization or even death. The CDC also recommends everyday preventive actions (such as staying away from people who are sick, covering coughs and sneezes and frequent handwashing) to help slow the spread of germs that cause respiratory (nose, throat, and lungs) illnesses, such as flu.

Diagnosing Flu
How Do I Know If I Have the Flu?

Your respiratory illness might be the flu if you have a fever, cough, sore throat, runny or stuffy nose, body aches, headache, chills, and fatigue. Some people may have vomiting and diarrhea. People may be infected with the flu and have respiratory symptoms without a fever. Flu viruses usually cause the most illness during the colder months of the year. However, influenza can also occur outside of the typical flu season. In addition, other viruses can also cause respiratory illness similar to the flu. So, it is impossible to tell for sure if you have the flu based on symptoms alone. If your doctor needs to know for sure whether you have the flu, there are laboratory tests that can be done.

What Kinds of Flu Tests Are There?

A number of flu tests are available to detect influenza viruses in respiratory specimens. The most common are called "rapid influenza diagnostic tests" (RIDTs). RIDTs work by detecting the parts of the virus (antigens) that stimulate an immune response. These tests can provide results within approximately 10 to 15 minutes, but they are not as accurate as other flu tests. Therefore, you could still have the flu even though your rapid test result is negative. Other flu tests are called "rapid molecular assays" that detect the genetic material of the virus. Rapid molecular assays produce results in 15 to 20 minutes and are more accurate than RIDTs. In addition, there are several more-accurate and sensitive flu tests available that must be performed in specialized laboratories, such as those found in hospitals or state public-health laboratories. All of these tests require that a healthcare provider swipe the inside of your nose or the back of your throat with a swab and then send the swab for testing. Results may take one hour or several hours.

How Well Can Rapid Tests Detect the Flu?

During an influenza outbreak, a positive rapid flu test is likely to indicate an influenza infection. However, rapid tests vary in their ability to detect flu viruses, depending on the type of rapid test used, and on the type of flu viruses circulating. Also, rapid tests appear to be better at detecting flu in children than in adults. This variation in ability to detect viruses can result in some people who are infected with the flu having a negative rapid test result. (This situation is called "a false negative test result.") Despite a negative rapid test result, your healthcare provider may diagnose you with flu based on your symptoms and their clinical judgment.

Treating Flu
Can Flu Be Treated?

Yes. There are prescription medications called "antiviral drugs" that can be used to treat flu illness. The CDC recommends prompt treatment for people who have flu infection or suspected flu infection and who are at a high risk of serious flu complications, such as people with asthma, diabetes (including gestational diabetes), or heart disease.

What Are Antiviral Drugs?

Antiviral drugs are prescription medicines (pills, liquid, an inhaled powder, or an intravenous (IV) solution) that fight against flu viruses in your body. Antiviral drugs are not sold over-the-counter (OTC). You can only get them if you have a prescription from a healthcare provider. Antiviral drugs are different from antibiotics, which fight against bacterial infections.

What Should I Do If I Think I Am Sick with Flu?

If you get sick with flu, antiviral drugs are a treatment option. Check with your doctor promptly if you are at a high risk of serious flu complications and you develop flu symptoms. Flu signs and symptoms can include feeling feverish or having a fever, cough, sore throat, runny or stuffy nose, body aches, headache, chills, and fatigue. Your doctor may prescribe antiviral drugs to treat your flu illness.

Should I Still Get a Flu Vaccine?

Yes. Antiviral drugs are not a substitute for getting a flu vaccine. While flu vaccine can vary in how well it works, a flu vaccine is the best way to help prevent seasonal flu and its potentially serious complications. Antiviral drugs are a second line of defense that can be used to treat flu (including seasonal flu and variant flu viruses) if you get sick.

Section 21.2

Pandemic Flu

This section includes text excerpted from "Pandemic Influenza (Flu)—Questions and Answers," Centers for Disease Control and Prevention (CDC), May 15, 2017.

What Is an Influenza Pandemic?

An influenza pandemic is a global outbreak of a new influenza A virus that is very different from current and recently circulating human seasonal influenza A viruses. Pandemics happen when new (novel) influenza A viruses emerge, which are able to infect people easily and spread from person to person in an efficient and sustained way. Because the virus is new to humans, very few people will have immunity against the pandemic virus, and a vaccine might not be widely available. The new virus will make a lot of people sick. How sick people get will depend on the characteristics of the virus whether or not people have any immunity to that virus and the health and age of the person being infected. With seasonal flu, for example, certain chronic health conditions are known to make those people more susceptible to serious flu infections. Influenza pandemics are uncommon and only occurred during the 20th century.

Where Do Pandemic Influenza Viruses Come From?

Different animals—including birds and pigs—are hosts to influenza A viruses that do not normally infect people. Influenza A viruses are constantly changing, making it possible on very rare occasions for nonhuman influenza viruses to change in such a way that they can infect people easily and spread efficiently from person to person.

How Do Influenza A Viruses Change to Cause a Pandemic?

Influenza A viruses are divided into subtypes based on 2 proteins on the surface of the virus: the hemagglutinin (H) and the neuraminidase (N). There are 18 different hemagglutinin subtypes and 11 different neuraminidase subtypes (H1 through H18 and N1 through N11). Theoretically, any combination of the 18 hemagglutinins and 11 neuraminidase proteins are possible, but not all have been found in animals and even fewer have been found to infect humans.

Influenza viruses can change in two different ways, one of which is called "antigenic shift" and can result in the emergence of a new influenza virus. The antigenic shift represents an abrupt, major change in an influenza A virus. This can result from direct infection of humans with a nonhuman influenza A virus, such as a virus circulating among birds or pigs. The antigenic shift also can happen when a nonhuman influenza A virus (for example, an avian influenza virus) exchanges genetic information with another influenza A viruses in a process called "genetic reassortment," and the resultant new virus is able to infect people. For example, an exchange of genes between a human influenza A virus and an avian influenza A virus can create a new influenza A virus with a hemagglutinin protein or both a hemagglutinin protein and a neuraminidase protein from an avian influenza A virus. If this new virus causes illness in infected people and can spread easily from person to person, an influenza pandemic can occur.

What Happens When a Pandemic Influenza Virus Emerges

When a pandemic influenza virus emerges, the virus can spread quickly because most people will not be immune and a vaccine might not be widely available to offer immediate protection. During the 2009 H1N1 pandemic, for example, a new H1N1 virus was first identified in April 2009. By June 2009, that novel H1N1 virus had spread worldwide and the World Health Organization (WHO) declared a pandemic. Spread of a pandemic influenza virus may occur in multiple disease "waves" that are separated by several months. As a pandemic influenza virus spreads, large numbers of people may need medical care worldwide. Schools, child care centers, workplaces, and other places for mass gatherings may experience more absenteeism. Public health and healthcare systems can become overloaded, with elevated rates of hospitalizations and deaths. Other critical infrastructure, such as law enforcement, emergency medical services, and the transportation industry, may also be affected.

Will Seasonal Flu Vaccines Protect against Pandemic Flu?

It is unlikely that seasonal flu vaccines would protect against a pandemic influenza virus. Seasonal flu vaccines that are used annually protect against currently circulating human influenza A and B viruses. They are not designed to protect against new influenza A viruses. A pandemic influenza virus would be very different from circulating seasonal influenza A viruses, and thus seasonal vaccines would not be expected to offer protection.

Are There Vaccines to Protect against Pandemic Flu?

The federal government has created a stockpile of some vaccines against select influenza A viruses with pandemic potential that could be used in the event of a pandemic, including vaccines against certain avian influenza A (e.g., H5N1 and H7N9) viruses. If a similar virus were to begin a pandemic, some vaccine would already be available.

The U.S. Department of Health and Human Services (HHS) is the lead agency for public health preparedness and medical response to an influenza pandemic. Within HHS, the Biomedical Advanced Research and Development Authority (BARDA) Influenza Division is charged with the advanced development and procurement of medical and non-pharmaceutical countermeasures for pandemic influenza preparedness and response.

How Long Would It Take to Develop a New Pandemic Vaccine?

If a new pandemic influenza virus (not included in the prepandemic vaccine stockpile) were to emerge, it is likely that a vaccine would have to be developed against that virus in order for a sufficient supply of the vaccine to become available for everyone who wishes to be vaccinated. How long it would take to produce a pandemic flu vaccine would depend on many factors, including how long it would take to create a candidate vaccine virus (CVV) and what vaccine manufacturing process would be used. For seasonal influenza vaccine, it usually takes at least six months to produce large quantities of flu vaccine. During the 2009 H1N1 pandemic, it took about the same amount of time. The Centers for Disease Control and Prevention (CDC) began developing a CVV to make monovalent (one component) H1N1pdm09 vaccine in mid-April. The first doses of this vaccine were administered in early October, and large quantities of the vaccine became available in late November. Efforts are underway now to shorten the time it takes to produce influenza vaccines, but because of the current amount of time needed to make the flu vaccine, early supplies of pandemic vaccine might not be enough to meet demand, especially if most people need two doses of vaccine for protective immunity.

How Many Doses of Pandemic Vaccine Would Each Person Need?

People with no immunity against a new influenza virus may need 2 doses to be fully protected against that virus. The first dose primes the immune system, and the second dose creates a protective response. During the 2009 H1N1 influenza pandemic, CDC recommended that 2 doses of the vaccine be given to children 6 months through 9 years of age in order to increase the immune response.

What Treatments Are Available for Pandemic Flu?

During a flu pandemic, antiviral drugs would be an important tool to treat and prevent the spread of influenza illness. Antiviral drugs are medicines (pills, liquid or an inhaled powder) that fight against the influenza viruses infecting the respiratory tract. Antiviral drugs are recommended to treat seasonal influenza in people who are very sick or who are at high risk of serious flu complications. These same drugs may be useful for treating pandemic influenza, depending upon whether the pandemic influenza virus is susceptible or resistant to available antiviral drugs. Antiviral drugs are prescription drugs (they are not sold over-the-counter (OTC)) and are different from prescription antibiotics that treat bacterial infections.

Are There Other Ways to Slow a Pandemic?

Nonpharmaceutical interventions (NPIs) are actions, apart from getting vaccinated and taking medicine, which people and communities can take to help slow the spread of respiratory illnesses, such as pandemic flu. Again, these actions do not include medicines, vaccines, or other pharmaceutical interventions. Given that it may take months to produce a pandemic flu vaccine (not included in the prepandemic vaccine stockpile) and that antiviral drugs may be reserved for treatment, NPIs will likely be the only prevention tools available during the early stages of a pandemic and, thus, critically important to help slow the spread of infection.

How Would Nonpharmaceutical Interventions Be Used during a Pandemic?

Nonpharmaceutical interventions, also known as "community mitigation strategies," may be more efficient when used early in a flu pandemic and in a layered fashion. Public health officials will recommend that people practice everyday preventive actions at all times. These actions include staying home when sick, covering coughs and sneezes with a tissue, washing hands often, and cleaning frequently touched surfaces and objects. During severe, very severe, or extreme flu pandemics, public health officials may recommend additional actions, such as using face masks when sick and in close contact with other people, temporarily dismissing child care facilities and schools, and increasing the space between people and decreasing the frequency of contact among people (that is, social distancing).

Section 21.3

H1N1 Flu

This section includes text excerpted from "H1N1 Flu—2009 H1N1
Flu ("Swine Flu") and You," Centers for Disease Control and
Prevention (CDC), February 9, 2010. Reviewed July 2019.

What Is H1N1 (Swine Flu)?

H1N1 (sometimes called "swine flu") is a new influenza virus causing illness in people. This new virus was first detected in people in the United States in April 2009. This virus is spreading from person-to-person worldwide, probably in much the same way that regular seasonal influenza viruses spread. On June 11, 2009, the World Health Organization (WHO) declared that a pandemic of H1N1 flu was underway.

Why Is the H1N1 Virus Sometimes Called "Swine Flu"?

This virus was originally referred to as "swine flu" because laboratory testing showed that many of the genes in the virus were very similar to influenza viruses that normally occur in pigs (swine) in North America. But, further study has shown that the H1N1 is very different from what normally circulates in North American pigs. It has two genes from flu viruses that normally circulate in pigs in Europe and Asia and bird (avian) genes and human genes. Scientists call this a "quadruple reassortant" virus.

Is the H1N1 Virus Contagious?

The H1N1 virus is contagious and is spread from human to human.

How Does the H1N1 Virus Spread?

The spread of the H1N1 virus is thought to occur in the same way that seasonal flu spreads. Flu viruses are spread mainly from person to person through coughing, sneezing, or talking by people with influenza. Sometimes, people may become infected by touching something—such as a surface or object—with flu viruses on it and then touching their mouth or nose.

Can I Get H1N1 More than Once?

Getting infected with any influenza virus, including H1N1, should cause your body to develop immune resistance to that virus so it is not likely that a person would be infected with the identical influenza virus more than once. (However, people with weakened immune systems might not develop full immunity after infection and might be more likely to get infected with the same influenza virus more than once.) However, it is also possible that a person could have a positive test result for flu infection more than once in an influenza season. This can occur for two reasons:

1. A person may be infected with different influenza viruses (for example, the first time with H1N1 and the second time with a regular seasonal flu virus). Most rapid tests cannot distinguish which influenza virus is responsible for the illness.

2. Influenza tests can occasionally give false positive and false negative results so it is possible that one of the test results were incorrect. This is more likely to happen when the diagnosis is made with the rapid flu tests.

What Are the Signs and Symptoms of H1N1 Virus in People?

The symptoms of H1N1 flu virus in people include fever, cough, sore throat, runny or stuffy nose, body aches, headache, chills, and fatigue. Some people may have vomiting and diarrhea. People may be infected with the flu, including H1N1, and have respiratory symptoms without a fever. Severe illnesses and deaths have occurred as a result of illness associated with this virus.

How Severe Is Illness Associated with H1N1 Flu Virus?

Illness with H1N1 virus has ranged from mild to severe. While most people who have been sick have recovered without needing medical treatment, hospitalizations and deaths from infection with this virus have occurred.

In seasonal flu, certain people are at a high risk of serious complications. This includes people 65 years of age and older, children younger than 5 years of age, pregnant women, and people of any age with certain chronic medical conditions. More than 70 percent of adults who have been hospitalized with the H1N1 virus have had one or more medical conditions previously recognized as placing people at a higher risk of serious seasonal flu-related complications. This includes pregnancy, diabetes, heart disease, asthma, and kidney disease. In one study, 57 percent of children who had been hospitalized as a result of H1N1 have had one or more higher risk medical conditions.

Young children are also at a high risk of serious complications from H1N1, just as they are from seasonal flu. And while people 65 years of age and older are less likely to be infected with H1N1 flu, if they get sick, they are also at a high risk of developing serious complications from their illness.

The Centers for Disease Control and Prevention (CDC) laboratory studies have shown that no children and very few adults younger than 60 years of age have existing antibody to the H1N1 flu virus; however, about one-third of adults older than 60 years of age may have antibodies against this virus. It is unknown how much, if any, protection may be afforded against H1N1 flu by any existing antibody.

Who Is at Higher Risk from Serious H1N1-Related Complications?

Most people who get the flu (either seasonal or H1N1) will have mild illness, will not need medical care or antiviral drugs, and will recover in less than two weeks. Some people, however, are more likely to get flu complications that result in being hospitalized and occasionally result in death. Pneumonia, bronchitis, sinus infections, and ear infections are examples of flu-related complications. The flu can also make chronic health problems worse. For example, people with asthma may experience asthma attacks while they have the flu, and people with chronic congestive heart failure may have worsening of this condition that is triggered by the flu. The list below includes the groups of people more likely to get flu-related complications if they get sick from influenza.

People at High Risk for Developing Flu-Related Complications

- Children younger than five years of age, but especially children younger than two years of age
- Adults 65 years of age and older
- Pregnant women

People who have medical conditions including:

- Asthma

- Neurological and neurodevelopmental conditions (including disorders of the brain, spinal cord, peripheral nerve, and muscle, such as cerebral palsy (CP); epilepsy (seizure disorders); stroke; intellectual disability (mental retardation); moderate to severe developmental delay; muscular dystrophy (MD); or spinal cord injury (SCI)).

- Chronic lung disease (such as chronic obstructive pulmonary disease (COPD) and cystic fibrosis (CF))

- Heart disease (such as congenital heart disease (CHD), congestive heart failure (CHF), and coronary artery disease (CAD))

- Blood disorders (such as sickle cell disease (SCD))

- Endocrine disorders (such as diabetes mellitus)

- Kidney disorders

- Liver disorders

- Metabolic disorders (such as inherited metabolic disorders and mitochondrial disorders)

- Weakened immune system due to disease or medication (such as people with human immunodeficiency virus (HIV), acquired immunodeficiency syndrome (AIDS), or cancer, or those on chronic steroids)

- People younger than 19 years of age who are receiving long-term aspirin therapy

In addition, some studies have shown that obese persons (body mass index more than 30) and particularly morbidly obese persons (body mass index more than 40) are at higher risk, perhaps because they have one of the higher risk conditions above but do not realize it.

How Long Can an Infected Person Spread This Virus to Others?

People infected with seasonal and H1N1 flu shed virus and may be able to infect others from one day before getting sick to five to seven days after. This can be longer in some people, especially children and people with weakened immune systems and in people infected with H1N1 viruses.

What Can I Do to Protect Myself from Getting Sick?

There is a seasonal flu vaccine to protect against seasonal flu viruses and an H1N1 vaccine to protect against the H1N1 influenza virus. A flu vaccine is by far the most important step in protecting against flu infection.

There are also everyday actions that can help prevent the spread of germs that cause respiratory illnesses like the flu.

Take These Everyday Steps to Protect Your Health

- Cover your nose and mouth with a tissue when you cough or sneeze. Throw the tissue in the trash after you use it.

- Wash your hands often with soap and water. If soap and water are not available, use an alcohol-based hand rub.

- Avoid touching your eyes, nose, or mouth. Germs spread this way.

- Try to avoid close contact with sick people.

- If you are sick with flu-like illness, the CDC recommends that you stay home for at least 24 hours after your fever is gone except to get medical care or for other necessities. (Your fever should be gone without the use of a fever-reducing medicine.) Keep away from others as much as possible to keep from making others sick.

Other Important Actions That You Can Take

- Follow public health advice regarding school closures, avoiding crowds, and other social distancing measures.

- Be prepared in case you get sick and need to stay home for a week or so; a supply of over-the-counter (OTC) medicines, alcohol-based hand rubs (for when soap and water are not available), tissues and other related items could help you to avoid the need to make trips out in public while you are sick and contagious.

Chapter 22

Measles

Measles starts with a fever, runny nose, cough, red eyes, and a sore throat. It is followed by a rash that spreads over the body. Measles is highly contagious and spreads through coughing and sneezing. Make sure you and your child are protected with the measles, mumps, and rubella (MMR) vaccine.

Prevaccine Era

In the ninth century, a Persian doctor published one of the first written accounts of measles disease.

Francis Home, a Scottish physician, demonstrated in 1757 that measles is caused by an infectious agent in the blood of patients.

In 1912, measles became a nationally notifiable disease in the United States, requiring the U.S. healthcare providers and laboratories to report all diagnosed cases. In the first decade of reporting, an average of 6,000 measles-related deaths were reported each year.

In the decade before 1963 when a vaccine became available, nearly all children got measles by the time they were 15 years of age. It is estimated 3 to 4 million people in the United States were infected each year. Also each year, among reported cases, an estimated 400 to 500 people died, 48,000 were hospitalized, and 1,000 suffered encephalitis (swelling of the brain) from measles.

This chapter includes text excerpted from "Measles (Rubeola)," Centers for Disease Control and Prevention (CDC), June 13, 2019.

Vaccine Development

In 1954, John F. Enders and Dr. Thomas C. Peebles collected blood samples from several ill students during a measles outbreak in Boston, Massachusetts. They wanted to isolate the measles virus in the student's blood and create a measles vaccine. They succeeded in isolating measles in 13-year-old David Edmonston's blood.

In 1963, John Enders and his colleagues transformed their Edmonston-B strain of measles virus into a vaccine and licensed it in the United States. In 1968, an improved and even weaker measles vaccine, developed by Maurice Hilleman and his colleagues, began to be distributed. This vaccine, called the "Edmonston-Enders" (formerly "Moraten") strain has been the only measles vaccine used in the United States since 1968. The measles vaccine is usually combined with a vaccine for mumps and rubella, or it is combined with mumps, rubella, and varicella (MMRV).

Measles Elimination

In 1978, the Centers for Disease Control and Prevention (CDC) set a goal to eliminate measles from the United States by 1982. Although this goal was not met, widespread use of the measles vaccine drastically reduced the disease rates. By 1981, the number of reported measles cases was 80 percent less than the previous year. However, a 1989 measles outbreak among vaccinated school-aged children prompted the Advisory Committee on Immunization Practices (ACIP), the American Academy of Pediatrics (AAP), and the American Academy of Family Physicians (AAFP) to recommend a second dose of the MMR vaccine for all children. Following widespread implementation of this recommendation and improvements in first-dose MMR vaccine coverage, reported measles cases declined even more.

Signs and Symptoms of Measles

Measles symptoms appear 7 to 14 days after contact with the virus and typically include high fever, cough, runny nose, and watery eyes. Measles rash appears 3 to 5 days after the first symptoms.

7 to 14 Days after a Measles Infection: Symptoms Show

Measles is not just a little rash. Measles can be dangerous, especially for babies and young children. Measles typically begins with:

- High fever (may spike to more than 104°F),
- Cough,
- Runny nose (coryza), and
- Red, watery eyes (conjunctivitis).

2 to 3 Days after Symptoms Begin: Koplik Spots

Tiny white spots (Koplik spots) may appear inside the mouth 2 to 3 days after symptoms begin.

3 to 5 Days after Symptoms Begin: Measles Rash

3 to 5 days after symptoms begin, a rash breaks out. It usually begins as flat red spots that appear on the face at the hairline and spread downward to the neck, trunk, arms, legs, and feet.

- Small raised bumps may also appear on top of the flat red spots.
- The spots may become joined together as they spread from the head to the rest of the body.
- When the rash appears, a person's fever may spike to more than 104°F.

Transmission of Measles

Measles is a highly contagious virus that lives in the nose and throat mucus of an infected person. It can spread to others through coughing and sneezing. Also, the measles virus can live for up to 2 hours in an airspace where the infected person coughed or sneezed. If other people breathe the contaminated air or touch the infected surface then touch their eyes, noses, or mouths, they can become infected. Measles is so contagious that if 1 person has it, up to 90 percent of the people close to that person who are not immune will also become infected.

Infected people can spread measles to others from four days before through four days after the rash appears.

Measles is a disease of humans; the measles virus is not spread by any other animal species.

Complications of Measles

Measles can be serious in all age groups. However, children younger than 5 years of age and adults older than 20 years of age are more likely to suffer from measles complications. Common complications are ear infections and diarrhea. Serious complications include pneumonia and encephalitis.

People and Groups at Risk of Measles Complications

Measles can be serious in all age groups. However, there are several groups that are more likely to suffer from measles complications:

- Children younger than 5 years of age
- Adults older than 20 years of age
- Pregnant women
- People with compromised immune systems, such as from leukemia or human immunodeficiency virus (HIV) infection

Common Complications

- Ear infections occur in about 1 out of every 10 children with measles and can result in permanent hearing loss.
- Diarrhea is reported in less than 1 out of 10 people with measles.

Severe Complications

Some people may suffer from severe complications, such as pneumonia (infection of the lungs) and encephalitis (swelling of the brain). They may need to be hospitalized and could die.

- About one out of five people who get measles will be hospitalized
- As many as 1 out of every 20 children with measles gets pneumonia, the most common cause of death from measles in young children.
- About 1 child out of every 1,000 who get measles will develop encephalitis (swelling of the brain) that can lead to convulsions and can leave the child deaf or with an intellectual disability.
- Nearly 1 to 3 of every 1,000 children who become infected with measles will die from respiratory and neurologic complications.
- Measles may cause pregnant women who have not had the MMR vaccine to give birth prematurely, or have a low-birth-weight baby.

Long-Term Complications

Subacute sclerosing panencephalitis (SSPE) is a very rare, but fatal disease of the central nervous system that results from a measles virus infection acquired earlier in life.

- Subacute sclerosing panencephalitis generally develops 7 to 10 years after a person has measles, even though the person seems to have fully recovered from the illness.

- Since measles was eliminated in 2000, SSPE is rarely reported in the United States.

- Among people who contracted measles during the resurgence in the United States from 1989 to 1991, 4 to 11 out of every 100,000 were estimated to be at risk for developing SSPE.

- The risk of developing SSPE may be higher for a person who gets measles before they are 2 years of age.

The Measles Vaccination

Prevent measles and talk to your doctor about the measles, mumps, and rubella (MMR) vaccine, especially if planning to travel.

Prevent Measles with MMR Vaccine

Measles can be prevented with MMR vaccine. The vaccine protects against three diseases: measles, mumps, and rubella. MMR vaccine is given later than some other childhood vaccines because antibodies transferred from the mother to the baby can provide some protection from disease and make the MMR vaccine less effective until about one year of age.

Table 22.1. Schedule for MMR Vaccine

	First Dose	Second Dose
Children*	Age 12 to 15 months	Age 4 to 6 years
Teenagers and adults with no evidence of immunity**	As soon as possible	N/A

The CDC recommends this schedule for children 12 months and older. Infants younger than 12 months old and children traveling outside the United States should follow another schedule.

** *Acceptable evidence of immunity against measles includes at least one of the following: written documentation of adequate vaccination, laboratory evidence of immunity, laboratory confirmation of measles, or birth in the United States before 1957.*

197

If you have children, see if they are due for MMR vaccine:

- Check your child's vaccination record,

- Contact their healthcare provider, or

- Visit the immunization scheduler for newborn to 6-year-old children

Measles, Mumps, and Rubella Vaccine Is Safe

Measles, mumps, and rubella (MMR) vaccine is very safe and effective. Two doses of MMR vaccine are about 97 percent effective at preventing measles; one dose is about 93 percent effective.

Is There a Link between the MMR Shot and Autism?

No. Scientists in the United States and other countries have carefully studied the MMR shot. None has found a link between autism and the MMR shot.

Measles Can Also Be Prevented with MMRV Vaccine

Children may also get MMRV vaccine, which protects against measles, mumps, rubella, and varicella (chickenpox). This vaccine is only licensed for use in children who are 12 months through 12 years of age.

Paying for the Measles Vaccine

Most health insurance plans cover the cost of vaccines. But you may want to check with your health insurance provider before going to the doctor.

If you have a child and do not have insurance or if your insurance does not cover vaccines for your child, the Vaccines for Children Program (VFC) may be able to help. This program helps families of eligible children who might not otherwise have access to vaccines. To find out if your child is eligible, visit the VFC website or ask your child's doctor. You can also contact your state VFC coordinator.

Chapter 23

Viral Meningitis

What Is Viral Meningitis?

Viral meningitis is the most common type of meningitis, an inflammation of the tissue that covers the brain and spinal cord. It is often less severe than bacterial meningitis, and most people get better on their own (without treatment). However, it is very important for anyone with symptoms of meningitis to see a healthcare provider right away because some types of meningitis can be very serious. Only a doctor can determine if you have the disease, the type of meningitis, and the best treatment, which can sometimes be lifesaving. Babies younger than one month of age and people with weakened immune systems are more likely to have a severe illness from viral meningitis.

Causes of Viral Meningitis

Nonpolio enteroviruses are the most common cause of viral meningitis in the United States, especially from late spring to fall when these viruses spread most often. However, only a small number of people infected with enteroviruses will actually develop meningitis.

Other viruses that can cause meningitis are:

• Mumps virus

This chapter includes text excerpted from "Viral Meningitis," Centers for Disease Control and Prevention (CDC), April 15, 2016.

- Herpesviruses, including, herpes simplex viruses, and varicella-zoster virus (which causes chickenpox and shingles)

- Measles virus

- Influenza virus

- Arboviruses, such as West Nile Virus (VNV)

- Lymphocytic choriomeningitis virus (LCMV)

People at Risk

You can get viral meningitis at any age. However, some people have a higher risk of getting the disease, including:

- Children younger than five years of age

- People with weakened immune systems caused by diseases, medications (such as chemotherapy), and recent organ or bone marrow transplantations

Babies younger than one month of age and people with weakened immune systems are more likely to have severe illness.

How It Spreads

If you have close contact with a person who has viral meningitis, you may become infected with the virus that made that person sick. However, you are not likely to develop meningitis. That is because only a small number of people who get infected with the viruses that cause meningitis will actually develop viral meningitis.

Viruses that can cause meningitis spread in different ways.

- Nonpolio enteroviruses

- Mumps virus

- Herpesviruses, including Epstein-Barr virus (EBV), herpes simplex viruses, and varicella-zoster virus (VZV)

- Measles virus (MeV)

- Influenza virus

- Arboviruses (spread through mosquitoes and other insects)

- Lymphocytic choriomeningitis virus (LCMV)

Symptoms of Viral Meningitis
Common Symptoms in Babies

- Fever
- Irritability
- Poor eating
- Sleepiness or trouble waking up from sleep
- Lethargy (a lack of energy)

Common Symptoms in Children and Adults

- Fever
- Headache
- Stiff neck
- Sensitivity to bright light
- Sleepiness or trouble waking up from sleep
- Nausea
- Irritability
- Vomiting
- Lack of appetite
- Lethargy (a lack of energy)

Most people with mild viral meningitis usually get better on their own within 7 to 10 days.

Initial symptoms of viral meningitis are similar to those for bacterial meningitis. However, bacterial meningitis is usually severe and can cause serious complications, such as brain damage, hearing loss, or learning disabilities. The pathogens (germs) that cause bacterial meningitis can also be associated with another serious illness, sepsis. Sepsis is the body's overwhelming and life-threatening response to infection that can cause tissue damage, organ failure, and death.

It is very important to see a healthcare provider right away if you think you or your child might have meningitis. A doctor can determine if you have the disease, the type of meningitis, and the best treatment.

Diagnosis of Viral Meningitis

Meningitis is only diagnosed by doing specific lab tests on specimens from a person suspected of having meningitis. If your doctor thinks you might have meningitis, she or he may collect samples for testing by:

- Swabbing your nose and/or throat
- Obtaining a stool sample
- Taking some blood
- Drawing fluid from around your spinal cord

Treatment of Viral Meningitis

In most cases, there is no specific treatment for viral meningitis. Most people who get mild viral meningitis completely recover on their own usually within 7 to 10 days. However, people with meningitis caused by certain viruses such as herpesvirus and influenza will usually need and get better from treatment such as antiviral medicine.

Antibiotics do not help viral infections, so they are not useful in the treatment of viral meningitis. However, antibiotics do fight bacteria, so they are very important when treating bacterial meningitis.

People who develop severe illness, or those who are at risk for developing severe illness, such as babies, and people with weakened immune systems may need to be hospitalized.

Prevention of Viral Meningitis

There are no vaccines to protect against nonpolio enteroviruses, which are the most common cause of viral meningitis. You can take the following steps to help lower your chances of getting infected with nonpolio enteroviruses or spreading them to other people:

- Wash your hands often with soap and water, especially after changing diapers, using the toilet, or coughing or blowing your nose.
- Avoid touching your face with unwashed hands.
- Avoid close contact such as kissing, hugging, or sharing cups or eating utensils with people who are sick.
- Cover your coughs and sneezes with a tissue or your upper shirt sleeve, not your hands.

- Clean and disinfect frequently touched surfaces, such as toys and doorknobs, especially if someone is sick.

- Stay home when you are sick.

Some vaccinations can protect against diseases such as measles, mumps, chickenpox, and influenza that can lead to viral meningitis. Make sure you and your child are vaccinated on schedule.

Avoid bites from mosquitoes and other insects that carry diseases that can infect humans.

Control mice and rats.

Chapter 24

Mumps

Mumps is a contagious disease that is caused by a virus. It typically starts with a few days of fever, headache, muscle aches, tiredness, and loss of appetite. Then, most people will have swelling of their salivary glands. This is what causes the puffy cheeks and a tender, swollen jaw.

Signs and Symptoms of Mumps

Mumps is best known for the puffy cheeks and tender, swollen jaw that it causes. This is a result of swollen salivary glands under the ears on one or both sides, often referred to as "parotitis."

Other symptoms that might begin a few days before parotitis include:

- Fever

- Headache

- Muscle aches

- Tiredness

- Loss of appetite

Symptoms typically appear 16 to 18 days after infection, but this period can range from 12 to 25 days after infection.

This chapter includes text excerpted from "Mumps," Centers for Disease Control and Prevention (CDC), March 8, 2019.

Some people who get mumps have very mild symptoms (similar to a cold) or no symptoms at all, and they may not know that they have the disease.

In rare cases, mumps can cause more severe complications.

Most people with mumps recover completely within two weeks.

Transmission of Mumps

Mumps is a contagious disease caused by a virus. It spreads through direct contact with saliva or respiratory droplets from the mouth, nose, or throat. An infected person can spread the virus by:

- Coughing, sneezing, or talking

- Sharing items that may have saliva on them, such as water bottles or cups

- Participating in close-contact activities with others, such as playing sports, dancing, or kissing

- Touching objects or surfaces with unwashed hands that are then touched by others

An infected person can likely spread mumps from a few days before their salivary glands begin to swell to up to five days after the swelling begins. A person with mumps should limit their contact with others during this time. For example, stay home from school and do not attend social events.

Complications of Mumps

Mumps can occasionally cause complications, especially in adults. Complications can include:

- Inflammation of the testicles (orchitis) in males who have reached puberty; this may lead to a decrease in testicular size (testicular atrophy).

- Inflammation of the ovaries (oophoritis) and/or breast tissue (mastitis)

- Inflammation in the pancreas (pancreatitis)

- Inflammation of the brain (encephalitis)

- Inflammation of the tissue covering the brain and spinal cord (meningitis)

- Deafness

Neither inflammation of the testicles nor inflammation of the ovaries caused by mumps has been shown to lead to infertility.

Chapter 25

Nonpolio Enterovirus

Nonpolio enteroviruses are very common viruses. They cause about 10 to 15 million infections in the United States each year. Tens of thousands of people are hospitalized each year for illnesses caused by enteroviruses.

Anyone can get infected with nonpolio enteroviruses. But infants, children, and teenagers are more likely to get infected and become sick. That is because they do not yet have immunity (protection) from previous exposures to the viruses.

Most people who get infected with nonpolio enteroviruses do not get sick. Or, they may have a mild illness, like the common cold. But, some people can get very sick and have an infection of their heart or brain or even become paralyzed. Infants and people with weakened immune systems have a greater chance of having these complications.

You can get infected with nonpolio enteroviruses by having close contact with an infected person. You can also get infected by touching objects or surfaces that have the virus on them then touching your mouth, nose, or eyes.

In the United States, people are more likely to get infected with nonpolio enteroviruses in the summer and fall.

This chapter includes text excerpted from "Non-Polio Enterovirus," Centers for Disease Control and Prevention (CDC), September 19, 2014. Reviewed July 2019.

Symptoms of Nonpolio Enterovirus

Most people who get infected with nonpolio enteroviruses do not get sick, or they only have a mild illness Infants, children, and teenagers are more likely than adults to get infected and become sick because they do not yet have immunity (protection) from previous exposures to the viruses. Adults can get infected too, but they are less likely to have symptoms, or their symptoms may be milder. Symptoms of mild illness may include:

- Fever

- Runny nose, sneezing, cough

- Skin rash

- Mouth blisters

- Body and muscle aches

Some nonpolio enterovirus infections can cause:

- Viral conjunctivitis

- Hand, foot, and mouth disease (HFMD)

- Viral meningitis (infection of the covering of the spinal cord and/or brain)

- Viral encephalitis (infection of the brain)

- Myocarditis (infection of the heart)

- Pericarditis (infection of the sac around the heart)

- Acute flaccid paralysis (sudden onset of weakness in one or more arms or legs)

- Inflammatory muscle disease (slow, progressive muscle weakness)

Infants and people with weakened immune systems have a greater chance of having these complications.

People who develop myocarditis may have heart failure and require long-term care. Some people who develop encephalitis or paralysis may not fully recover.

Newborns infected with a nonpolio enterovirus may develop sepsis (the body's overwhelming response to infection, which can lead to tissue damage, organ failure, and death). But this is very rare.

Nonpolio enterovirus infections may play a role in the development of type 1 diabetes in children.

Transmission of Nonpolio Enterovirus

Nonpolio enteroviruses can be found in an infected person's:

- Feces
- Eye, nose, and mouth secretions (such as saliva, nasal mucus, or sputum)
- Blister fluid

You can get exposed to the virus by:

- Having close contact, such as touching or shaking hands, with an infected person
- Touching objects or surfaces that have the virus on them, then touching your eyes, nose, or mouth before washing your hands
- Changing diapers of an infected person, then touching your eyes, nose, or mouth before washing your hands
- Drinking water that has the virus in it

Once infected, you can shed (pass from your body into the environment) the virus for several weeks, even if you do not have symptoms.

Pregnant women who get infected with a nonpolio enterovirus shortly before delivery can pass the virus to their babies.

Mothers who are breastfeeding should talk with their doctor if they are sick or think they may have an infection.

Treatment of Nonpolio Enterovirus

There is no specific treatment for nonpolio enterovirus infection. People with a mild illness caused by nonpolio enterovirus infection typically only need to treat their symptoms. This includes drinking enough water to stay hydrated and taking over-the-counter (OTC) cold medications as needed. Most people recover completely. However, some illnesses caused by nonpolio enteroviruses can be severe enough to require hospitalization.

If you are concerned about your symptoms, you should contact your healthcare provider.

Prevention of Nonpolio Enterovirus

Many people who get infected with nonpolio enteroviruses do not have symptoms, but they can still spread the virus to other people.

This makes it is difficult to prevent them from spreading. The best way to help protect yourself and others from nonpolio enterovirus infections is to:

- Wash your hands often with soap and water for 20 seconds, especially after using the toilet or changing diapers.

- Avoid close contact, such as touching and shaking hands, with people who are sick.

- Clean and disinfect frequently touched surfaces.

There is no vaccine to protect you from nonpolio enterovirus infection.

Chapter 26

Norovirus

Norovirus is a very contagious virus that causes vomiting and diarrhea. People of all ages can get infected and sick with norovirus.

You can get norovirus from:

- Having direct contact with an infected person

- Consuming contaminated food or water

- Touching contaminated surfaces and then putting your unwashed hands in your mouth

You can get norovirus illness many times in your life because there are many different types of noroviruses. Infection with one type of norovirus may not protect you against other types. It is possible to develop immunity to (protection against) specific types. But, it is not known exactly how long immunity lasts. This may explain why so many people of all ages get infected during norovirus outbreaks. Also, whether you are susceptible to norovirus infection is also determined in part by your genes.

Symptoms of Norovirus

Norovirus is a common virus that is not related to the flu. Norovirus is the most common cause of foodborne diarrhea and vomiting.

This chapter includes text excerpted from "About Norovirus," Centers for Disease Control and Prevention (CDC), June 1, 2018.

The most common symptoms of norovirus are:

- Diarrhea

- Vomiting

- Nausea

- Stomach pain

Other symptoms include:

- Fever

- Headache

- Body aches

Norovirus causes inflammation of the stomach or intestines. This is called "acute gastroenteritis."

A person usually develops symptoms 12 to 48 hours after being exposed to norovirus. Most people with norovirus illness get better within 1 to 3 days.

If you have norovirus illness, you can feel extremely ill and vomit or have diarrhea many times a day. This can lead to dehydration, especially in young children, older adults, and people with other illnesses.

Symptoms of dehydration include:

- Decrease in urination

- Dry mouth and throat

- Feeling dizzy when standing up

Children who are dehydrated may cry with few or no tears and be unusually sleepy or fussy.

Transmission of Norovirus

Norovirus spreads very easily and quickly in different ways.

You can get norovirus by accidentally getting tiny particles of poop or vomit from an infected person in your mouth.

This can happen if you:

- Eat food or drink liquids that are contaminated with norovirus

- Touch surfaces or objects contaminated with norovirus then put your fingers in your mouth

- Have direct contact with someone who is infected with norovirus, such as by caring for them or sharing food or eating utensils with them

If you get norovirus illness, you can shed billions of norovirus particles that you cannot see without a microscope. Only a few norovirus particles can make other people sick. You are most contagious:

- When you have symptoms of norovirus illness, especially vomiting

- During the first few days after you recover from norovirus illness

However, studies have shown that you can still spread norovirus for two weeks or more after you feel better.

Norovirus Spreads through Contaminated Food

Norovirus can easily contaminate food and water because it only takes a very small amount of virus particles to make you sick. Food and water can get contaminated with norovirus in many ways, including when:

- An infected person touches food with their bare hands that have poop or vomit particles on them.

- Food is placed on a counter or surface that has poop or vomit particles on it.

- Tiny drops of vomit from an infected person spray through the air and land on the food.

- The food is grown or harvested with contaminated water, such as oysters harvested from contaminated water, or fruit and vegetables irrigated with contaminated water in the field.

Norovirus Spreads through Contaminated Water

Recreational or drinking water can get contaminated with norovirus and make you sick or contaminate your food. This can happen:

- At the source such as when a septic tank leaks into a well

- When an infected person vomits or poops in the water

- When water is not treated properly, such as not having enough chlorine

Norovirus Spreads through Sick People and Contaminated Surfaces

Surfaces can get contaminated with norovirus in many ways, including when:

- An infected person touches the surface with their bare hands that have poop or vomit particles on them.

- An infected person vomits or has diarrhea that splatters onto surfaces.

- Food, water, or objects that are contaminated with norovirus are placed on surfaces.

How You Treat Norovirus

There is no specific medicine to treat people with norovirus illness. Antibiotic drugs will not help because they fight bacteria, not viruses.

If you have norovirus illness, you should drink plenty of liquids to replace fluid lost from vomiting and diarrhea. This will help prevent dehydration.

Dehydration can lead to serious problems. Severe dehydration may require hospitalization for treatment with fluids given through your vein (intravenous or IV fluids).

Watch for signs of dehydration in children who have norovirus illness. Children who are dehydrated may cry with few or no tears and be unusually sleepy or fussy.

If you think you or someone you are caring for is severely dehydrated, call the doctor.

Prevention of Norovirus

You can help protect yourself and others from norovirus by washing your hands thoroughly with soap and water and following other simple prevention tips.

There is currently no vaccine to prevent norovirus; although, this is an area of active research.

Practice Proper Hand Hygiene

Wash your hands thoroughly with soap and water:

- Especially after using the toilet or changing diapers

- Always before eating, preparing, or handling food
- Before giving yourself or someone else medicine

Norovirus can be found in your vomit or poop even before you start feeling sick. The virus can stay in your poop for two weeks or more after you feel better. It is important to continue washing your hands often during this time.

You can use alcohol-based hand sanitizers in addition to hand washing. But, you should not use hand sanitizer as a substitute for washing your hands with soap and water. Hand sanitizers are not as effective as washing hands with soap and water at removing norovirus particles.

Handle and Prepare Food Safely

Carefully wash fruits and vegetables before preparing and eating them. Cook oysters and other shellfish thoroughly before eating them.

Be aware that noroviruses are relatively resistant to heat. They can survive temperatures as high as 145°F and quick steaming processes that are often used for cooking shellfish.

Food that might be contaminated with norovirus should be thrown out.

Keep sick infants and children out of areas where food is being handled and prepared.

When You Are Sick, Do Not Prepare Food or Care for Others

You should not prepare food for others or provide healthcare while you are sick and for at least two days after symptoms stop. This also applies to sick workers in restaurants, schools, day-care centers, long-term care facilities, and other places where they may expose people to norovirus.

Clean and Disinfect Surfaces

After someone vomits or has diarrhea, always thoroughly clean and disinfect the entire area immediately. Put on rubber or disposable gloves, and wipe the entire area with paper towels, then disinfect the area using a bleach-based household cleaner as directed on the product label. Leave the bleach disinfectant on the affected area for at least five minutes, then clean the entire area again with soap and hot water. Finish by cleaning soiled laundry, taking out the trash, and washing your hands.

To help make sure that food is safe from norovirus, routinely clean and sanitize kitchen utensils, counters, and surfaces before preparing food.

You should use a chlorine bleach solution with a concentration of 1000 to 5000 ppm (5 to 25 tablespoons of household bleach (5 percent to 8 percent) per gallon of water) or other disinfectant registered as effective against norovirus by the U.S. Environmental Protection Agency (EPA).

Wash Laundry Thoroughly

Immediately remove and wash clothes or linens that may be contaminated with vomit or poop.

You should:

- Handle soiled items carefully without agitating them.

- Wear rubber or disposable gloves while handling soiled items, and wash your hands after.

- Wash the items with detergent and hot water at the maximum available cycle length, then machine dry them at the highest heat setting.

Chapter 27

Polio

Polio, or poliomyelitis, is a crippling and potentially deadly infectious disease. It is caused by poliovirus. The virus spreads from person-to-person and can invade an infected person's brain and spinal cord, causing paralysis (cannot move parts of the body).

Symptoms of Polio

Most people who get infected with poliovirus (about 72 out of 100) will not have any visible symptoms.

About one out of four people with poliovirus infection will have flu-like symptoms that may include:

- Sore throat
- Fever
- Tiredness
- Nausea
- Headache
- Stomach pain

These symptoms usually last two to five days then go away on their own.

This chapter includes text excerpted from "What Is Polio?" Centers for Disease Control and Prevention (CDC), July 25, 2017.

A smaller proportion of people with poliovirus infection will develop other more serious symptoms that affect the brain and spinal cord:

- Paresthesia (feeling of pins and needles in the legs)

- Meningitis (infection of the covering of the spinal cord and/or brain) occurs in about 1 out of 25 people with poliovirus infection

- Paralysis (cannot move parts of the body) or weakness in the arms, legs, or both occurs in about 1 out of 200 people with poliovirus infection

Paralysis is the most severe symptom associated with polio because it can lead to permanent disability and death. Between 2 and 10 out of 100 people who have paralysis from poliovirus infection die because the virus affects the muscles that help them breathe.

Even children who seem to fully recover can develop new muscle pain, weakness, or paralysis as adults, 15 to 40 years later. This is called "postpolio syndrome."

Note that "poliomyelitis" (or "polio" for short) is defined as the paralytic disease. Therefore, only people with paralytic infection are considered to have the disease.

Transmission of Polio

Poliovirus only infects humans. It is very contagious and spreads through person-to-person contact. The virus lives in an infected person's throat and intestines. It enters the body through the mouth and spreads through contact with the feces of an infected person and, though less common, through droplets from a sneeze or cough. You can get infected with poliovirus if you have feces on your hands and you touch your mouth. Also, you can get infected if you put objects, such as toys, that are contaminated with feces in your mouth.

An infected person may spread the virus to others immediately before and about one to two weeks after symptoms appear. The virus can live in an infected person's feces for many weeks. It can contaminate food and water in unsanitary conditions.

People who do not have symptoms can still pass the virus to others and make them sick.

Prevention of Polio

The polio vaccine protects children by preparing their bodies to fight the polio virus. Almost all children (99 children out of 100) who get all the recommended doses of vaccine will be protected from polio.

There are two types of vaccine that can prevent polio: inactivated poliovirus vaccine (IPV) and oral poliovirus vaccine (OPV). Only IPV has been used in the United States since 2000; OPV is still used throughout much of the world.

Chapter 28

Respiratory Syncytial Virus Infection

Respiratory syncytial virus (RSV) is a common respiratory virus that usually causes mild cold-like symptoms. Most people recover in a week or two, but RSV can be serious, especially for infants and older adults. In fact, RSV is the most common cause of bronchiolitis (inflammation of the small airways in the lung) and pneumonia (infection of the lungs) in children younger than one year of age in the United States. It is also a significant cause of respiratory illness in older adults.

Symptoms

Symptoms of RSV infection usually include:

- Runny nose
- Decrease in appetite
- Coughing
- Sneezing
- Fever
- Wheezing

This chapter includes text excerpted from "Respiratory Syncytial Virus Infection (RSV)," Centers for Disease Control and Prevention (CDC), June 26, 2018.

These symptoms usually appear in stages and not all at once. In very young infants with RSV, the only symptoms may be irritability, decreased activity, and breathing difficulties.

Respiratory syncytial virus can also cause more severe infections, such as bronchiolitis, an inflammation of the small airways in the lung, and pneumonia, an infection of the lungs. It is the most common cause of bronchiolitis and pneumonia in children younger than one year of age.

Almost all children will have had an RSV infection by their second birthday. People infected with RSV usually show symptoms within four to six days after getting infected.

Care

Most RSV infections go away on their own in a week or two. You can manage fever and pain with over-the-counter (OTC) fever reducers and pain relievers, such as acetaminophen or ibuprofen. Talk to your healthcare provider before giving your child nonprescription cold medicines since some medicines contain ingredients that are not recommended for children. It is important for people with RSV infection to drink enough fluids to prevent dehydration (loss of body fluids).

Healthy infants and adults infected with RSV do not usually need to be hospitalized. But some people with RSV infection, especially infants younger than six months of age and older adults, may need to be hospitalized if they are having trouble breathing or are dehydrated. In most of these cases, hospitalization only lasts a few days.

Visits to a healthcare provider for an RSV infection are very common. During such visits, the healthcare provider will evaluate how severe the person's RSV infection is to determine if the patient should be hospitalized. In the most severe cases, a person may require additional oxygen or intubation (have a breathing tube inserted through the mouth and down to the airway) with mechanical ventilation (a machine to help a person breathe).

There is no specific treatment for RSV infection, though researchers are working to develop vaccines and antivirals (medicines that fight viruses).

Transmission

Respiratory syncytial virus can spread when an infected person coughs or sneezes. You can get infected if you get droplets from the cough or sneeze in your eyes, nose, or mouth, or if you touch a surface that has the virus on it, such as a doorknob, and then touch your face before washing your hands. Additionally, it can spread through direct contact with the virus, such as kissing the face of a child with RSV.

People infected with RSV are usually contagious for three to eight days. However, some infants and people with weakened immune systems can continue to spread the virus even after they stop showing symptoms, for as long as four weeks. Children are often exposed to and infected with RSV outside the home, such as in school or child care centers. They can then transmit the virus to other members of the family.

Respiratory syncytial virus can survive for many hours on hard surfaces, such as tables and crib rails. It typically lives on soft surfaces, such as tissues and hands, for shorter amounts of time.

People of any age can get another RSV infection, but infections later in life are generally less severe. People at highest risk for severe disease include:

- Premature infants

- Young children with congenital (from birth) heart or chronic lung disease

- Young children with compromised (weakened) immune systems due to a medical condition or medical treatment

- Adults with compromised immune systems

- Older adults, especially those with underlying heart or lung disease

In the United States and other areas with similar climates, RSV infections generally occur during the Fall, Winter, and Spring. The timing and severity of RSV circulation in a given community can vary from year to year.

Prevention

There are steps you can take to help prevent the spread of RSV. Specifically, if you have cold-like symptoms you should:

- Cover your coughs and sneezes with a tissue or your upper shirt sleeve, not your hands.

- Wash your hands often with soap and water for 20 seconds.

- Avoid close contact, such as kissing, shaking hands, and sharing cups and eating utensils, with others.

225

In addition, cleaning contaminated surfaces (such as doorknobs) may help stop the spread of RSV.

Ideally, people with cold-like symptoms should not interact with children at high risk for severe RSV disease, including premature infants, children younger than two years of age with chronic lung or heart conditions, and children with weakened immune systems. If this is not possible, they should carefully follow the prevention steps mentioned above and wash their hands before interacting with such children. They should also refrain from kissing high-risk children while they have cold-like symptoms.

Parents of children at high risk for developing severe RSV disease should help their child, when possible, and do the following:

- Avoid close contact with sick people

- Wash their hands often with soap and water

- Avoid touching their face with unwashed hands

- Limit the time they spend in child care centers or other potentially contagious settings, especially during Fall, Winter, and Spring. This may help prevent infection and spread of the virus during the RSV season

Researchers are working to develop RSV vaccines, but none are available yet. A drug called "palivizumab" is available to prevent severe RSV illness in certain infants and children who are at high risk for severe disease. The drug can help prevent serious RSV disease; but, it cannot help cure or treat children already suffering from serious RSV disease, and it cannot prevent infection with RSV. If your child is at high risk for severe RSV disease, talk to your healthcare provider to see if palivizumab can be used as a preventive measure.

Chapter 29

Rubella

Rubella is a contagious disease caused by a virus. Most people who get rubella usually have a mild illness with symptoms that can include a low-grade fever, sore throat, and a rash that starts on the face and spreads to the rest of the body. Rubella can cause a miscarriage or serious birth defects if a woman is infected while she is pregnant. The best protection against rubella is the measles, mumps, and rubella (MMR) vaccine.

Rubella in the United States

Rubella is also called "German measles," but it is caused by a different virus than measles. Rubella was eliminated from the United States in 2004. Rubella elimination is defined as the absence of continuous disease transmission for 12 months or more in a specific geographic area. Rubella is no longer endemic (constantly present) in the United States. However, rubella remains a problem in other parts of the world. It can still be brought into the United States by people who get infected in other countries.

Before the rubella vaccination program started in 1969, rubella was a common and widespread infection in the United States. During the last major rubella epidemic in the United States from 1964 to 1965, an

---

This chapter includes text excerpted from "Rubella (German Measles, Three-Day Measles)," Centers for Disease Control and Prevention (CDC), September 15, 2017.

estimated 12.5 million people got rubella, 11,000 pregnant women lost their babies, 2,100 newborns died, and 20,000 babies were born with congenital rubella syndrome (CRS). Once the vaccine became widely used, the number of people infected with rubella in the United States dropped dramatically.

Today, less than 10 people in the United States are reported as having rubella each year. Since 2012, all rubella cases had evidence that they were infected when they were living or traveling outside the United States. To maintain rubella elimination, it is important that children and women of childbearing age are vaccinated against rubella.

Signs and Symptoms of Rubella

In children, rubella is usually mild and with few noticeable symptoms. For children who do have symptoms, a red rash is typically the first sign. The rash generally first appears on the face and then spreads to the rest of the body, and it lasts about three days. Other symptoms that may occur one to five days before the rash appears include:

- A low-grade fever
- Headache
- Mild pink eye (redness or swelling of the white of the eye)
- General discomfort
- Swollen and enlarged lymph nodes
- Cough
- Runny nose

Most adults who get rubella usually have a mild illness with low-grade fever, sore throat, and a rash that starts on the face and spreads to the rest of the body.

Some adults may also have a headache, pink eye, and general discomfort before the rash appears.

About 25 to 50 percent of people infected with rubella will not experience any symptoms.

Complications of Rubella

Up to 70 percent of women who get rubella may experience arthritis; this is rare in children and men. In rare cases, rubella can cause serious problems, including brain infections and bleeding problems.

The most serious complication from rubella infection is the harm it can cause a fetus. If an unvaccinated pregnant woman gets infected with rubella virus, she can have a miscarriage or her baby can die just after birth. Also, she can pass the virus to the fetus, which can then develop into serious birth defects, such as:

- Heart problems
- Loss of hearing and eyesight
- Intellectual disability
- Liver or spleen damage

Serious birth defects are more common if a woman is infected early in her pregnancy, especially in the first trimester. These severe birth defects are known as "congenital rubella syndrome" (CRS).

Transmission of Rubella

Rubella spreads when an infected person coughs or sneezes.

A person with rubella may spread the disease to others up to 1 week before the rash appears and remain contagious up to 7 days after. However, 25 to 50 percent of people infected with rubella do not develop a rash or have any symptoms.

People infected with rubella should tell their friends; their family; and the people they work with, especially pregnant women, if they have rubella. If your child has rubella, it is important to tell your child's school or day care provider.

Treatment of Rubella

There is no specific medicine to treat rubella or make the disease go away faster. In many cases, symptoms are mild. For others, mild symptoms can be managed with bed rest and medicines for fever, such as acetaminophen.

If you are concerned about your symptoms or your child's symptoms, contact your doctor.

Chapter 30

Smallpox

What Is Smallpox?

Before smallpox was eradicated, it was a serious infectious disease caused by the variola virus. It was contagious, meaning that it spread from one person to another. People who had smallpox had a fever and a distinctive, progressive skin rash.

Most people with smallpox recover, but about 3 out of every 10 people with the disease died. Many smallpox survivors have permanent scars over large areas of their body, especially their faces. Some are left blind.

Thanks to the success of vaccination, smallpox was eradicated, and no cases of naturally occurring smallpox have happened since 1977. The last natural outbreak of smallpox in the United States occurred in 1949.

Signs and Symptoms of Smallpox

A person with smallpox goes through several stages as the disease progresses. Each stage has its own signs and symptoms.

Incubation Period

This stage can last anywhere from 7 to 19 days (although the average length is 10 to 14 days).

This chapter includes text excerpted from "What Is Smallpox?" Centers for Disease Control and Prevention (CDC), June 7, 2016.

Contagious? *No*

The incubation period is the length of time the virus is in a person's body before they look or feel sick. During this period, a person usually has no symptoms and may feel fine.

Initial Symptoms

This stage lasts anywhere from two to four days.

Contagious? *Sometimes*. Smallpox may be contagious during this phase, but is most contagious during the next two stages (early rash and pustular rash and scabs).

The first symptoms include:

- High fever

- Head and body aches

- Sometimes vomiting

At this time, people are usually too sick to carry on their normal activities.

Early Rash

This stage lasts about four days.

Contagious? *Yes*. At this time, the person is at their most contagious.

A rash starts as small red spots on the tongue and in the mouth. These spots change into sores that break open and spread large amounts of the virus into the mouth and throat. The person continues to have a fever.

Once the sores in the mouth start breaking down, a rash appears on the skin, starting on the face and spreading to the arms and legs, and then to the hands and feet. Usually, it spreads to all parts of the body within 24 hours. As this rash appears, the fever begins to decline, and the person may start to feel better.

By the fourth day, the skin sores fill with a thick, opaque fluid and often have a dent in the center.

Once the skin sores fill with fluid, the fever may rise again and remain high until scabs form over the bumps.

Pustular Rash and Scabs

This stage lasts about 10 days.

Contagious? *Yes*

The sores become pustules (sharply raised, usually round and firm to the touch, like peas under the skin).

After about five days, the pustules begin to form a crust and then scab.

By the end of the second week, after the rash appears, most of the sores have scabbed over.

Scabs Fall Off

This stage lasts about six days.
Contagious? *Yes*
The scabs begin to fall off, leaving marks on the skin.
Three weeks after the rash appears, most scabs will have fallen off.

No Scabs

Contagious? *No*.
Four weeks after the rash appears, all scabs should have fallen off. Once all scabs have fallen off, the person is no longer contagious.

Transmission of Smallpox
How Does Smallpox Spread?

Before smallpox was eradicated, it was mainly spread by direct and fairly prolonged face-to-face contact between people. Smallpox patients became contagious once the first sores appeared in their mouth and throat (early rash stage). They spread the virus when they coughed or sneezed, and droplets from their nose or mouth spread to other people. They remained contagious until their last smallpox scab fell off.

These scabs and the fluid found in the patient's sores also contained the variola virus. The virus can spread through these materials or through the objects contaminated by them, such as bedding or clothing. People who cared for smallpox patients and washed their bedding or clothing had to wear gloves and take care to not get infected.

Rarely, smallpox has spread through the air in enclosed settings, such as a building (airborne route).

Smallpox can be spread by humans only. Scientists have no evidence that smallpox can be spread by insects or animals.

Prevention and Treatment of Smallpox

There is a vaccine to protect people from smallpox. If there were a smallpox outbreak, health officials would use the smallpox vaccine to control it. While some antiviral drugs may help treat it or prevent the smallpox disease from getting worse, there is no treatment for it that has been proven effective in people sick with the disease.

Smallpox Vaccine

Smallpox can be prevented by the smallpox vaccine. If you get the vaccine:

- **Before contact with the virus,** the vaccine can protect you from getting sick.

- **Within three days of being exposed to the virus,** the vaccine might protect you from getting the disease. If you still get the disease, you might get much less sick than an unvaccinated person would.

- **Within four to seven days of being exposed to the virus,** the vaccine likely gives you some protection from the disease. If you still get the disease, you might not get as sick as an unvaccinated person would.

Once you have developed the smallpox rash, the vaccine will not protect you.

Currently, the smallpox vaccine is not available to the general public because smallpox has been eradicated, and the virus no longer exists in nature. However, there is enough smallpox vaccine to vaccinate every person in the United States if a smallpox outbreak were to occur.

Antiviral Drugs

- In July 2018, the U.S. Food and Drug Administration (FDA) approved tecovirimat (TPOXX) for the treatment of smallpox. In laboratory tests, tecovirimat has been shown to be effective against the virus that causes smallpox. In laboratory settings, this drug was effective in treating animals that had diseases similar to smallpox. Tecovirimat has not been tested in people who are sick with smallpox, but it has been given to healthy people. Test results showed that it is safe and causes only minor side effects.

- In laboratory tests, cidofovir and brincidofovir have been shown to be effective against the virus that causes smallpox. In laboratory settings, these drugs were effective in treating animals that had diseases similar to smallpox. Cidofovir and brincidofovir have not been tested in people who are sick with smallpox, but they have been tested in healthy people and in those with other viral illnesses. These drugs continue to be evaluated for effectiveness and toxicity.

Because these drugs were not tested in people sick with smallpox, it is not known if a person with smallpox would benefit from treatment with them. However, their use may be considered if there ever is an outbreak of smallpox.

Tecovirimat and cidofovir are currently stockpiled by the Centers for Disease Control and Prevention's (CDC) Strategic National Stockpile (SNS), which has medicine and medical supplies to protect the American public if there is a public health emergency, including one involving smallpox.

Chapter 31

Zika Virus

Zika is spread mostly by the bite of an infected *Aedes* species mosquito (*Ae. aegypti* and *Ae. albopictus*). These mosquitoes bite during the day and night.

Zika can be passed from a pregnant woman to the fetus. Infection during pregnancy can cause certain birth defects.

There is no vaccine or medicine for Zika.

What Are the Symptoms of Zika?

Many people infected with Zika virus do not have symptoms or will only have mild symptoms. The most common symptoms of Zika are:

- Fever
- Rash
- Headache
- Joint pain
- Red eyes
- Muscle pain

Symptoms can last for several days to a week. People usually do not get sick enough to go to the hospital, and they very rarely die of

This chapter includes text excerpted from "About Zika," Centers for Disease Control and Prevention (CDC), May 20, 2019.

Zika. Once a person has been infected with Zika, they are likely to be protected from future infections.

How Long Symptoms Last

Zika is usually mild with symptoms lasting for several days to a week. People usually don't get sick enough to go to the hospital, and they very rarely die of Zika. For this reason, many people might not realize they have been infected. Symptoms of Zika are similar to other viruses spread through mosquito bites, like dengue and chikungunya.

How Soon You Should Be Tested

Zika virus usually remains in the blood of an infected person for about a week. See your doctor or other healthcare provider if you develop symptoms and you live in or have recently traveled to an area with risk of Zika. Your doctor or other healthcare provider may order blood or urine tests to help determine if you have Zika. Once a person has been infected, she or he is likely to be protected from future infections.

When to See a Doctor or Healthcare Provider

See your doctor or other healthcare provider if you have the symptoms described above and have visited an area with risk of Zika. This is especially important if you are pregnant. Be sure to tell your doctor or other healthcare provider where you traveled.

Why Zika Is Risky for Some People?

Zika infection during pregnancy can cause a birth defect of the brain called "microcephaly" and other severe brain defects. It is also linked to other problems, such as miscarriage, stillbirth, and other birth defects. There have also been increased reports of Guillain-Barré syndrome, an uncommon sickness of the nervous system, in areas affected by Zika.

How Zika Is Transmitted?

Zika can be transmitted:

- Through mosquito bites
- From a pregnant woman to the fetus

- Through sex

- Through blood transfusion (very likely but not confirmed)

Through Mosquito Bites

Zika virus is transmitted to people primarily through the bite of an infected *Aedes* species mosquito (*Ae. aegypti* and *Ae. albopictus*). These are the same mosquitoes that spread dengue and chikungunya viruses.

- These mosquitoes typically lay eggs in or near standing water in things like buckets, bowls, animal dishes, flower pots, and vases. They prefer to bite people, and live indoors and outdoors near people.

  - Mosquitoes that spread chikungunya, dengue, and Zika bite during the day and night.

- Mosquitoes become infected when they feed on a person already infected with the virus. Infected mosquitoes can then spread the virus to other people through bites.

From Mother to Child

- A pregnant woman can pass Zika virus to her fetus during pregnancy. Zika is a cause of microcephaly and other severe fetal brain defects. The full range of other potential health problems that Zika virus infection during pregnancy may cause is being studied.

- A pregnant woman already infected with Zika virus can pass the virus to her fetus during the pregnancy or around the time of birth.

- Zika virus has been found in breast milk. Possible Zika virus infections have been identified in breastfeeding babies, but Zika virus transmission through breast milk has not been confirmed. Additionally, the long-term effects of Zika virus on young infants infected after birth are not yet known. Because current evidence suggests that the benefits of breastfeeding outweigh the risk of Zika virus spreading through breast milk, CDC continues to encourage mothers to breastfeed, even if they were infected or lived in or traveled to an area with risk of Zika. CDC continues to study Zika virus and the ways it can spread and will update recommendations as new information becomes available.

Through Sex

- Zika can be passed through sex from a person who has Zika to his or her partners. Zika can be passed through sex, even if the infected person does not have symptoms at the time. Learn how to protect yourself during sex.

  - It can be passed from a person with Zika before their symptoms start, while they have symptoms, and after their symptoms end.

    - Though not well documented, the virus may also be passed by a person who carries the virus but never develops symptoms.

- Studies are underway to find out how long Zika stays in the semen and vaginal fluids of people who have Zika, and how long it can be passed to sex partners. It is known that Zika can remain in semen longer than in other body fluids, including vaginal fluids, urine, and blood.

Through Blood Transfusion

- To date, there have not been any confirmed blood transfusion transmission cases in the United States.

- There have been multiple reports of possible blood transfusion transmission cases in Brazil.

- During the French Polynesian outbreak, 2.8 percent of blood donors tested positive for Zika and in previous outbreaks, the virus has been found in blood donors.

Through Laboratory and Healthcare Setting Exposure

- There are reports of laboratory-acquired Zika virus infections, although the route of transmission was not clearly established in all cases.

- To date, no cases of Zika virus transmission in healthcare settings have been identified in the United States. Recommendations are available for healthcare providers to help prevent exposure to Zika virus in healthcare settings.

Risks

- Anyone who lives in or travels to an area with risk of Zika and has not already been infected with Zika virus can get it from mosquito bites. Once a person has been infected, he or she is likely to be protected from future infections.

How to Prevent Zika

There is no vaccine to prevent Zika. The best way to prevent diseases that are spread by mosquitoes is to protect yourself and your family from mosquito bites.

Clothing

- Wear long-sleeved shirts and long pants.
- Treat your clothing and gear with permethrin, or buy pretreated items.

Insect Repellent

- Use U.S. Environmental Protection Agency (EPA)-registered insect repellents with one of the following active ingredients:
  - N,N-diethyl-meta-toluamide (DEET), picaridin, IR3535, oil of lemon eucalyptus or para-menthane-diol, or 2-undecanone. Always follow the product label instructions.
- When used as directed, these insect repellents are proven safe and effective even for pregnant and breastfeeding women.
- Do not use insect repellents on babies younger than two months of age.
- Do not use products containing oil of lemon eucalyptus or para-menthane-diol on children younger than three years of age.

At Home

- Stay in places with air conditioning and window and door screens to keep mosquitoes outside.
- Take steps to control mosquitoes inside and outside your home.
- Mosquito netting can be used to cover babies younger than two months of age in carriers, strollers, or cribs.

- Sleep under a mosquito bed net if air-conditioned or screened rooms are not available or if sleeping outdoors.

Sexual Transmission

- Prevent sexual transmission of Zika by using condoms or not having sex.

How Zika Is Diagnosed?

- A diagnosis of Zika is based on a person's recent travel history, symptoms, and test results.
- A blood or urine test can confirm a Zika infection.
- Symptoms of Zika are similar to other illnesses that are spread through mosquito bites, such as dengue and chikungunya.
- Your doctor or other healthcare providers may order tests to look for several types of infections.

Only Some People Need Zika Testing

Zika virus testing is recommended only for certain people. If you have questions or think you should be tested, talk to your healthcare provider.

If You Have Symptoms

Zika testing is recommended if you have symptoms of Zika and

- You live in or traveled to an area with risk of Zika or
- You had sex without a condom with a partner who lives in or traveled to an area with risk of Zika.

Pregnant Women

Zika testing is recommended for pregnant women who don't have Zika symptoms in certain cases. You should be tested for Zika if you are pregnant and

- You have ongoing exposure to Zika because you live in or frequently travel to an area with risk of Zika or
- Your doctor sees Zika-associated abnormalities on an ultrasound or you deliver a baby with birth defects that may be related to Zika.

If You Have Tested Positive for Zika

- If you are pregnant, you can pass Zika to your fetus. For information for pregnant women, please see Zika and Pregnancy.

- You can pass Zika to your sex partner(s). Learn how you can prevent passing Zika to your partner.

- You can pass Zika to mosquitoes, which can bite you, get infected with Zika virus, and spread the virus to other people. Learn how you can prevent mosquito bites.

What Are the Treatments for Zika?

There is no specific medicine or vaccine for Zika virus.

- Treat the symptoms.
- Get plenty of rest.
- Drink fluids to prevent dehydration.
- Take medicines such as acetaminophen (Tylenol®) to reduce fever and pain.
- Do not take aspirin and other nonsteroidal anti-inflammatory drugs (NSAIDs) until dengue can be ruled out to reduce the risk of bleeding.
- If you are taking medicine for another medical condition, talk to your healthcare provider before taking additional medication.

If You Think You May Have or Had Zika

Tell your doctor or healthcare provider, and take these steps to protect others.

If You Are Caring for a Person with Zika

Take steps to protect yourself from exposure to the person's blood and bodily fluids (urine, stool, vomit). If you are pregnant, you can care for someone with Zika if you follow these steps.

- Do not touch blood or bodily fluids or surfaces with these fluids on them with exposed skin.
- Wash your hands with soap and water immediately after providing care.

- Immediately remove and wash your clothes if they get blood or bodily fluids on them. Use laundry detergent and the water temperature specified on the garment label. Using bleach is not necessary.

- Clean the sick person's environment daily using household cleaners according to the label instructions.

- Immediately clean surfaces that have blood or other bodily fluids on them using household cleaners and disinfectants according to the label instructions.

If you visit a family member or friend with Zika in a hospital, you should avoid contact with the person's blood and bodily fluids and surfaces with these fluids on them. Helping the person sit up or walk should not expose you. Make sure to wash your hands before and after touching the person.

Part Three

Bacterial Contagious Diseases

Chapter 32

Chancroid

The prevalence of chancroid has declined in the United States. When infection does occur, it is usually associated with sporadic outbreaks. Worldwide, chancroid appears to have declined as well, although infection might still occur in some regions of Africa and the Caribbean. Such as genital herpes and syphilis, chancroid is a risk factor in the transmission and acquisition of human immunodeficiency virus (HIV) infection.

Diagnostic Considerations

A definitive diagnosis of chancroid requires the identification of *Haemophilus ducreyi* (*H. ducreyi*) on special culture media that is not widely available from commercial sources; even when these media are used, sensitivity is less than 80 percent. No U.S. Food and Drug Administration (FDA)-cleared polymerase chain reaction (PCR) test for *H. ducreyi* is available in the United States, but such testing can be performed by clinical laboratories that have developed their own PCR test and have conducted Clinical Laboratory Improvement Amendments (CLIA) verification studies in genital specimens.

The combination of a painful genital ulcer and tender suppurative inguinal adenopathy suggests the diagnosis of chancroid. For both clinical and surveillance purposes, a probable diagnosis of chancroid can be made if all of the following criteria are met:

This chapter includes text excerpted from "Chancroid," Centers for Disease Control and Prevention (CDC), June 4, 2015. Reviewed July 2019.

- The patient has one or more painful genital ulcers.

- The clinical presentation, the appearance of genital ulcers, and, if present, regional lymphadenopathy are typical for chancroid.

- The patient has no evidence of *Treponema pallidum* infection by dark-field examination of ulcer exudate or by a serologic test for syphilis performed at least seven days after onset of ulcers.

- A herpes simplex virus (HSV) PCR test or HSV culture performed on the ulcer exudate is negative.

Treatment

Successful treatment for chancroid cures the infection, resolves the clinical symptoms, and prevents transmission to others. In advanced cases, scarring can result despite successful therapy.

Recommended Regimens

Azithromycin 1 g orally in a single dose
OR
Ceftriaxone 250 mg IM in a single dose
OR
Ciprofloxacin 500 mg orally twice a day for 3 days
OR
Erythromycin base 500 mg orally three times a day for 7 days

Azithromycin and ceftriaxone offer the advantage of single-dose therapy. Worldwide, several isolates with intermediate resistance to either ciprofloxacin or erythromycin have been reported. However, because cultures are not routinely performed, data are limited regarding the current prevalence of antimicrobial resistance.

Other Management Considerations

Men who are uncircumcised and patients with HIV infection do not respond as well to treatment as persons who are circumcised or HIV-negative. Patients should be tested for HIV infection at the time chancroid is diagnosed. If the initial test results were negative, a serologic test for syphilis and HIV infection should be performed three months after the diagnosis of chancroid.

Follow-Up

Patients should be reexamined three to seven days after the initiation of therapy. If treatment is successful, ulcers usually improve symptomatically within three days and objectively within seven days after therapy. If no clinical improvement is evident, the clinician must consider whether:

- The diagnosis is correct.

- The patient is coinfected with another sexually transmitted disease.

- The patient is infected with HIV.

- The treatment was not used as instructed.

- The *H. ducreyi* strain causing the infection is resistant to the prescribed antimicrobial.

The time required for complete healing depends on the size of the ulcer; large ulcers might require more than two weeks. In addition, healing is slower for some uncircumcised men who have ulcers under the foreskin. Clinical resolution of fluctuant lymphadenopathy is slower than that of ulcers and might require needle aspiration or incision and drainage, despite otherwise successful therapy. Although needle aspiration of buboes is a simpler procedure, incision and drainage might be preferred because of the reduced need for subsequent drainage procedures.

Management of Sex Partners

Regardless of whether symptoms of the disease are present, sex partners of patients who have chancroid should be examined and treated if they had sexual contact with the patient during the 10 days preceding the patient's onset of symptoms.

Special Considerations
Pregnancy

Data suggest ciprofloxacin presents a low risk to the fetus during pregnancy, with a potential for toxicity during breastfeeding. Alternate drugs should be used during pregnancy and lactation. No adverse effects of chancroid on pregnancy outcome have been reported.

Human Immunodeficiency Virus Infection

Persons with HIV infection who have chancroid should be monitored closely because they are more likely to experience treatment failure and to have ulcers that heal slowly. Persons with HIV infection might require repeated or longer courses of therapy, and treatment failures can occur with any regimen. Data are limited concerning the therapeutic efficacy of the recommended single-dose azithromycin and ceftriaxone regimens in persons with HIV infection.

Chapter 33

Chlamydia and Lymphogranuloma Venereum

About Chlamydia

Chlamydia is a common sexually transmitted disease (STD) caused by infection with *Chlamydia trachomatis*. It can cause cervicitis in women and urethritis and proctitis in both women and men. Chlamydial infections in women can lead to serious consequences, including pelvic inflammatory disease (PID), tubal factor infertility, ectopic pregnancy, and chronic pelvic pain. Lymphogranuloma venereum (LGV), another type of an STD caused by different serovars of the same bacterium, occurs commonly in the developing world and has emerged as a cause of outbreaks of proctitis among men who have sex with men (MSM) worldwide.

How Common Is Chlamydia?

Chlamydia is the most frequently reported bacterial sexually transmitted infection (STI) in the United States. In 2017, 1,708,569 cases of

This chapter contains text excerpted from the following sources: Text under the heading "About Chlamydia" is excerpted from "Chlamydia—CDC Fact Sheet (Detailed)," Centers for Disease Control and Prevention (CDC), October 4, 2016; Text under the heading "About Lymphogranuloma Venereum" is excerpted from "Lymphogranuloma Venereum (LGV)," Centers for Disease Control and Prevention (CDC), June 4, 2015. Reviewed July 2019.

chlamydia were reported to the Centers for Disease Control and Prevention (CDC) from 50 states and the District of Columbia, but an estimated 2.86 million infections occur annually. A large number of cases are not reported because most people with chlamydia are asymptomatic and do not seek testing. Chlamydia is most common among young people. Almost two-thirds of new chlamydia infections occur among youth between 15 and 24 years of age. It is estimated that 1 in 20 sexually active young women between 14 to 24 years of age has chlamydia.

Substantial racial/ethnic disparities in chlamydial infection exist, with prevalence among non-Hispanic Blacks 5.6 times the prevalence among non-Hispanic Whites. Chlamydia is also common among men who have sex with men. Among MSM screened for rectal chlamydial infection, positivity has ranged from 3.0 to 10.5 percent. Among MSM screened for pharyngeal chlamydial infection, positivity has ranged from 0.5 to 2.3 percent.

How Do People Get Chlamydia?

Chlamydia is transmitted through sexual contact with the penis, vagina, mouth, or anus of an infected partner. Ejaculation does not have to occur for chlamydia to be transmitted or acquired. Chlamydia can also be spread perinatally from an untreated mother to her baby during childbirth, resulting in ophthalmia neonatorum (conjunctivitis) or pneumonia in some exposed infants. In published prospective studies, chlamydial conjunctivitis has been identified in 18 to 44 percent and chlamydial pneumonia in 3 to 16 percent of infants born to women with untreated chlamydial cervical infection at the time of delivery. While rectal or genital chlamydial infection has been shown to persist 1 year or longer in infants infected at birth, the possibility of sexual abuse should be considered in prepubertal children beyond the neonatal period with a vaginal, urethral, or rectal chlamydial infection.

People who have had chlamydia and have been treated may get infected again if they have sexual contact with a person infected with chlamydia.

Who Is at Risk for Chlamydia?

Any sexually active person can be infected with chlamydia. It is a very common STD, especially among young people.

Sexually active young people are at high risk of acquiring chlamydia for a combination of behavioral, biological, and cultural reasons. Some young people do not use condoms consistently. Some adolescents may move from one monogamous relationship to the next more rapidly than the likely infectivity period of chlamydia, thus increasing risk of transmission. Teenage girls and young women may have cervical ectopy (where cells from the endocervix are present on the ectocervix). Cervical ectopy may increase susceptibility to chlamydial infection. The higher prevalence of chlamydia among young people also may reflect multiple barriers to accessing STD prevention services, such as lack of transportation, cost, and perceived stigma.

Men who have sex with men are also at risk for chlamydial infection since chlamydia can be transmitted by oral or anal sex. Among MSM screened for rectal chlamydial infection, positivity has ranged from 3.0 to 10.5 percent. Among MSM screened for pharyngeal chlamydial infection, positivity has ranged from 0.5 to 2.3 percent.

What Are the Symptoms of Chlamydia?

Chlamydia is known as a "silent" infection because most infected people are asymptomatic and lack abnormal physical examination findings. Estimates of the proportion of chlamydia-infected people who develop symptoms vary by setting and study methodology; 2 published studies that incorporated modeling techniques to address limitations of point prevalence surveys estimated that only about 10 percent of men and 5 to 30 percent of women with laboratory-confirmed chlamydial infection develop symptoms. The incubation period of chlamydia is poorly defined. However, given the relatively slow replication cycle of the organism, symptoms may not appear until several weeks after exposure in those persons who develop symptoms.

In women, the bacteria initially infect the cervix, where the infection may cause signs and symptoms of cervicitis (e.g., mucopurulent endocervical discharge, easily induced endocervical bleeding), and sometimes the urethra, which may result in signs and symptoms of urethritis (e.g., pyuria, dysuria, urinary frequency). Infection can spread from the cervix to the upper reproductive tract (i.e., uterus, fallopian tubes), causing pelvic inflammatory disease (PID), which may be asymptomatic ("subclinical PID") or acute, with typical symptoms of abdominal and/or pelvic pain, along with signs of cervical motion tenderness and uterine or adnexal tenderness on examination.

Men who are symptomatic typically have urethritis, with a mucoid or watery urethral discharge and dysuria. A minority of infected men develop epididymitis (with or without symptomatic urethritis), presenting with unilateral testicular pain, tenderness, and swelling.

Chlamydia can infect the rectum in men and women, either directly (through receptive anal sex), or possibly via spread from the cervix and vagina in a woman with a cervical chlamydial infection. While these infections are often asymptomatic, they can cause symptoms of proctitis (e.g., rectal pain, discharge, and/or bleeding).

Sexually acquired chlamydial conjunctivitis can occur in both men and women through contact with infected genital secretions.

While chlamydia can also be found in the throats of women and men having oral sex with an infected partner, it is typically asymptomatic and not thought to be an important cause of pharyngitis.

What Complications Can Result from Chlamydial Infection?

The initial damage that chlamydia causes often goes unnoticed. However, chlamydial infections can lead to serious health problems with both short- and long-term consequences.

In women, untreated chlamydia can spread into the uterus or fallopian tubes and cause PID. Symptomatic PID occurs in about 10 to 15 percent of women with untreated chlamydia. However, chlamydia can also cause subclinical PID. Both acute and subclinical PID can cause permanent damage to the fallopian tubes, uterus, and surrounding tissues. The damage can lead to chronic pelvic pain, tubal factor infertility, and potentially fatal ectopic pregnancy.

Some patients with chlamydial PID develop perihepatitis, or "Fitz-Hugh-Curtis syndrome," an inflammation of the liver capsule and surrounding peritoneum, which is associated with right upper quadrant pain.

In pregnant women, untreated chlamydia has been associated with preterm delivery, as well as ophthalmia neonatorum and pneumonia in the newborn.

Reactive arthritis can occur in men and women following symptomatic or asymptomatic chlamydial infection, sometimes as part of a triad of symptoms (with urethritis and conjunctivitis) formerly referred to as "Reiter syndrome."

What about Chlamydia and Human Immunodeficiency Virus?

Untreated chlamydia may increase a person's chances of acquiring or transmitting the human immunodeficiency virus (HIV)—the virus that causes acquired immunodeficiency syndrome (AIDS).

How Does Chlamydia Affect a Pregnant Woman and Her Baby?

In pregnant women, untreated chlamydia has been associated with preterm delivery, as well as ophthalmia neonatorum and pneumonia in the newborn. In published prospective studies, chlamydial conjunctivitis has been identified in 18 to 44 percent and chlamydial pneumonia in 3 to 16 percent of infants born to women with untreated chlamydial cervical infection at the time of delivery. Neonatal prophylaxis against gonococcal conjunctivitis routinely performed at birth does not effectively prevent chlamydial conjunctivitis.

Screening and treatment of chlamydia in pregnant women is the best method for preventing neonatal chlamydial disease. All pregnant women should be screened for chlamydia at their first prenatal visit. Pregnant women under 25 years of age and those at an increased risk for chlamydia (e.g., women who have a new or more than one sex partner) should be screened again in their third trimester. Pregnant women with chlamydial infection should be retested 3 weeks and 3 months after completion of recommended therapy.

Who Should Be Tested for Chlamydia?

Any sexually active person can be infected with chlamydia. Anyone with genital symptoms, such as discharge, burning during urination, unusual sores, or rash, should refrain from having sex until they are able to see a healthcare provider about their symptoms.

Also, anyone with an oral, anal, or vaginal sex partner who has been recently diagnosed with an STD should see a healthcare provider for evaluation.

Because chlamydia is usually asymptomatic, screening is necessary to identify most infections. Screening programs have been demonstrated to reduce rates of adverse sequelae in women. The CDC recommends yearly chlamydia screening of all sexually active women younger than 25 years of age, as well as older women with risk factors such as new or multiple partners, or a sex partner who has an STI. Pregnant women under the age of 25 or older pregnant women at an increased risk for chlamydia (e.g., women who have a new or more than 1 sex partner) should be screened during their first prenatal visit and again during their third trimester. Women diagnosed with chlamydial infection should be retested approximately 3 months after treatment. Any woman who is sexually active should discuss her risk factors with a healthcare provider who can then determine if more frequent screening is necessary.

255

Routine screening is not recommended for men. However, the screening of sexually active young men should be considered in clinical settings with a high prevalence of chlamydia (e.g., adolescent clinics, correctional facilities, and STD clinics) when resources permit and do not hinder screening efforts in women.

Sexually active men who have sex with men who had insertive intercourse should be screened for urethral chlamydial infection, and MSM who had receptive anal intercourse should be screened for rectal infection at least annually; screening for pharyngeal infection is not recommended. More frequent chlamydia screening at three-month intervals is indicated for MSM, including those with HIV infection, if risk behaviors persist or if they or their sexual partners have multiple partners.

At the initial HIV care visit, providers should test all sexually active persons with HIV infection for chlamydia and perform testing at least annually during the course of HIV care. A patient's healthcare provider might determine if more frequent screening is necessary, based on the patient's risk factors.

How Is Chlamydia Diagnosed?

There are a number of diagnostic tests for chlamydia, including nucleic acid amplification tests (NAATs), cell culture, and others. NAATs are the most sensitive tests and can be performed on easily obtainable specimens, such as vaginal swabs (either clinician- or patient-collected) or urine.

Vaginal swabs, either patient- or clinician-collected, are the optimal specimen to screen for genital chlamydia using NAATs in women; urine is the specimen of choice for men and is an effective alternative specimen type for women. Self-collected vaginal swab specimens perform at least as well as other approved specimens using NAATs. In addition, patients may prefer self-collected vaginal swabs or urine-based screening to more invasive endocervical or urethral swab specimens. Adolescent girls may be particularly good candidates for self-collected vaginal swab- or urine-based screening because pelvic exams are not indicated if they are asymptomatic.

Chlamydial culture can be used for rectal or pharyngeal specimens, but it is not widely available. NAATs have demonstrated improved sensitivity and specificity compared with culture for the detection of *C. trachomatis* at nongenital sites. Most tests, including NAATs, are not U.S. Food and Drug Administration (FDA)-cleared for use with rectal or pharyngeal swab specimens; however, NAATS have demonstrated improved sensitivity and specificity when compared with culture for the detection of *C. trachomatis* at rectal sites; however, some laboratories have met regulatory requirements and have validated NAAT testing on rectal and pharyngeal swab specimens.

What Is the Treatment for Chlamydia?

Chlamydia can be easily cured with antibiotics. HIV-positive persons with chlamydia should receive the same treatment as those who are HIV-negative.

Persons with chlamydia should abstain from sexual activity for seven days after single-dose antibiotics or until completion of a seven-day course of antibiotics, to prevent spreading the infection to partners. It is important to take all of the medication prescribed to cure chlamydia. Medication for chlamydia should not be shared with anyone. Although medication will cure the infection, it will not repair any permanent damage done by the disease. If a person's symptoms continue for more than a few days after receiving treatment, she or he should return to a healthcare provider to be reevaluated.

Repeat infection with chlamydia is common. Women whose sex partners have not been appropriately treated are at high risk for reinfection. Having multiple chlamydial infections increases a woman's risk of serious reproductive health complications, including pelvic inflammatory disease and ectopic pregnancy. Women and men with chlamydia should be retested about three months after treatment of an initial infection, regardless of whether they believe that their sex partners were successfully treated.

Infants infected with chlamydia may develop ophthalmia neonatorum and/or pneumonia. Chlamydial infection in infants can be treated with antibiotics.

What about Partners

If a person has been diagnosed and treated for chlamydia, she or he should tell all recent anal, vaginal, or oral sex partners (all sex partners within 60 days before the onset of symptoms or diagnosis), so they can see a healthcare provider and be treated. This will reduce the risk that the sex partners will develop serious complications from chlamydia and will also reduce the person's risk of becoming reinfected. A person with chlamydia and all of her or his sex partners must avoid having sex until they have completed their treatment for chlamydia (i.e., seven days after single-dose antibiotics or until completion of a seven-day course of antibiotics) and until they no longer have symptoms.

To help get partners treated quickly, healthcare providers in some states may give infected individuals extra medicine or prescriptions to give to their sex partners. This is called "expedited partner therapy" or "EPT." In published clinical trials comparing EPT to traditional patient referral (i.e., asking the patient to refer their partners in for treatment), EPT was associated with fewer persistent or recurrent chlamydial infections in the index patient, and a larger reported number of partners treated. For providers, EPT represents an additional strategy for partner management of persons with chlamydial infection; partners should still be encouraged to seek medical evaluation, regardless of whether they receive EPT.

How Can Chlamydia Be Prevented?

Latex male condoms, when used consistently and correctly, can reduce the risk of getting or giving chlamydia. The surest way to avoid chlamydia is to abstain from vaginal, anal, and oral sex, or to be in a long-term mutually monogamous relationship with a partner who has been tested and is known to be uninfected.

About Lymphogranuloma Venereum

Lymphogranuloma venereum (LGV) is caused by *C. trachomatis* serovars L1, L2, or L3. The most common clinical manifestation of LGV among heterosexuals is tender inguinal and/or femoral lymphadenopathy that is typically unilateral. A self-limited genital ulcer or papule sometimes occurs at the site of inoculation. However, by the time patients seek care, the lesions have often disappeared. Rectal exposure in women or MSM can result in proctocolitis mimicking inflammatory bowel disease (IBD), and clinical findings may include mucoid and/or hemorrhagic rectal discharge, anal pain, constipation, fever, and/or tenesmus. Outbreaks of LGV proctocolitis have been reported among MSM. LGV can be an invasive, systemic infection, and if it is not treated early, LGV proctocolitis can lead to chronic colorectal fistulas and strictures; reactive arthropathy has also been reported. However, reports indicate that rectal LGV can be asymptomatic. Persons with genital and colorectal LGV lesions can also develop a secondary bacterial infection or can be coinfected with other sexually and nonsexually transmitted pathogens.

Diagnostic Considerations of Lymphogranuloma Venereum

Diagnosis is based on clinical suspicion; epidemiologic information; and the exclusion of other etiologies for proctocolitis, inguinal lymphadenopathy, or genital or rectal ulcers. Genital lesions, rectal specimens, and lymph node specimens (i.e., lesion swab or bubo aspirate) can be tested for *C. trachomatis* by culture, direct immunofluorescence, or nucleic acid detection. NAATs for *C. trachomatis* perform well on rectal specimens but are not FDA-cleared for this purpose. Many laboratories have performed the Clinical Laboratory Improvement Amendments (CLIA) validation studies needed to provide results from rectal specimens for clinical management. MSM presenting with proctocolitis should be tested for chlamydia; NAAT performed on rectal specimens is the preferred approach to testing.

Additional molecular procedures (e.g., polymerase chain reaction (PCR) based genotyping) can be used to differentiate LGV from non-LGV *C. trachomatis* in rectal specimens. However, they are not widely available, and results are not available in a timeframe that would influence clinical management.

Chlamydia serology (complement fixation titers >1:64 or microimmunofluorescence titers >1:256) might support the diagnosis of LGV in the appropriate clinical context. Comparative data between types of serologic tests are lacking, and the diagnostic utility of these older serologic methods has not been established. Serologic test interpretation for LGV is not standardized, tests have not been validated for clinical proctitis presentations, and *C. trachomatis* serovar-specific serologic tests are not widely available.

Treatment of Lymphogranuloma Venereum

At the time of the initial visit (before diagnostic tests for chlamydia are available), persons with a clinical syndrome consistent with LGV, including proctocolitis or genital ulcer disease with lymphadenopathy, should be presumptively treated for LGV. As required by state law, these cases should be reported to the health department.

Treatment cures infection and prevents ongoing tissue damage; although, tissue reaction to the infection can result in scarring. Buboes might require aspiration through intact skin or incision and drainage to prevent the formation of inguinal/femoral ulcerations.

Recommended Regimen

Doxycycline 100 mg orally twice a day for 21 days

Alternative Regimen

Erythromycin base 500 mg orally 4 times a day for 21 days

Although clinical data are lacking, azithromycin 1 g orally once weekly for 3 weeks is probably effective based on its chlamydial antimicrobial activity. Fluoroquinolone-based treatments also might be effective, but the optimal duration of treatment has not been evaluated.

Other Management Considerations of Lymphogranuloma Venereum

Patients should be followed clinically until signs and symptoms have resolved. Persons who receive an LGV diagnosis should be tested for other STDs, especially HIV, gonorrhea, and syphilis. Those who test positive for another infection should be referred for or provided with appropriate care and treatment.

Follow-Up

Patients should be followed clinically until signs and symptoms resolve.

Management of Sex Partners

Persons who have had sexual contact with a patient who has LGV within the 60 days before the onset of the patient's symptoms should be examined and tested for urethral, cervical, or rectal chlamydial infection depending on anatomic site of exposure. They should be presumptively treated with a chlamydia regimen (azithromycin 1 g orally single dose or doxycycline 100 mg orally twice a day for 7 days).

Pregnancy

Pregnant and lactating women should be treated with erythromycin. Doxycycline should be avoided in the second and third trimester of pregnancy because of the risk for discoloration of teeth and bones, but it is compatible with breastfeeding. Azithromycin might prove useful for the treatment of LGV in pregnancy, but no published data are available regarding an effective dose and duration of treatment.

Human Immunodeficiency Virus Infection

Persons with both LGV and HIV infection should receive the same regimens as those who are HIV negative. Prolonged therapy might be required, and delay in resolution of symptoms might occur.

Chapter 34

Cholera

Cholera, caused by the bacterium *Vibrio cholerae*, is rare in the United States and other industrialized nations. However, globally, cholera cases have increased steadily since 2005, and the disease still occurs in many places, including Africa, Southeast Asia, and Haiti. The Centers for Disease Control and Prevention (CDC) responds to cholera outbreaks across the world using its Global Water, Sanitation, and Hygiene (WASH) expertise.

Cholera can be life-threatening, but it is easily prevented and treated. Travelers, public health and medical professionals, and outbreak responders should be aware of areas with high rates of cholera, know how the disease spreads, and what to do to prevent it.

What Is Cholera?

Cholera is an acute, diarrheal illness caused by infection of the intestine with the toxigenic bacterium *Vibrio cholerae* serogroup O1 or O139. An estimated 2.9 million cases and 95,000 deaths occur each year around the world.

Where Is Cholera Found?

The cholera bacterium is usually found in water or food sources that have been contaminated by feces from a person infected with

This chapter includes text excerpted from "Cholera—*Vibrio cholerae* infection," Centers for Disease Control and Prevention (CDC), May 3, 2018.

cholera. Cholera is most likely to be found and spread in places with inadequate water treatment, poor sanitation, and inadequate hygiene.

The cholera bacterium may also live in the environment in brackish rivers and coastal waters. Shellfish eaten raw have been a source of cholera, and few people in the United States have contracted cholera after eating raw or undercooked shellfish from the Gulf of Mexico.

How Does a Person Get Cholera?

A person can get cholera by drinking water or eating food contaminated with the cholera bacterium. In an epidemic, the source of the contamination is usually the feces of an infected person that contaminates water and/or food. The disease can spread rapidly in areas with inadequate treatment of sewage and drinking water. The disease is not likely to spread directly from one person to another; therefore, casual contact with an infected person is not a risk for becoming ill.

What Are the Symptoms of Cholera?

Cholera infection is often mild or without symptoms, but it can sometimes be severe. Approximately 1 in 10 (10%) infected persons will have severe disease characterized by profuse watery diarrhea, vomiting, and leg cramps. In these people, rapid loss of body fluids leads to dehydration and shock. Without treatment, death can occur within hours.

How Long after Infection Do the Symptoms Appear?

The infection can take anywhere from a few hours to five days for symptoms to appear after infection. Symptoms typically appear in two to three days.

Who Is More Likely to Get Cholera?

Individuals living in places with unsafe drinking water, poor sanitation, and inadequate hygiene are at a greater risk for cholera.

What Should I Do If I Think a Family Member Has or I Have Cholera?

If you think you or a member of your family may have cholera, seek medical attention immediately. Dehydration can be rapid, so fluid replacement is essential. If you have an oral rehydration solution (ORS), a prepackaged mixture of sugar and salts to be mixed with one liter of water, the ill person should start taking it immediately; it can save a life. She or he should continue to drink the ORS at home and during travel to get medical treatment. If you have an infant who has watery diarrhea, continue to breastfeed.

How Is Cholera Diagnosed?

To test for cholera, doctors must take a stool sample or a rectal swab and send it to a laboratory to look for the cholera bacterium.

What Is the Treatment for Cholera?

Cholera can be simply and successfully treated by immediate replacement of the fluid and salts lost through diarrhea. Patients can be treated with an ORS. This solution is used throughout the world to treat diarrhea. Severe cases also require intravenous fluid replacement. With prompt appropriate rehydration, fewer than one percent of cholera patients die.

Antibiotics shorten the course and diminish the severity of the illness, but they are not as important as receiving rehydration. Persons who develop severe diarrhea and vomiting in countries where cholera occurs should seek medical attention promptly.

Should I Be Worried about Getting Cholera from Others?

The disease is not likely to spread directly from one person to another; therefore, casual contact with an infected person is not a risk for becoming ill.

How Can I Avoid Getting Cholera?

The risk for cholera is very low for people visiting areas with epidemic cholera. When simple precautions are observed, contracting the disease is unlikely.

All people (visitors or residents) in areas where cholera is occurring or has occurred should observe the following recommendations:

- Drink only bottled, boiled, or chemically treated water and bottled or canned carbonated beverages. When using bottled drinks, make sure that the seal has not been broken.

- To disinfect your own water: boil for 1 minute or filter the water and add 2 drops of household bleach or ½ an iodine tablet per liter of water.

- Avoid tap water, fountain drinks, and ice cubes.

- Wash your hands often with soap and clean water.

- If no water and soap are available, use an alcohol-based hand cleaner (with at least 60% alcohol).

  - Clean your hands especially before you eat or prepare food and after using the bathroom.

- Use bottled, boiled, or chemically treated water to wash dishes, brush your teeth, wash and prepare food, or make ice.

- Eat foods that are packaged or that are freshly cooked and served hot.

  - Do not eat raw or undercooked meat and seafood or raw or undercooked fruits and vegetables unless they are peeled.

- Dispose of feces in a sanitary manner to prevent contamination of water and food sources.

Is a Vaccine Available to Prevent Cholera?

The FDA approved a single-dose live oral cholera vaccine called "Vaxchora®" (lyophilized CVD 103-HgR) for adults between 18 and 64 years of age who are traveling to an area of active cholera transmission with toxigenic *Vibrio cholerae* O1 (the bacteria strain that most commonly causes cholera). The vaccine is not routinely recommended for most travelers from the United States, as most people do not visit areas of active cholera transmission. Three other oral inactivated, or nonlive cholera vaccines—Dukoral®, ShanChol®, and Euvichol-Plus®/Euvichol®—are World Health Organization (WHO)-prequalified, but these vaccines are not available in the United States. No cholera vaccine is 100 percent protective, and vaccination against cholera is not a substitute for standard prevention and control measures, including the precautions for food and water as outlined above.

What Is the Risk for Cholera in the United States?

In the United States, cholera was prevalent in the 1800s, but water-related spread has been eliminated by modern water and sewage treatment systems. Very rarely, persons in the United States acquire cholera from shellfish consumed raw or inadequately cooked.

However, U.S. travelers to areas with epidemic cholera (for example, parts of Africa, Asia, or Latin America) may be exposed to the cholera bacterium. In addition, travelers may bring contaminated seafood back to the United States; foodborne outbreaks of cholera have been caused by contaminated seafood brought into the United States by travelers.

Where Can a Traveller Get Information about Cholera?

The global picture of cholera changes periodically, so travelers should seek updated information on countries of interest. The CDC has a Travelers' Health website that contains information on cholera and other diseases of concern to travelers.

What Is the U.S. Government Doing to Combat Cholera?

The U.S. and international public health authorities are working to enhance surveillance for cholera, investigate cholera outbreaks, and design and implement preventive measures across the globe. The CDC investigates epidemic cholera wherever it occurs at the invitation of the affected country and trains laboratory workers in proper techniques for identification of *Vibrio cholerae*. In addition, the CDC provides information on the diagnosis, treatment, and prevention of cholera to public health officials and educates the public about effective preventive measures.

The U.S. Agency for International Development (USAID) sponsors some of the international U.S. government activities and provides medical supplies and water, sanitation, and hygiene supplies to affected countries.

The U.S. Food and Drug Administration (FDA) tests imported and domestic shellfish for *V. cholerae* and monitors the safety of U.S. shellfish beds through the shellfish sanitation program.

With cooperation at the state and local, national, and international levels, assistance will be provided to countries where cholera is present. The risk to the U.S. residents remains small.

Chapter 35

Clostridium difficile *Infection*

What Is Clostridium difficile?

Clostridioides difficile is formerly known as *"Clostridium difficile"* and often called *"C. difficile* or *C. diff." C. diff* is a bacterium (germ) that causes diarrhea and colitis (an inflammation of the colon).

Most cases of *C. diff* occur while you are taking antibiotics or soon after you have finished taking antibiotics. *C. diff* can be deadly.

It is estimated to cause almost half a million illnesses in the United States each year.

About 1 in 5 patients who get *C. diff* will get it again.

Within a month of diagnosis, 1 in 11 people over age 65 died of a healthcare-associated *C. diff* infection.

Your Risk of Clostridium difficile
Can I Get Clostridium difficile *in the Hospital?*

C. diff bacteria is commonly found in the environment, but most cases of *C. diff* occur while you're taking antibiotics or not long after you have finished taking antibiotics. People on antibiotics are 7 to 10 times more likely to get *C. diff* while on the drugs and during the month after.

This chapter includes text excerpted from *"Clostridioides difficile (C. diff)"* Centers for Disease Control and Prevention (CDC), December 17, 2018.

That's because antibiotics affect your microbiome by wiping out bad germs but also the good germs that protect your body against infections.

The effect of antibiotics can last as long as several months. If you come in contact with *C. diff* germs during this time, you can get sick.

If you have been taking antibiotics for more than a week, you could be even more susceptible.

Here are more *C. diff* risk factors:

- Age (more than 80 percent of *C. diff* deaths happen among those 65 and older)

- Complicated medical care and extended stays in healthcare settings, especially hospitals and nursing homes

- Certain antibiotics, such as fluoroquinolones

- A weakened immune system

- Previous infection with *C. diff* or known exposure to the germs

But you can get *C. diff* even if none of these apply.

Talk with your healthcare provider about your risk for developing *C. diff*.

What Is the Microbiome?

The microbiome is the neighborhood of good and bad germs that live in or on your body—including your stomach and intestines, your mouth, and your urinary tract—and on your skin.

Some of those germs can cause illness, but others are very important in keeping you healthy. A healthy microbiome helps protect you from infection, but antibiotics disrupt your microbiome, wiping out both the good and the bad bacteria.

What Are the Complications of Clostridium difficile?

The most common complications include:

- Dehydration

- Inflammation of the colon, known as colitis

- Severe diarrhea

Rare complications include:

- Serious intestinal conditions, such as toxic megacolon

- Sepsis, the body's extreme response to an infection

- Death

Is Clostridium difficile *Contagious?*

Yes, but most healthy adults who come in contact with *C. diff* won't get sick. They won't pick up the germs or be affected by them at all.

What Is Colonization?

Sometimes when healthy people come into contact with *C. diff*, they will begin to carry *C. diff* germs in or on their body, but they won't get sick.

In medical terms, they are said to be "colonized" with *C. diff*. This is also sometimes called "*C. diff* carriage," and a person might be said to be a "*C. diff* carrier."

Someone who is colonized has no signs or symptoms.

Colonization is more common than *C. diff* infection and does not require treatment. Once your body is colonized, you can remain colonized for several months.

If you are colonized with *C. diff*, you can spread the infection to others.

Some reasons you might become colonized are:

- You have recently recovered from *C. diff*.

- You have a history of taking antibiotics.

- You have recently been hospitalized.

Once your body is colonized with *C. diff*, you can remain colonized for several months. Colonization is more common than *C. diff* infection and does not require treatment.

Because it is possible to spread *C. diff* to others while you are colonized, it is important to always practice good hand hygiene, making sure to wash your hands well with soap and water before eating and after using the bathroom.

Can I Get Clostridium difficile *in the Hospital?*

Yes. *C. diff* is more common in healthcare settings, such as hospitals and nursing homes. This is because many people colonized with *C. diff* are staying or being treated there.

Symptoms of Clostridium difficile

Symptoms might develop within a few days after you begin taking antibiotics.

- Diarrhea including loose, watery stools (poop) or frequent bowel movements for several days

- Fever

- Stomach tenderness or pain

- Loss of appetite

- Nausea

What If I Have Symptoms?

If you have been taking antibiotics recently and have symptoms of *C. diff*, you should see a doctor.

- Developing diarrhea is fairly common while on, or after taking antibiotics, but in only a few cases will that diarrhea caused by *C. diff*. If your diarrhea is very severe, do not delay getting medical care.

- Your doctor will review your symptoms and order a lab test of a stool (poop) sample.

- If the test is positive, you will take an antibiotic (e.g., vancomycin or fidaxomicin) for at least 10 days. If you were already taking an antibiotic, your healthcare provider might ask you to stop taking it if they think it is safe to do so.

- Your doctor might decide to admit you to the hospital, in which case your healthcare providers will use certain precautions, such as wearing gowns and gloves, to prevent the spread of *C. diff* to themselves and to other patients.

Prevent the Spread of Clostridium difficile
Information for Patients

C. diff germs are carried from person to person in poop.

If someone with *C. diff* (or caring for someone with *C. diff*) does not clean their hands with soap and water after using the bathroom, they can spread the germs to everything they touch.

And if someone with *C. diff* cannot take a shower with soap and water, they can end up with *C. diff* germs on their skin.

Then, when someone else touches the skin of that person, or the surfaces that person touched, they can pick up the germs on their hands.

C. diff germs are so small relative to our size that if you were the size of the state of California, a germ would be the size of a baseball home plate. There is no way you can see C. diff germs on your hands, but that does not mean they are not there.

Washing with soap and water is the only way to prevent the spread from person to person.

Remember: you can come in contact with *C. diff* germs—and even carry them on, or in, your body—and not get sick. But that does not mean you cannot infect others.

How Long Can Clostridium difficile *Germs Live?*

When *C. diff* germs are outside the body, they become spores. These spores are an inactive form of the germ and have a protective coating allowing them to live for months or sometimes years on surfaces and in the soil.

The germs become active again when these spores are swallowed and reach the intestines.

Healthy people will often not be infected even if the spores reach their intestines, but if your immune system is weakened or you have recently taken antibiotics, you could get sick.

How Do I Make Sure I Do Not Spread Clostridium difficile*?*
In a Healthcare Setting

Make sure all doctors, nurses, and other healthcare providers clean their hands before and after caring for you. If you do not see your providers clean their hands, ask them to do so.

While caring for you and other patients with *C. diff*, doctors, nurses and other healthcare providers will use certain precautions, such as gowns and gloves, to prevent the spread of *C. diff* to themselves and to other patients.

If you are in the hospital, wash your hands with soap and water every time you use the bathroom and always before you eat. Remind relatives and friends taking care of you to do the same.

At Home

Wash your hands with soap and water every time you use the bathroom and always before you eat. Remind relatives and friends taking care of you to do the same.

Try to use a separate bathroom if you have diarrhea. If you cannot, be sure the bathroom is well cleaned before others use it.

Take showers and wash with soap to remove any C. diff germs you could be carrying on your body.

How Do I Kill Clostridium difficile *Germs at Home?*

Finding *C. diff* germs in the home is not unusual, even when no one in the home has been ill with *C. diff*. Most healthy adults who come in contact with *C. diff* in the home won't get sick.

Hospitals use special cleaning products to kill *C. diff*, but you can make a cleaner at home. Mix 1 part bleach to 10 parts water (for example, ¼ cup bleach poured into 2½ cups water).

Surfaces

When you are cleaning, focus on items that are touched by hands:

- Doorknobs
- Electronics (be careful because bleach can damage many electronics and plastics)
- Refrigerator handles
- Shared cups
- Toilet flushers and toilet seats

Laundry

If someone in your house has *C. diff*, wash items they touch before others use them. These include but are not limited to:

- Bed linens
- Towels
- Household linens
- Clothing, especially underwear

If these things have visible poop, rinse them well before washing.

Then launder in a washer and dryer, using the hottest water that is safe for those items. Use chlorine bleach if the items can be safely washed with it.

Wash your hands with soap and water after you handle the dirty laundry.

It is ok to take clothes to a dry cleaner that were worn by a patient infected with *C. diff*. However, dry cleaning is not as effective as other methods of killing the spores. So this option should be used only for clothes that cannot be machine-washed.

Life after Clostridium difficile
When Can I Go Back to Work? When Can My Children Go Back to School?

You and your children should return to work or school only when your symptoms are gone.

Can I Still Spread Clostridium difficile *after Treatment?*

The risk of spreading *C. diff* after completing treatment is low. But if you are colonized (see the "Your Risk of *C. diff*" page), you can still spread it to others.

So always wash your hands with soap and water before you eat and after you use the bathroom. Showering and washing with soap is the best way to remove any *C. diff* germs you might be carrying on your body.

After Treatment, Can I Be Tested Again to Make Sure I'm Cured?

No, because once you recover from your *C. diff* infection, you could still be carrying the germs.

A test would only show the germs are still there, but not whether you're likely to become sick again.

Will I Get Clostridium difficile *Again?*

One in 5 people who've had *C. diff* will get infected again. This can be a relapse of their original infection, or it can happen when they come in contact with *C. diff* again.

The best way to be sure you do not get *C. diff* again is to avoid taking unnecessary antibiotics and to wash your hands with soap and water every time you use the bathroom and before you eat anything.

If you have had a *C. diff* infection, tell all of your healthcare providers. This important information will help them make the best decisions when prescribing antibiotics in the future.

This is as important at your dentist's office as it is when you see your primary care doctor.

Should I Report My **Clostridium difficile** *Infection to the Centers for Disease Control and Prevention?*

No. Hospitals are required to report *C. diff* infections to the Centers for Disease Control and Prevention's (CDC) National Healthcare Safety Network (NHSN). Some states also require other healthcare facilities to report *C. diff* infections, and the requirements vary from state to state. Contact your local or state health department for information specific to your state.

Chapter 36

Diphtheria

Starting in the 1920s, diphtheria rates dropped quickly in the United States and other countries with the widespread use of vaccines. In the past decade, there were less than 5 cases of diphtheria in the United States reported to the Centers for Disease Control and Prevention (CDC). However, the disease continues to cause illness globally. In 2016, countries reported about 7,100 cases of diphtheria to the World Health Organization (WHO), but there are likely many more cases.

Causes of Diphtheria

Diphtheria is an infection caused by the *Corynebacterium diphtheriae* bacterium.

Transmission of Diphtheria

Diphtheria spreads (transmits) from person to person, usually through respiratory droplets, such as coughing or sneezing. Rarely, people can get sick from touching open sores (skin lesions) or clothes that touched open sores of someone sick with diphtheria. A person also can get diphtheria by coming in contact with an object, such as a toy, that has the diphtheria-causing bacteria on it.

This chapter includes text excerpted from "About Diphtheria," Centers for Disease Control and Prevention (CDC), December 17, 2018.

Symptoms of Diphtheria

Bacteria that cause diphtheria can get into and attach to the lining of the respiratory system, which includes parts of the body that help you breathe. When this happens, the bacteria can produce a poison (toxin) that can cause:

- Weakness
- Sore throat
- Fever
- Swollen glands in the neck

The poison destroys healthy tissues in the respiratory system. Within two to three days, the dead tissue forms a thick, gray coating that can build up in the throat or nose. Medical experts call this thick gray coating a "pseudomembrane." It can cover tissues in the nose, tonsils, voice box, and throat, making it very hard to breathe and swallow.

The poison may also get into the bloodstream and cause damage to the heart, nerves, and kidneys.

Complications of Diphtheria

Complications from diphtheria may include:

- Blocking of the airway
- Damage to the heart muscle (myocarditis)
- Nerve damage (polyneuropathy)
- Loss of the ability to move (paralysis)
- Lung infection (respiratory failure or pneumonia)

For some people, diphtheria can lead to death. Even with treatment, about 1 in 10 diphtheria patients die. Without treatment, up to half of the patients can die from the disease.

Diagnosis of Diphtheria

Doctors usually decide if a person has diphtheria by looking for common signs and symptoms. They can use a swab from the back of the throat and test it for the bacteria that cause diphtheria. A doctor can also take a sample from a skin lesion and try and grow the bacteria. If the bacteria grow, the doctor can be sure that a patient has diphtheria.

Treatment of Diphtheria

It is important to start treatment right away if a doctor suspects diphtheria and not to wait for laboratory confirmation. In the United States, before there was a treatment for diphtheria, up to half of the people who got the disease died from it.

Diphtheria treatment involves:

- Using diphtheria antitoxin to stop the poison produced by the bacteria from damaging the body

- Using antibiotics to kill and get rid of the bacteria

Even with treatment, about 1 in 10 people who get diphtheria will die.

People with diphtheria are usually no longer able to infect others 48 hours after they begin taking antibiotics. However, it is important to finish taking the full course of antibiotics to make sure the bacteria are completely removed from the body. After the patient finishes the full treatment, the doctor will run tests to make sure that the bacteria are not in the patient's body anymore.

Prevention of Diphtheria

Getting vaccinated is the best way to prevent diphtheria. In the United States, there are four vaccines used to prevent diphtheria: DTaP, Tdap, DT, and Td. Each of these vaccines prevents diphtheria and tetanus; DTaP and Tdap also help prevent pertussis (whooping cough). Healthcare professionals give DTaP and DT to children younger than seven years of age, while older children, teens, and adults get Tdap and Td.

Babies and Children

The online childhood immunization schedule for diphtheria, which is offered by the Centers for Disease Control and Prevention (CDC), includes five doses of DTaP for children younger than seven years of age.

Preteens and Teens

The CDC's online adolescent immunization schedule recommends that preteens get a booster dose of Tdap at 11 or 12 years of age. Teens who did not get Tdap when they were 11 or 12 years of age should get a dose the next time they see their doctor.

Adults

Adults should get a dose of Td every 10 years, according to the adult immunization schedule. For added protection against whooping cough, any adult who never received a dose of Tdap should get one as soon as possible. The dose of Tdap takes the place of one of the Td shots.

Chapter 37

Hansen Disease (Leprosy)

What Is Hansen Disease?

Hansen disease (also known as "leprosy") is an infection caused by bacteria called "*Mycobacterium leprae*." These bacteria grow very slowly, and it may take up to 20 years to develop signs of the infection.

The disease can affect the nerves, skin, eyes, and lining of the nose (nasal mucosa). The bacteria attack the nerves, which can become swollen under the skin. This can cause the affected areas to lose the ability to sense touch and pain, which can lead to injuries, such as cuts and burns. Usually, the affected skin changes color and either becomes:

- Lighter or darker, often dry or flaky, with loss of feeling

or

- Reddish, due to inflammation of the skin

Other signs of advanced Hansen disease may include loss of eyebrows and saddle-nose deformity resulting from damage to the nasal septum.

Early diagnosis and treatment usually prevent disability that can result from the disease, and people with Hansen disease can continue to work and lead an active life. Once treatment is started, the person is no longer contagious. However, it is very important to finish the entire course of treatment as directed by the doctor.

This chapter includes text excerpted from "What Is Hansen Disease?" Centers for Disease Control and Prevention (CDC), February 10, 2017.

Each year, about 150 people in the United States and 250,000 around the world get the illness. In the past, Hansen disease was feared as a highly contagious, devastating disease, but now it is known that it is hard to spread and it is easily treatable once recognized. Still, a lot of stigma and prejudice remains about the disease, and those suffering from it are isolated and discriminated against in many places where the disease is seen. Continued commitment to fighting the stigma through education and improving access to treatment will lead to a world free of this completely treatable disease.

Signs and Symptoms of Hansen Disease

Symptoms mainly affect the skin, nerves, and mucous membranes (the soft, moist areas just inside the body's openings).

The disease can cause skin symptoms such as:

- Discolored patches of skin, usually flat, that may be numb and look faded (lighter than the skin around)

- Growths (nodules) on the skin

- Thick, stiff, or dry skin

- Painless ulcers on the soles of feet

- Painless swelling or lumps on the face or earlobes

- Loss of eyebrows or eyelashes

Symptoms caused by damage to the nerves are:

- Numbness of affected areas of the skin

- Muscle weakness or paralysis (especially in the hands and feet)

- Enlarged nerves (especially those around the elbow and knee and in the sides of the neck)

- Eye problems that may lead to blindness (when facial nerves are affected)

Symptoms caused by the disease in the mucous membranes are:

- A stuffy nose

- Nosebleeds

Since Hansen disease affects the nerves, loss of feeling or sensation can occur. When loss of sensation occurs, injuries such as burns may go unnoticed. Because you may not feel the pain that can warn you of harm to your body, take extra caution to ensure the affected parts of your body are not injured.

If left untreated, the signs of advanced leprosy can include:

- Paralysis and crippling of the hands and feet
- Shortening of the toes and fingers due to reabsorption
- Chronic nonhealing ulcers on the bottoms of the feet
- Blindness
- Loss of eyebrows
- Nose disfigurement

Other complications that may sometimes occur are:

- Painful or tender nerves
- Redness and pain around the affected area
- Burning sensation on the skin

Transmission of Hansen Disease
How Do People Get Hansen Disease?

It is not known exactly how Hansen disease spreads between people. Scientists think it may happen when a person with Hansen disease coughs or sneezes, and a healthy person breathes in the droplets containing the bacteria. Prolonged, close contact with someone with untreated leprosy over many months is needed to catch the disease.

You cannot get leprosy from casual contact with a person who has Hansen disease such as:

- Shaking hands or hugging
- Sitting next to each other on the bus
- Sitting together at a meal

Hansen disease is also not passed on from a mother to the fetus during pregnancy, and it is also not spread through sexual contact.

Due to the slow-growing nature of the bacteria and the long time it takes to develop signs of the disease, it is often very difficult to find the source of infection.

In the southern United States, some armadillos are naturally infected with the bacteria that cause Hansen disease in people, and it may be possible that they can spread it to people. However, the risk is very low, and most people who come into contact with armadillos are unlikely to get Hansen disease.

For general health reasons, avoid contact with armadillos whenever possible. If you had a contact with an armadillo and are worried about getting Hansen disease, talk to your healthcare provider. Your doctor will follow up with you over time and perform periodic skin examinations to see if you develop the disease. In the unlikely event that you have Hansen disease, your doctor can help you get treatment.

Who Is at Risk?

In the United States, Hansen disease is rare. Around the world, as many as two million people are permanently disabled as a result of Hansen disease.

Overall, the risk of getting Hansen disease for any adult around the world is very low. That is because more than 95 percent of all people have a natural immunity to the disease.

You may be at risk for the disease if you live in a country where the disease is widespread. Countries that reported more than 1,000 new cases of Hansen disease to the World Health Organization (WHO) between 2011 and 2015 are:

- **Africa:** Democratic Republic of Congo, Ethiopia, Madagascar, Mozambique, Nigeria, and the United Republic of Tanzania

- **Asia:** Bangladesh, India, Indonesia, Myanmar, Nepal, the Philippines, and Sri Lanka

- **Americas:** Brazil

You may also be at risk if you are in prolonged close contact with people who have untreated Hansen disease. If they have not been treated, you could get the bacteria that cause Hansen disease. However, as soon as patients start treatment, they are no longer able to spread the disease.

Diagnosis and Treatment of Hansen Disease
How Is the Disease Diagnosed?

Hansen disease can be recognized by the appearance of patches of skin that may look lighter or darker than the normal skin. Sometimes the affected skin areas may be reddish. Loss of feeling in these skin patches is common. You may not feel a light touch or a prick with a needle.

To confirm the diagnosis, your doctor will take a sample of your skin or nerve (through a skin or nerve biopsy) to look for the bacteria under the microscope, and they may also do tests to rule out other skin diseases.

How Is the Disease Treated?

Hansen disease is treated with a combination of antibiotics. Typically, two or three antibiotics are used at the same time. These are dapsone with rifampicin, and clofazimine is added for some types of the disease. This is called "multidrug therapy." This strategy helps prevent the development of antibiotic resistance by the bacteria, which may otherwise occur due to length of the treatment.

Treatment usually lasts between one to two years. The illness can be cured if treatment is completed as prescribed.

If you are treated for Hansen disease, it is important to:

- Tell your doctor if you experience numbness or a loss of feeling in certain parts of the body or in patches on the skin. This may be caused by nerve damage from the infection. If you have numbness and loss of feeling, take extra care to prevent injuries that may occur, such as burns and cuts.

- Take the antibiotics until your doctor says your treatment is complete. If you stop earlier, the bacteria may start growing again, and you may get sick again.

- Tell your doctor if the affected skin patches become red and painful, nerves become painful or swollen, or you develop a fever, as these may be complications of Hansen disease that may require more intensive treatment with medicines that can reduce inflammation.

If left untreated, the nerve damage can result in paralysis and crippling of the hands and feet. In very advanced cases, the person may have multiple injuries due to lack of sensation, and eventually, the body may reabsorb the affected digits over time, resulting in the apparent loss of toes and fingers. Corneal ulcers or blindness can also occur if facial nerves are affected, due to loss of sensation of the cornea (outside) of the eye.

Antibiotics used during the treatment will kill the bacteria that cause leprosy. But, while the treatment can cure the disease and prevent it from getting worse, it does not reverse nerve damage or physical disfiguration that may have occurred before the diagnosis. Thus, it is very important that the disease be diagnosed as early as possible before any permanent nerve damage occurs.

Chapter 38

Hib Disease

What Is Hib Disease?

Hib disease is a serious illness caused by the bacteria *Haemophilus influenzae type b* (Hib). Babies and children younger than five years of age are most at risk for Hib disease. It can cause lifelong disability, and it can be deadly.

What Are the Symptoms of Hib Disease?

Hib disease causes different symptoms depending on which part of the body it affects. The most common type of Hib disease is meningitis. This is an infection of the covering of the brain and spinal cord.

It causes the following:

- High fever
- Confusion
- Headache or stiff neck
- Pain from bright lights
- Poor eating and drinking, low alertness, or vomiting (in babies)

This chapter includes text excerpted from "Hib Disease and the Vaccine (Shot) to Prevent It," Centers for Disease Control and Prevention (CDC), April 2017.

Hib disease can also cause the following:

- Throat swelling that makes it hard to breathe
- Joint infection
- Skin infection
- Pneumonia (lung infection)
- Bone infection

Is It Serious?

Hib disease is very serious. Most children with Hib disease need care in the hospital. Even with treatment, as many as 1 out of 20 children with Hib meningitis dies. As many as 1 out of 5 children who survive Hib meningitis will have brain damage or become deaf.

How Does Hib Bacteria Spread?

Hib bacteria spread when an infected person coughs or sneezes. Usually, the Hib bacteria stay in a person's nose and throat, and it does not cause illness. But if the bacteria spread into the lungs or blood, the person will get very sick.

Why Should My Child Get the Hib Shot?

The Hib vaccine:

- Protects your child from Hib disease, which can cause lifelong disability and be deadly
- Protects your child from the most common type of Hib disease, meningitis
- Keeps your child from missing school or child care (and keeps you from missing work to care for your sick child)

Is the Hib Shot Safe?

Yes. The Hib vaccine is very safe, and it is effective at preventing Hib disease. Vaccines, as with any medicine, can have side effects. Most children do not have any side effects from the vaccine.

What Are the Side Effects?

When side effects do occur, they are usually mild and last two or three days.

They include:

- Redness, swelling, warmth, or pain where the shot was given

- Fever

Chapter 39

Impetigo

It is a scary sight when your child comes home from day care or elementary school with red sores and oozing fluid-filled blisters. Do not be alarmed if it is impetigo. Impetigo—one of the most common childhood diseases—can be treated with medications approved by the U.S. Food and Drug Administration (FDA).

Impetigo is a common bacterial skin infection that can produce blisters or sores anywhere on the body, but they usually appear on the face (around the nose and mouth), neck, hands, and diaper area. It is contagious, preventable, and manageable with antibiotics, says pediatrician Thomas D. Smith, M.D., of the FDA.

What Causes Impetigo

Two types of bacteria found on our skin cause impetigo: *Staphylococcus aureus* and *Streptococcus pyogenes* (which also causes strep throat). Most of us go about our lives carrying around these bacteria without a problem, Smith says. But then a minor cut, scrape, or insect bite allows the bacteria to cause an infection, resulting in impetigo.

Anyone can get impetigo—and more than once, Smith says. Although impetigo is a year-round disease, it occurs most often during the warm weather months. There are more than three million cases of impetigo in the United States every year.

This chapter includes text excerpted from "How to Treat Impetigo and Control This Common Skin Infection," U.S. Food and Drug Administration (FDA), November 1, 2016.

"We typically see impetigo with kids two to six years old, probably because they get more cuts and scrapes and scratch more. And that spreads the bacteria," Smith says.

Treating Impetigo

Look for these signs of impetigo:

- Itchy red sores that fill with fluid and then burst open, forming a yellow crust
- Itchy rash
- Fluid-filled blisters

If you see these symptoms, visit your healthcare provider. Impetigo is usually treated with topical or oral antibiotics. If you have multiple lesions or if there is an outbreak, your doctor might prescribe an oral antibiotic. There is no over-the-counter (OTC) treatment for impetigo.

Controlling and Preventing Impetigo

Left untreated, impetigo often clears up on its own after a few days or weeks, Smith says. The key is to keep the infected area clean with soap and water and to not to scratch it. The downside of not treating impetigo is that some people might develop more lesions that spread to other areas of their body.

And, you can infect others. "To spread impetigo, you need fairly close contact—not casual contact—with the infected person or the objects they touched," he says. Avoid spreading impetigo to other people or other parts of your body by:

- Cleaning the infected areas with soap and water
- Loosely covering scabs and sores until they heal
- Gently removing crusty scabs
- Washing your hands with soap and water after touching infected areas or infected persons

Because impetigo spreads by skin-to-skin contact, there often are small outbreaks within a family or a classroom, Smith says. Avoid touching objects that someone with impetigo has used, such as utensils, towels, sheets, clothing, and toys. If you have impetigo, keep your fingernails short so the bacteria cannot live under your nails and spread. Also, do not scratch the sores.

Call your healthcare provider if the symptoms do not go away or if there are signs that the infection has worsened, such as fever, pain, or increased swelling.

Chapter 40

Bacterial Meningitis

What Is Bacterial Meningitis?

Bacterial meningitis is very serious and can be deadly. Death can occur in as little as a few hours. Most people recover from meningitis. However, permanent disabilities (such as brain damage, hearing loss, and learning disabilities) can result from the infection.

There are several types of bacteria that can cause meningitis. Leading causes in the United States include:

- *Streptococcus pneumoniae*

- Group B Streptococcus

- *Neisseria meningitidis*

- *Haemophilus influenzae*

- *Listeria monocytogenes*

On average, bacterial meningitis caused about 4,100 cases and 500 deaths in the United States each year between 2003 and 2007.

These bacteria can also be associated with another serious illness, sepsis. Sepsis is the body's overwhelming and life-threatening response to infection that can cause tissue damage, organ failure, and death.

This chapter includes text excerpted from "Bacterial Meningitis," Centers for Disease Control and Prevention (CDC), January 25, 2017.

Causes of Bacterial Meningitis

Common causes of bacterial meningitis vary by age group:

- **Newborns:** Group B Streptococcus, *Streptococcus pneumoniae, Listeria monocytogenes, Escherichia coli*

- **Babies and children:** *Streptococcus pneumoniae, Neisseria meningitidis, Haemophilus influenzae type b* (Hib), group B Streptococcus

- **Teens and young adults:** *Neisseria meningitidis, Streptococcus pneumoniae*

- **Older adults:** *Streptococcus pneumoniae, Neisseria meningitidis, Haemophilus influenzae type b* (Hib), group B Streptococcus, *Listeria monocytogenes*

Risk Factors of Bacterial Meningitis

Certain people are at increased risk for bacterial meningitis. Some risk factors include:

- Age
  - Babies are at an increased risk for bacterial meningitis when compared to people in other age groups. However, people of any age can develop bacterial meningitis.

- Community setting
  - Infectious diseases tend to spread where large groups of people gather together. College campuses have reported outbreaks of meningococcal disease, caused by *N. meningitidis*.

- Certain medical conditions
  - There are certain medical conditions, medications, and surgical procedures that put people at increased risk for meningitis.

- Working with meningitis-causing pathogens
  - Microbiologists routinely exposed to meningitis-causing bacteria are at an increased risk for meningitis.

- Travel
  - Travelers may be at an increased risk for meningococcal disease, caused by *N. meningitidis*, if they travel to certain places, such as:
    - The meningitis belt in sub-Saharan Africa, particularly during the dry season
    - Mecca during the annual Hajj and Umrah pilgrimage

How It Spreads

Generally, the germs that cause bacterial meningitis spread from one person to another. Certain germs, such as *Listeria monocytogenes*, can spread through food.

How people spread germs often depends on the type of bacteria. It is also important to know that people can carry these bacteria in or on their bodies without being sick. These people are "carriers." Most carriers never become sick, but they can still spread the bacteria to others.

Here are some of the most common examples of how people spread each type of bacteria to each other:

- Mothers can pass group B Streptococcus and *Escherichia coli* to their babies during labor and birth.

- People spread Hib and *Streptococcus pneumoniae* by coughing or sneezing while in close contact with others who breathe in the bacteria.

- People spread *Neisseria meningitidis* by sharing respiratory or throat secretions (saliva or spit). This typically occurs during close (coughing or kissing) or lengthy (living in the same household) contact.

- People can get *Escherichia coli* by eating food prepared by people who did not wash their hands well after using the toilet.

People usually get sick from *Escherichia coli* and *Listeria monocytogenes* by eating contaminated food.

Signs and Symptoms of Bacterial Meningitis

Meningitis symptoms include sudden onset of fever, headache, and stiff neck.

There are often other symptoms, such as

- Nausea

- Vomiting

- Photophobia (increased sensitivity to light)

- Altered mental status (confusion)

In newborns and babies, the meningitis symptoms of fever, headache, and neck stiffness may be absent or difficult to notice. The baby may be irritable, vomit, feed poorly, or appear to be slow or inactive. In young babies, doctors may also look for a bulging fontanelle (soft spot on infant's head) or abnormal reflexes. If you think that your baby or child has any of these symptoms, call the doctor right away.

Symptoms of bacterial meningitis can appear quickly or over several days. Typically, they develop within three to seven days after exposure

Later symptoms of bacterial meningitis can be very serious (e.g., seizures, coma). For this reason, anyone who thinks that they may have meningitis should see a doctor as soon as possible.

Diagnosis of Bacterial Meningitis

If a doctor thinks you have meningitis, they will collect samples of blood or cerebrospinal fluid (fluid near the spinal cord). A laboratory will test the samples to see what is causing the infection. It is important to know the specific cause of meningitis so the doctors know how to treat it.

Treatment of Bacterial Meningitis

Doctors treat bacterial meningitis with a number of antibiotics. It is important to start treatment as soon as possible.

Prevention of Bacterial Meningitis

The most effective way to protect you and your child against certain types of bacterial meningitis is to get vaccinated. There are vaccines for three types of bacteria that can cause meningitis:

- *Neisseria meningitidis*

- *Streptococcus pneumoniae*

- Hib

Make sure you and your child are vaccinated on schedule.

As with any vaccine, the vaccines that protect against these bacteria are not 100 percent effective. The vaccines also do not protect against all the types (strains) of each bacteria. For these reasons, there is still a chance you can develop bacterial meningitis even if you were vaccinated.

Pregnant women should talk to their doctor or midwife about getting tested for group B Streptococcus. Women receive the test when they are 35 to 37 weeks pregnant. Doctors give antibiotics (during labor) to women who test positive in order to prevent passing group B strep to their newborns.

Pregnant women can also reduce their risk of meningitis caused by *Listeria monocytogenes*. Women should avoid certain foods during pregnancy and safely prepare others.

If someone has bacterial meningitis, a doctor may recommend antibiotics to help prevent other people from getting sick. Doctors call this "prophylaxis." The Centers for Disease Control and Prevention (CDC) recommends prophylaxis for:

- Close contacts of someone with meningitis caused by *Neisseria meningitidis*

- Family members, especially if they are at increased risk, of someone with a serious Hib infection

Your doctor or local health department will tell you if you or someone in your house need prophylaxis.

You can also help protect yourself and others from bacterial meningitis by maintaining healthy habits:

- Do not smoke, and avoid cigarette smoke.

- Get plenty of rest.

- Avoid close contact with people who are sick.

This is especially important for people at increased risk for disease, including:

- Young babies

- Older adults

- People with weak immune systems

- People without a spleen or a spleen that does not work the way it should (functional asplenia)

Chapter 41

Methicillin-Resistant Staphylococcus aureus

Methicillin-Resistant Staphylococcus aureus: *An Overview*

During the past four decades, a type of bacteria has evolved from a controllable nuisance into a serious public health concern. This bacterium is known as "methicillin-resistant *Staphylococcus aureus*" (MRSA). About one-third of people in the world have *S. aureus* bacteria on their bodies at any given time, primarily in the nose and on the skin. The bacteria can be present without causing an active infection. Of the people with *S. aureus* present, about one percent has MRSA, according to the Centers for Disease Control and Prevention (CDC).

Methicillin-resistant *Staphylococcus aureus* can be categorized according to where the infection was acquired: hospital-Acquired MRSA (HA-MRSA) or community-associated MRSA (CA-MRSA).

Hospital-Acquired Methicillin-Resistant Staphylococcus aureus

Hospital-acquired methicillin-resistant *Staphylococcus aureus* is acquired in the hospital setting and is one of many hospital-acquired

This chapter includes text excerpted from "Methicillin-Resistant *Staphylococcus aureus* (MRSA)," National Institute of Allergy and Infectious Diseases (NIAID), June 22, 2015. Reviewed July 2019.

infections exhibiting increased antimicrobial resistance. HA-MRSA has increased during the past decade due to a number of factors including an increased number of immunocompromised and elderly patients; an increase in the number of invasive procedures, such as advanced surgical operations and life support treatments; and failures in infection control measures, such as hand washing prior to patient contact and removal of nonessential catheters.

Community-Associated Methicillin-Resistant Staphylococcus aureus

Community-associated methicillin-resistant *Staphylococcus aureus* is caused by newly emerging strains unlike those responsible for HA-MRSA and can cause infections in otherwise healthy persons with no links to healthcare systems. CA-MRSA infections typically occur as skin or soft tissue infections, but they can develop into more invasive, life-threatening infections. CA-MRSA is occurring with increasing frequency in the United States and around the world, and it tends to occur in conditions where people are in close physical contact, such as athletes involved in football and wrestling, soldiers kept in close quarters, inmates, child care workers, and residents of long-term care facilities.

Methicillin-resistant *Staphylococcus aureus* has attracted the attention of the medical research community, illustrating the urgent need to develop better ways to diagnose and treat bacterial infections.

History of Methicillin-Resistant Staphylococcus aureus

The *Staphylococcus aureus* bacterium, commonly known as "staph," was discovered in the 1880s. During this era, *S. aureus* infection commonly caused painful skin and soft tissue conditions, such as boils, scalded-skin syndrome, and impetigo. More serious forms of *S. aureus* infection can progress to bacterial pneumonia and bacteria in the bloodstream—both of which can be fatal. *S. aureus* acquired from improperly prepared or stored food can also cause a form of food poisoning.

In the 1940s, medical treatment for *S. aureus* infections became routine and successful with the discovery and introduction of antibiotic medicine, such as penicillin.

From that point on, however, the use of antibiotics—including misuse and overuse—has aided natural bacterial evolution by helping the microbes become resistant to drugs designed to help fight these infections.

In the late 1940s and throughout the 1950s, *S. aureus* developed resistance to penicillin. Methicillin, a form of penicillin, was introduced to counter the increasing problem of penicillin-resistant *S. aureus*. Methicillin was one of the most common types of antibiotics used to treat *S. aureus* infections; but, in 1961, British scientists identified the first strains of *S. aureus* bacteria that resisted methicillin. This was the so-called birth of MRSA.

The first reported human case of MRSA in the United States came in 1968. Subsequently, new strains of bacteria have developed that can now resist previously effective drugs, such as methicillin and most related antibiotics.

Methicillin-resistant *Staphylococcus aureus* is actually resistant to an entire class of penicillin-like antibiotics called "beta-lactams." This class of antibiotics includes penicillin, amoxicillin, oxacillin, methicillin, and others.

S. aureus is evolving even more and has begun to show resistance to additional antibiotics. In 2002, physicians in the United States documented the first *S. aureus* strains resistant to the antibiotic, vancomycin, which had been one of a handful of antibiotics of last resort for use against *S. aureus*. Though it is feared that this could quickly become a major issue in antibiotic resistance, thus far, vancomycin-resistant strains are still rare.

Transmission of Methicillin-Resistant Staphylococcus aureus

S. aureus has evolved to the point where experts refer to MRSA in terms ranging from a considerable public-health burden to a crisis. The bacteria have been classified into two categories based on where the infection is first acquired.

Diagnosis of Methicillin-Resistant Staphylococcus aureus

To diagnose *S. aureus*, a sample is obtained from the infection site and sent to a microbiology laboratory for testing. If *S. aureus* is found, the organism should be further tested to determine which antibiotic would be effective for treatment.

Doctors often diagnose MRSA by checking a tissue sample or nasal secretions for signs of drug-resistant bacteria. Current diagnostic procedures involve sending a sample to a lab where it is placed in a dish of nutrients that encourage bacterial growth (a culture). It takes about 48 hours for the bacteria to grow. However, newer tests that can detect staph DNA in a matter of hours are now becoming more widely available. This will help healthcare providers decide on the proper treatment regimen for a patient more quickly after an official diagnosis has been made.

In the hospital, you might be tested for MRSA if you show signs of infection or if you are transferred to a hospital from another healthcare setting where MRSA is known to be present. You also might be tested if you have had a previous history of MRSA.

Treatment of Methicillin-Resistant Staphylococcus aureus

Healthcare providers can treat many *S. aureus* skin infections by draining the abscess or boil and may not need to use antibiotics. Draining of skin boils or abscesses should only be done by a healthcare provider.

For mild to moderate skin infections, incision and drainage by a healthcare provider is the first-line treatment. Before prescribing antibiotics, your provider will consider the potential for antibiotic resistance. Thus, if MRSA is suspected, your provider will avoid treating you with beta-lactam antibiotics, a class of antibiotic observed not to be effective in killing the staph bacteria.

For severe infection, doctors will typically use vancomycin intravenously.

Prevention of Methicillin-Resistant Staphylococcus aureus

The best defense against spreading MRSA is to practice good hygiene, as follows:

- Keep your hands clean by washing thoroughly with soap and water. Scrub them briskly for at least 15 seconds, then dry them with a disposable towel and use another towel to turn off the faucet. When you do not have access to soap and water, carry a small bottle of hand sanitizer containing at least 62 percent alcohol.

- Always shower promptly after exercising.

- Keep cuts and scrapes clean and covered with a bandage until healed. Keep wounds that are draining or have pus covered with clean, dry bandages. Follow your healthcare provider's instructions on proper care of the wound. Pus from infected wounds can contain *S. aureus* and MRSA, so keeping the infection covered will help prevent the spread to others. Bandages or tape can be discarded with regular trash.

- Avoid contact with other people's wounds or bandages.

- Avoid sharing personal items, such as towels, washcloths, razors, clothes, or uniforms.

- Wash sheets, towels, and clothes that become soiled with water and laundry detergent; use bleach and hot water if possible. Drying clothes in a hot dryer, rather than air-drying, also helps kill bacteria in clothes.

Tell any healthcare providers who treat you if you have or had an *S. aureus* or MRSA skin infection. If you have a skin infection that requires treatment, ask your healthcare provider if you should be tested for MRSA. Many healthcare providers prescribe drugs that are not effective against antibiotic-resistant staph, which delays treatment and creates more resistant germs.

Healthcare providers are fighting back against MRSA infection by tracking bacterial outbreaks and by investing in products, such as antibiotic-coated catheters and gloves that release disinfectants.

Chapter 42

Pneumonia

Pneumonia is a bacterial, viral, or fungal infection of one or both sides of the lungs that causes the air sacs, or alveoli, of the lungs to fill up with fluid or pus. Symptoms can be mild or severe and may include a cough with phlegm (a slimy substance), fever, chills, and trouble breathing. Many factors affect how serious pneumonia is, such as the type of germ causing the lung infection, your age, and your overall health. Pneumonia tends to be more serious for children under the age of 5; adults over the age of 65; people with certain conditions, such as heart failure, diabetes, or chronic obstructive pulmonary disease (COPD); or people who have weak immune systems due to human immunodeficiency virus/acquired immunodeficiency syndrome (HIV/AIDS), chemotherapy (a treatment for cancer), or organ or blood and marrow stem cell transplant procedures.

To diagnose pneumonia, your doctor will review your medical history, perform a physical exam, and order diagnostic tests. This information can help your doctor determine what type of pneumonia you have. If your doctor suspects you got your infection while in a hospital, you may be diagnosed with hospital-acquired pneumonia. If you have been on a ventilator to help you breathe, you may have ventilator-associated pneumonia. The most common form of pneumonia is community-acquired pneumonia, which is when you get an infection outside of a hospital.

This chapter includes text excerpted from "Pneumonia," National Heart, Lung, and Blood Institute (NHLBI), September 27, 2016.

Treatment depends on whether bacteria, viruses, or fungi are causing your pneumonia. If bacteria are causing your pneumonia, you usually are treated at home with oral antibiotics. Most people respond quickly to treatment. If your symptoms worsen, you should see a doctor right away. If you have severe symptoms or underlying health problems, you may need to be treated in a hospital. It may take several weeks to recover from pneumonia.

Causes of Pneumonia

Bacteria, viruses, and fungi infections can cause pneumonia. These infections cause inflammation in the air sacs, or alveoli, of the lungs. This inflammation causes the air sacs to fill with fluid and pus.

Bacteria

Bacteria are the most common cause of pneumonia in adults. Many types of bacteria can cause bacterial pneumonia. *Streptococcus pneumoniae* or pneumococcus bacteria are the most common cause of bacterial pneumonia in the United States.

If your pneumonia is caused by one of the following types of bacteria, it is called "atypical pneumonia."

- *Legionella pneumophila.* This type of pneumonia sometimes is called "Legionnaires' disease," and it has caused serious outbreaks. Outbreaks have been linked to exposure to cooling towers, whirlpool spas, and decorative fountains.

- *Mycoplasma pneumoniae.* This is a common type of pneumonia that usually affects people younger than 40 years of age. People who live or work in crowded places, such as schools, homeless shelters, and prisons, are at higher risk for this type of pneumonia. It is usually mild and responds well to treatment with antibiotics. However, *Mycoplasma pneumoniae* can be very serious. It may be associated with a skin rash and hemolysis. This type of bacteria is a common cause of "walking pneumonia."

- *Chlamydia pneumoniae.* This type of pneumonia can occur all year and often is mild. The infection is most common in people between 65 and 79 years of age.

Bacterial pneumonia can occur on its own or develop after you have had a viral cold or the flu. Bacterial pneumonia often affects just one lobe, or area, of a lung. When this happens, the condition is called "lobar pneumonia."

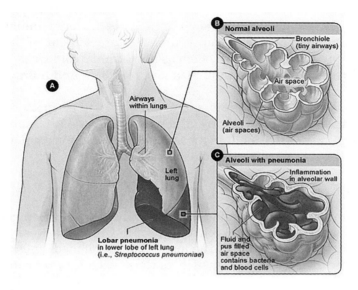

Figure 42.1. *Lobar Bacterial Pneumonia*

This figure shows pneumonia affecting the single lower lobe of the left lung. Figure A shows the location of the lungs and airways in the body. Figure B shows normal alveoli. Figure C shows infected alveoli or air sacs.

Most of the time, the body filters bacteria out of the air that we breathe to protect the lungs from infection. Your immune system; the shape of your nose and throat; your ability to cough; and fine, hair-like structures called "cilia" help stop the germs from reaching your lungs.

Sometimes, bacteria manage to enter the lungs and cause infections. This is more likely to occur if:

- Your immune system is weak.

- A germ is very strong.

- Your body fails to filter out the bacteria from the air that you breathe. For example, if you cannot cough because you have had a stroke or are sedated, bacteria may remain in your airways.

When bacteria reach your lungs, your immune system goes into action. It sends many kinds of cells to attack the bacteria. These cells cause inflammation in alveoli (air sacs) and can cause these spaces to fill up with fluid and pus. This causes the symptoms of pneumonia.

Virus

Viruses that infect the respiratory tract may cause pneumonia. Influenza, or flu virus, is the most common cause of viral pneumonia in adults. Respiratory syncytial virus (RSV) is the most common cause of viral pneumonia in children younger than one year of age. Other viruses can cause pneumonia, such as the common cold virus known as "rhinovirus," human parainfluenza virus (HPIV), and human metapneumovirus (HMPV).

Most cases of viral pneumonia are mild. They get better in about one to three weeks without treatment. Some cases are more serious and may require treatment in a hospital. If you have viral pneumonia, you run the risk of getting bacterial pneumonia.

Fungi

Pneumocystis pneumonia is a serious fungal infection caused by *Pneumocystis jirovecii*. It occurs in people who have weak immune systems due to HIV/AIDS or the long-term use of medicines that suppress their immune systems, such as those used to treat cancer or as part of organ or blood and marrow stem cell transplant procedures.

Other fungal infections also can lead to pneumonia. The following are three fungi that occur in the soil in some parts of the United States and can cause some people to get pneumonia.

- **Coccidioidomycosis.** This fungus is found in Southern California and the desert Southwest. It is the cause of valley fever.

- **Histoplasmosis.** This fungus is found in the Ohio and Mississippi River Valleys.

- **Cryptococcus.** This fungus is found throughout the United States in bird droppings and soil contaminated with bird droppings.

Risk Factors of Pneumonia

Many factors, such as age, smoking, and other medical conditions, can increase your chances of getting pneumonia and having more severe pneumonia.

Age

Pneumonia can affect people of all ages. However, two age groups are at a greater risk of developing pneumonia and having more severe pneumonia:

- Infants who are 2 years of age or younger because their immune systems are still developing during the first few years of life.

- People who are 65 years of age or older because their immune systems begin to change as a normal part of aging.

Environment

Your risk for pneumonia may increase if you have been exposed to certain chemicals, pollutants, or toxic fumes.

Lifestyle Habits

Smoking cigarettes, excessive use of alcohol, or being undernourished also increases your risk for pneumonia.

Other Medical Conditions

Other conditions and factors also increase your risk of pneumonia. Your risk also goes up if you:

- Have trouble coughing because of a stroke or other condition, or have problems swallowing

- Cannot move around much or are sedated

- Recently had a cold or the flu

- Have a lung disease or other serious disease, including cystic fibrosis, asthma, COPD, bronchiectasis, diabetes, heart failure, or sickle cell disease (SCD)

- Are in a hospital intensive-care unit (ICU), especially if you using a ventilator to help you breathe

- Have a weak or suppressed immune system due to HIV/AIDS, organ transplant or blood and marrow stem cell transplant, chemotherapy, or long-term steroid use

Screening and Prevention of Pneumonia

Pneumonia can be very serious and even life-threatening. Vaccines can help prevent certain types of pneumonia. Practicing good hygiene, quitting smoking, and keeping your immune system strong by exercising and healthy eating are other ways to prevent pneumonia.

Vaccines

Vaccines are available to prevent pneumonia caused by pneumococcal bacteria or the flu virus. Vaccines cannot prevent all cases of infection. However, compared to people who do not get vaccinated, those who are vaccinated and still get pneumonia tend to have:

- Milder infections
- Pneumonia that does not last as long
- Fewer serious complications

Pneumococcal Pneumonia Vaccines

Two vaccines are available to prevent pneumococcal pneumonia and potentially fatal complications, such as bacteremia and meningitis. Pneumococcal vaccines are particularly important for:

- Adults who are 65 years of age or older
- People who have chronic (ongoing) diseases, serious long-term health problems, or weak immune systems. For example, this may include people who have cancer, HIV/AIDS, asthma, sickle cell disease, or damaged or removed spleens.
- People who smoke
- Children who are younger than 5 years of age
- Children older than 5 years of age with certain medical conditions, such as heart or lung diseases or cancer

The Centers for Disease Control and Prevention (CDC) recommends that adults who are 65 years of age and older should have 2 pneumococcal vaccinations.

Influenza Vaccine

Because many people get pneumonia after having influenza or the flu, your yearly flu vaccine can help you and your family not get pneumonia. The flu vaccine is usually given in September through November before the months when influenza or the flu is most frequently spread.

Haemophilus Influenzae *Type B Vaccine*

Haemophilus influenzae type b (Hib) is a type of bacteria that can cause pneumonia and meningitis. The Hib vaccine is given to children to help prevent these infections. The vaccine is recommended for all children in the United States who are younger than five years of age. The vaccine often is given to infants starting at two months of age.

Other Ways to Help Prevent Pneumonia

You also can take the following steps to help prevent pneumonia:

- **Wash your hands** with soap and water or alcohol-based rubs to kill germs.

- **Do not smoke.** Smoking damages your lungs' ability to filter out and defend against germs.

- **Keep your immune system strong.** Get plenty of rest and physical activity, and follow a healthy diet.

Signs, Symptoms, and Complications of Pneumonia

The signs and symptoms of pneumonia vary from mild to severe. But, some people are at risk for developing more severe pneumonia or potentially fatal complications.

Signs and Symptoms

See your doctor promptly if you have the following signs and symptoms:

- Have a high fever
- Have shaking chills
- Have a cough with phlegm, which does not improve or worsens
- Develop shortness of breath with normal daily activities
- Have chest pain when you breathe or cough
- Feel suddenly worse after a cold or the flu

If you have pneumonia, you also may have other symptoms, including nausea (feeling sick to the stomach), vomiting, and diarrhea.

Symptoms may vary in certain populations. Newborns and infants may not show any signs of the infection. Or, they may vomit; have a fever and cough; or appear restless, sick, or tired and without energy.

Older adults and people who have serious illnesses or weak immune systems may have fewer and milder symptoms. They may even have a lower-than-normal temperature. If they already have a lung disease, it may get worse. Older adults who have pneumonia sometimes have sudden changes in mental awareness.

Complications

Often, people who have pneumonia can be successfully treated and do not have complications. Possible complications of pneumonia may include:

- **Bacteremia and septic shock.** Bacteremia is a serious complication in which bacteria from the initial site of infection spread into the blood. It may lead to septic shock, a potentially fatal complication.

- **Lung abscesses.** Lung abscesses usually are treated with antibiotics. Sometimes surgery or drainage with a needle is needed to remove the pus.

- **Pleural effusions, empyema, and pleurisy.** These painful or even potentially fatal complications can occur if pneumonia is not treated. The pleura is a membrane that consists of two large, thin layers of tissue. One layer wraps around the outside of your lungs, and the other layer lines the inside of your chest cavity. Pleurisy is when the two layers of the pleura become irritated and inflamed, causing sharp pain each time you breathe in. The pleural space is a very thin space between the two pleura. Pleural effusions are the buildup of fluid in the pleural space. If the fluid becomes infected, it is called "empyema." If this happens, you may need to have the fluid drained through a chest tube or removed with surgery.

- **Renal failure**

- **Respiratory failure**

Diagnosis of Pneumonia

Sometimes pneumonia is hard to diagnose because it may cause symptoms commonly seen in people with colds or the flu. You may not realize it is more serious until it lasts longer than these other conditions. Your doctor will diagnose pneumonia based on your medical history, a physical exam, and test results. Your doctor may be able to diagnose you with a certain type of pneumonia based on how you got your infection and the type of germ causing your infection.

Medical History

Your doctor will ask about your signs and symptoms and how and when they began. To find out whether you have bacterial, viral, or fungal pneumonia, your doctor also may ask about:

- Any recent traveling you have done
- Your hobbies
- Your exposure to animals
- Your exposure to sick people at home, school, or work
- Your past and current medical conditions, and whether any have gotten worse recently
- Any medicines you take
- Whether you smoke
- Whether you have had flu or pneumonia vaccinations

Physical Exam

Your doctor will listen to your lungs with a stethoscope. If you have pneumonia, your lungs may make crackling, bubbling, and rumbling sounds when you inhale. Your doctor also may hear wheezing. Your doctor may find it hard to hear sounds of breathing in some areas of your chest.

Diagnostic Tests

If your doctor thinks you have pneumonia, she or he may recommend one or more of the following tests.

- **Chest X-ray** to look for inflammation in your lungs. A chest X-ray is the best test for diagnosing pneumonia. However, this test would not tell your doctor what kind of germ is causing pneumonia.
- **Blood tests**, such as a complete blood count (CBC), to see if your immune system is actively fighting an infection.
- **Blood culture** to find out whether you have a bacterial infection that has spread to your bloodstream. If so, your doctor can decide how to treat the infection.

Your doctor may recommend other tests if you are in the hospital, have serious symptoms, are older, or have other health problems.

315

- **Sputum test**. Your doctor may collect a sample of sputum (spit) or phlegm that was produced from one of your deep coughs and send the sample to the lab for testing. This may help your doctor find out if bacteria are causing your pneumonia. Then, she or he can plan your treatment.

- **Chest computed tomography (CT) scan** to see how much of your lungs is affected by your condition or to see if you have complications, such as lung abscesses or pleural effusions. A CT scan shows more detail than a chest X-ray.

- **Pleural fluid culture**. For this test, a fluid sample is taken from the pleural space (a thin space between two layers of tissue that line the lungs and chest cavity). Doctors use a procedure called "thoracentesis" to collect the fluid sample. The fluid is studied for bacteria that may cause pneumonia.

- **Pulse oximetry**. For this test, a small sensor is attached to your finger or ear. The sensor uses light to estimate how much oxygen is in your blood. Pneumonia can keep your lungs from moving enough oxygen into your bloodstream. If you are very sick, your doctor may need to measure the level of oxygen in your blood using a blood sample. The sample is taken from an artery, usually in your wrist. This test is called an "arterial blood gas (ABG) test"

- **Bronchoscopy** is a procedure used to look inside the lungs' airways. If you are in the hospital and treatment with antibiotics is not working well, your doctor may use this procedure. Your doctor passes a thin, flexible tube through your nose or mouth, down your throat, and into the airways. The tube has a light and small camera that allow your doctor to see your windpipe and airways and take pictures. Your doctor can see whether something is blocking your airways or whether another factor is contributing to your pneumonia. Your doctor may use this procedure to collect samples of fluid from the site of pneumonia (called "bronchoalveolar lavage" (BAL)) or to take small biopsies of lung tissue to help find the cause of your pneumonia.

Types of Pneumonia

Your doctor may also diagnose you with a certain type of pneumonia. Pneumonia is named for the way in which a person gets the infection or for the germ that causes the infection.

- **Community-acquired pneumonia (CAP)** is the most common type of pneumonia and is usually caused by pneumococcus bacteria. Most cases occur during the winter. CAP occurs outside of hospitals and other healthcare settings. Most people get CAP by breathing in germs (especially while sleeping) that live in the mouth, nose, or throat.

- **Hospital-acquired pneumonia (HAP)** is when people catch pneumonia during a hospital stay for another illness. HAP tends to be more serious than the CAP because you are already sick. Also, hospitals tend to have more germs that are resistant to antibiotics that are used to treat bacterial pneumonia.

- **Ventilator-associated pneumonia (VAP)** is when people who are on a ventilator machine to help them breathe get pneumonia.

- **Atypical pneumonia** is a type of CAP. It is caused by lung infections with less common bacteria than the pneumococcus bacteria that cause CAP. Atypical bacteria include *Legionella pneumophila*, *Mycoplasma pneumoniae*, or *Chlamydia pneumoniae*.

- **Aspiration pneumonia** can occur if you inhale food, drink, vomit, or saliva from your mouth into your lungs. This may happen if something disturbs your normal gag reflex, such as a brain injury, swallowing problem, or excessive use of alcohol or drugs. Aspiration pneumonia can cause lung abscesses.

Treatment of Pneumonia

Treatment for pneumonia depends on the type of pneumonia you have, the germ causing your infection, and how severe your pneumonia is. Most people who have community-acquired pneumonia—the most common type of pneumonia—are treated at home. The goals of treatment are to cure the infection and prevent complications.

Bacterial Pneumonia

Bacterial pneumonia is treated with medicines called "antibiotics." You should take antibiotics as your doctor prescribes. You may start to feel better before you finish the medicine, but you should continue taking it as prescribed. If you stop too soon, pneumonia may come back.

317

Most people begin to improve after one to three days of antibiotic treatment. This means that they should feel better and have fewer symptoms, such as cough and fever.

Viral Pneumonia

Antibiotics do not work when the cause of pneumonia is a virus. If you have viral pneumonia, your doctor may prescribe an antiviral medicine to treat it. Viral pneumonia usually improves in one to three weeks.

Treating Severe Symptoms

You may need to be treated in a hospital if:

- Your symptoms are severe.

- You are at risk for complications because of other health problems.

If the level of oxygen in your bloodstream is low, you may receive oxygen therapy. If you have bacterial pneumonia, your doctor may give you antibiotics through an intravenous (IV) line inserted into a vein.

General Treatment Advice and Follow-Up Care

If you have pneumonia, follow your treatment plan, take all medicines as prescribed, and get follow-up medical care.

Living with Pneumonia

If you have pneumonia, you can take steps to recover from the infection and prevent complications.

- Get plenty of rest.

- Follow your treatment plan as your doctor advises.

- Take all medicines as your doctor prescribes. If you are using antibiotics, continue to take the medicine until it is all gone. You may start to feel better before you finish the medicine, but you should continue to take it. If you stop too soon, the bacterial infection and your pneumonia may come back.

- Ask your doctor when you should schedule follow-up care. Your doctor may recommend a chest X-ray to make sure the infection is gone.

It may take time to recover from pneumonia. Some people feel better and are able to return to their normal routines within a week. For other people, it can take a month or more. Most people continue to feel tired for about a month. Talk with your doctor about when you can go back to your normal routine.

If you have pneumonia, limit contact with family and friends. Cover your nose and mouth while coughing or sneezing, get rid of used tissues right away, and wash your hands. These actions help keep the infection from spreading to other people.

Chapter 43

Shigellosis

Shigellosis is an infectious disease caused by a group of bacteria called *"Shigella."* Most who are infected with *Shigella* develop diarrhea, fever, and stomach cramps starting a day or two after they are exposed to the bacteria. Shigellosis usually resolves in five to seven days. Some people who are infected may have no symptoms at all, but they may still pass the *Shigella* bacteria to others. The spread of *Shigella* can be stopped by frequent and careful handwashing with soap and taking other hygiene measures.

Symptoms of Shigellosis

People who are sick from *Shigella* infection usually start experiencing symptoms one to two days after contact with the germ. Symptoms of shigellosis include:

- Diarrhea (sometimes bloody)
- Fever
- Stomach pain
- Feeling the need to pass stool even when the bowels are empty

Some people with shigellosis will not have any symptoms.

This chapter includes text excerpted from *"Shigella*—Shigellosis," Centers for Disease Control and Prevention (CDC), January 17, 2018.

Symptoms usually last five to seven days, but some people may experience symptoms anywhere from a few days to four or more weeks. In some cases, it may take several months before bowel habits (for example, how often someone passes stool and the consistency of their stool) are entirely normal.

When to Contact Your Doctor

People with diarrhea should contact their healthcare provider if they have any of these symptoms:

- Fever

- Bloody diarrhea

- Severe stomach cramping or tenderness

- Dehydrated

- Feel very sick

People who are in poor health or who have immune systems weakened from diseases, such as human immunodeficiency virus (HIV)/acquired immunodeficiency syndrome (AIDS) or chemotherapy for cancer, are more likely to get sick for a longer period of time if they have shigellosis. They should contact their healthcare provider if they think they have shigellosis to determine the best course of treatment.

Sources of Infection and Risk Factors

People who are sick with shigellosis have *Shigella* germs in their stool while they have diarrhea and for up to a week or two after diarrhea has gone away. *Shigella* is very contagious; just a small amount of germs can make someone sick. People could get sick by:

- Getting *Shigella* germs on their hands and then touching their food or mouth. This may happen after:

  - Touching surfaces contaminated with germs from stool from a sick person, such as toys, bathroom fixtures, changing tables or diaper pails

  - Changing the diaper of a sick child or caring for a sick person

- Eating food that was prepared by someone who is sick with shigellosis

- Foods that are consumed raw are more likely to be contaminated with *Shigella* germs.

- *Shigella* germs can contaminate fruits and vegetables if the fields where they grow contain human waste.

- Swallowing recreational water (for example, lake or river water) while swimming or drinking water that is contaminated with stool containing the germ

- Having exposure to stool during sexual contact with someone who is sick or recent (several weeks) recovered from shigellosis

Groups of People Who Are Most Likely to Get Shigellosis

- Young children are the most likely to get shigellosis, but people of all ages can get this disease. Many outbreaks are related to child care settings and schools. Illness commonly spreads from young children to their family members and others in their communities because it is so contagious.

- Travelers to developing countries may be more likely to get shigellosis, and to become infected with strains of *Shigella* bacteria that cannot be treated effectively by important antibiotics. Travelers may get sick from food, drinking water, recreational water, and surfaces containing *Shigella* germs. Travelers can protect themselves by sticking to safe eating and drinking habits, and washing their hands often with soap and water.

- Gay or bisexual men and other men who have sex with men are more likely to get shigellosis than other adults. *Shigella* germs pass from stools or soiled fingers of one person to the mouth of another person, which can happen during sexual activity. Many shigellosis outbreaks among gay and bisexual men have been reported in the United States, Canada, Tokyo, and Europe since 1999.

- People whose immune systems are weakened due to illness (such as human immunodeficiency virus (HIV)) or medical treatment (such as chemotherapy for cancer) can get a more serious illness. A severe shigellosis illness may involve the infection spreading into the blood, which can be life-threatening.

- Large outbreaks of shigellosis often start in child care settings and spread among small social groups, such as in traditionally

323

observant Jewish communities. Similar outbreaks could occur among any race, ethnicity, or community social circle because *Shigella* germs can spread easily from one person to another.

Diagnosis of Shigellosis

Many kinds of germs can cause diarrhea. Knowing which germ is causing an illness is important to help guide appropriate treatment. Healthcare providers can order laboratory tests to identify *Shigella* germs in the stool of someone who is sick.

Treatment of Shigellosis

Most people will recover from shigellosis without treatment in five to seven days. People who have shigellosis should drink plenty of fluids to prevent dehydration. Contact your healthcare provider if you or one of your family members have a fever, bloody diarrhea, severe stomach cramping or tenderness; are dehydrated; or feel very sick. People who are in poor health or who have weakened immune systems, such as from HIV/AIDS or chemotherapy treatment for cancer, also should contact their healthcare provider because they are more likely to get sick for a longer period of time.

- In some people, bismuth subsalicylate (for example, Pepto-Bismol) can help to relieve symptoms.

- People with shigellosis should not use antidiarrheal medication, such as loperamide (for example, Imodium) or diphenoxylate with atropine (for example, Lomotil). These medications may make symptoms worse.

- Healthcare providers may prescribe antibiotics for some people who have severe cases of shigellosis. Antibiotics, such as ciprofloxacin (common treatment for adults), and azithromycin (common treatment for children), are useful for severe cases of shigellosis because they can help people get better faster. However, some antibiotics are not effective against certain types of *Shigella* bacteria. Healthcare providers can order laboratory tests to determine which antibiotics are likely to work.

People who have shigellosis should follow their healthcare provider's advice. If your healthcare provider prescribes antibiotics, let them know if you do not get better within a couple of days after starting the medication. They can do more tests to learn whether your type of

Shigella bacteria can be treated effectively with the antibiotic you are taking. If not, your doctor may prescribe another type of antibiotic.

Prevention of Shigellosis

Shigella germs spread easily from one person to another; just a small amount of *Shigella* germs can make someone sick. Understanding how to prevent the spread of *Shigella* germs can help you protect yourself and your loved ones from getting sick.

How Can I Avoid Getting Sick from Shigella Bacteria?

People usually get sick from *Shigella* bacteria after putting something in their mouth or swallowing something that has come into contact with the stool of someone else who is sick from *Shigella* bacteria. There is no vaccine to prevent shigellosis. However, you can reduce your chance of getting shigellosis by:

- Carefully washing your hands with soap and water during key times:
  - Before eating or preparing food for others
  - After changing a diaper or helping to clean another person who went to the bathroom
- If you care for a child in diapers who has shigellosis, promptly throw away soiled diapers in a covered, lined garbage can. Wash your hands and the child's hands carefully with soap and water immediately after changing the diapers. Clean up any leaks or spills of diaper contents immediately.
- Avoid swallowing water from ponds, lakes, or untreated swimming pools.
- When traveling internationally, follow safe food and water guidelines and wash your hands often with soap and water.
- Avoid sexual activity with those who have diarrhea or who recently (several weeks) recovered from shigellosis.

If you are sick with shigellosis you can prevent others from getting sick by:

- Washing your hands often, especially
- Before preparing food or eating

- After using the bathroom or changing diapers

- Not preparing food if you are sick

- Not sharing food with anyone if you or your family members are sick

- Not swimming

- Not having sex (vaginal, anal, and oral) for one week after you no longer have diarrhea. Because *Shigella* germs may be in the stool for several weeks, follow safe sexual practices, or ideally avoid having sex, for several weeks after you have recovered.

- Staying home from school or from healthcare, food service, or child care jobs while sick or until your health department says it is safe to return

Chapter 44

Staph Infections: Group A

Chapter Contents

Section 44.1—Staphylococcal Infections.................................... 328

Section 44.2—*Staphylococcus aureus* and Pregnancy 331

Section 44.3—Vancomycin-Intermediate/Resistance
Staphylococcus aureus 335

Section 44.1

Staphylococcal Infections

This section includes text excerpted from "Staphylococcal Infections," MedlinePlus, National Institutes of Health (NIH), August 25, 2016.

What Are Staphylococcal (Staph) Infections?

Staphylococcus (staph) is a group of bacteria. There are more than 30 types. A type called "*Staphylococcus aureus*" causes most infections.

Staph bacteria can cause many different types of infections, including:

- Skin infections, which are the most common types of staph infections

- Bacteremia, an infection of the bloodstream. This can lead to sepsis, a very serious immune response to infection.

- Bone infections

- Endocarditis, an infection of the inner lining of the heart chambers and valves

- Food poisoning

- Pneumonia

- Toxic shock syndrome (TSS), a life-threatening condition caused by toxins from certain types of bacteria

What Causes Staph Infections

Some people carry staph bacteria on their skin or in their noses, but they do not get an infection. But if they get a cut or wound, the bacteria can enter the body and cause an infection.

Staph bacteria can spread from person-to-person. They can also spread on objects, such as towels, clothing, door handles, athletic equipment, and remotes. If you have staph and do not handle food properly when you are preparing it, you can also spread staph to others.

Who Is at Risk for Staph Infections?

Anyone can develop a staph infection, but certain people are at a greater risk, including those who:

- Have a chronic condition, such as diabetes, cancer, vascular disease, eczema, and lung disease

- Have a weakened immune system, such as from human immunodeficiency virus/acquired immunodeficiency syndrome (HIV/AIDS), medicines to prevent organ rejection, or chemotherapy

- Had surgery

- Use a catheter, breathing tube, or feeding tube

- Are on dialysis

- Inject illegal drugs

- Do contact sports, since you may have skin-to-skin contact with others or share equipment

What Are the Symptoms of Staph Infections?

The symptoms of a staph infection depend on the type of infection:

- Skin infections can look like pimples or boils. They may be red, swollen, and painful. Sometimes there is pus or other drainages. They can turn into impetigo, which turns into a crust on the skin, or cellulitis, a swollen, red area of skin that feels hot.

- Bone infections can cause pain, swelling, warmth, and redness in the infected area. You may also have chills and fever.

- Endocarditis causes some flu-like symptoms, including fever, chills, and fatigue. It also causes symptoms, such as rapid heartbeat, shortness of breath, and fluid buildup in your arms or legs.

- Food poisoning typically causes nausea and vomiting, diarrhea, and fever. If you lose too many fluids, you may also become dehydrated.

- Pneumonia symptoms include high fever, chills, and a cough that does not get better. You may also have chest pain and shortness of breath.

- Toxic shock syndrome causes high fever, sudden low blood pressure, vomiting, diarrhea, and confusion. You may have a sunburn-like rash somewhere on your body. TSS can lead to organ failure.

How Are Staph Infections Diagnosed?

Your healthcare provider will do a physical exam and ask about your symptoms. Often, providers can tell if you have a staph skin infection by looking at it. To check for other types of staph infections, providers may do a culture, with a skin scraping, tissue sample, stool sample, or throat or nasal swabs. There may be other tests, such as imaging tests, depending on the type of infection.

What Are the Treatments for Staph Infections?

Treatment for staph infections is antibiotics. Depending on the type of infection, you may get a cream, ointment, medicines (to swallow), or intravenous (IV). If you have an infected wound, your provider might drain it. Sometimes you may need surgery for bone infections.

Some staph infections, such as methicillin-resistant *Staphylococcus aureus* (MRSA), are resistant to many antibiotics. There are still certain antibiotics that can treat these infections.

Can Staph Infections Be Prevented?

Certain steps can help to prevent staph infections:

- Practice good hygiene, including washing your hands often.
- Do not share towels, sheets, or clothing with someone who has a staph infection.
- It is best not to share athletic equipment. If you do need to share, make sure that it properly cleaned and dried before you use it.
- Practice food safety, including not preparing food for others when you have a staph infection.
- If you have a cut or wound, keep it covered.

Section 44.2

Staphylococcus aureus *and Pregnancy*

"*Staphylococcus aureus* and Pregnancy,"
© 2017 Omnigraphics. Reviewed July 2019.

Staphylococcus aureus

Staphylococcus aureus is a type of bacteria that causes a condition known as staph infection. These bacteria are usually found on the surface of the skin or in the nasal passages and ears of even a healthy person and do not generally cause any harm. But an infection can occur if the skin is cut or wounded and the bacteria enter the wound, making it inflamed, red, and painful. These bacteria are quite hardy in nature and can survive for some time on hard surfaces, withstanding dryness, high levels of salt, and extremes of temperature until a person comes in contact with them. Approximately 500,000 patients in American hospitals are affected annually by *Staphylococcus*, making it one of the primary causes of infection after injury or surgery.

Symptoms of Staph Infection

Staph infection often affects the skin, in which case some of its symptoms include:

- Large blisters that ooze fluids (impetigo)
- Redness and swelling in layers of skin (cellulitis)
- Abscesses on the skin

Staph infection can also be transmitted through food. The symptoms in such cases include:

- Nausea and vomiting
- Dehydration
- Low blood pressure
- Diarrhea

Severe symptoms may occur when the bacteria enter the bloodstream.

Toxins produced by strains of staph bacteria may develop such symptoms as:

- High fever
- Low blood pressure
- Rashes on the palms and soles
- Muscle aches
- Abdominal pain
- Diarrhea
- Confusion

Staph infection may also cause coughing because of infection in the lungs (pneumonia).

Treatment for Staph Infection

Staph infection is treated mainly with antibiotics, such as methicillin, penicillin, oxacillin, and amoxicillin. For staph skin infection, treatment would likely also include draining the abscesses.

Methicillin-Resistant Staphylococcus aureus

Methicillin-resistant *Staphylococcus aureus* (MRSA) is a variant that resists the antibiotic methicillin. Improper or overuse of antibiotics can increase the chances of MRSA bacteria developing. It is more difficult to treat than normal staph bacteria since commonly used antibiotics for staph infection may not work for MRSA infection.

Transmission of Methicillin-Resistant Staphylococcus aureus

MRSA, which in recent years has become a major health concern, is transmitted through physical contact or by touching objects that carry the bacteria. It is generally classified into two types:

- **Hospital-Acquired Methicillin-resistant *Staphylococcus aureus* (HA-MRSA).** HA-MRSA primarily affects people who are in hospitals, nursing homes, or other medical care facilities. People who are most prone to getting HA-MRSA are the elderly, people with compromised immune systems, those who have undergone recent surgery, or people undergoing kidney dialysis or using venous catheters or prosthetics. Studies suggest that at least one percent of in-patients contract HA-MRSA.

- **Community-Associated Methicillin-resistant *Staphylococcus aureus* (CA-MRSA).** CA-MRSA has posed great threats to public health. The CA-MRSA often cannot be traced back to a specific place of origin, unlike the case with HA-MRSA, which is specific to healthcare settings. It tends to spread in overpopulated and unhygienic places, by physical touch or by sharing equipment or personal items. CA-MRSA can be more severe in children, as their immune systems are not fully developed. If a child's skin is infected because of insect-bite, cuts, or scrapes, a doctor needs to be consulted.

Treatment for Methicillin-Resistant Staphylococcus aureus Infection

Methicillin-resistant *Staphylococcus aureus* (MRSA) is not resistant to all antibiotics. Similar to any staph infection, MRSA may be treated with medication and by the draining of any boils by a healthcare provider. Antibiotics that may be prescribed include clindamycin, tetracycline, doxycycline, trimethoprim-sulfamethoxazole, linezolid, vancomycin, and ciprofloxacin.

Staph or Methicillin-Resistant Staphylococcus aureus Infection and Pregnancy

Reports suggest that staph or MRSA infections have very low probability of affecting an unborn child. However, these bacteria can make a pregnant woman more susceptible to other infections, so treatment is important to ensure a safer pregnancy.

If infected with staph or MRSA during pregnancy, a healthcare provider should be consulted. For staph infection, certain antibiotics may be prescribed, and for MRSA infection, in which antibiotics do not work, or for people allergic to these medications, other treatments may be recommended by the doctor. If the prescribed antibiotics result in symptoms like rashes, hives, or diarrhea, a healthcare provider must be contacted immediately.

Staph or Methicillin-Resistant Staphylococcus aureus *Infection While Breastfeeding*

If either a mother or child is infected with staph or MRSA, it is possible to transmit the infection whenever they come in contact with each other, including during breastfeeding. While a baby is breastfed, the bacteria in its nasal passages can spread to the mother, and that could cause mastitis (breast infection), especially if she has some nipple damage. Bacteria can also be spread to the baby through pumped breast milk if it is stored in contaminated containers or by using unsterilized pumping equipment. Hence, a thorough cleaning of storage containers and pumping materials is crucial to help prevent the infection.

Prevention of Staph or Methicillin-Resistant Staphylococcus aureus *Infection*

Practicing good hygiene is the best way to prevent staph or MRSA infection:

- Wash hands regularly with soap and water. After washing, wipe them dry with a clean towel or napkin. And it is always a good idea to use a hand sanitizer regularly.

- Take regular showers to help decrease the risk of infection.

- Do not share personal items, such as razors, towels, bedsheets, clothes, and sports equipment. Avoid touching other people's wounds and bandages.

- Regularly wash clothes, towels, and sheets, and dry them in the sun or hot dryer to destroy bacteria.

References

1. "Methicillin-Resistant *Staphylococcus aureus* (MRSA)," National Institute of Allergy and Infectious Diseases (NIAID), February 18, 2009.

2. "*Staphylococcus aureus* and Pregnancy," Organization of Teratology and Information Specialists, October 2007.

3. Davis, Charles Patrick. "Methicillin-Resistant *Staphylococcus aureus* (MRSA)," eMedicineHealth.com, January 20, 2016.

4. Mandal, Ananya. "What Is *Staphylococcus aureus*?" News Medical, December 9, 2012

5. Bernstein, Lisa. "Understanding MRSA Infection—The Basics," WebMD, March 18, 2015

6. "Staph Infections," Mayo Clinic, June 11, 2014.

7. Reichstetter. Sandra. "Staph Infection and Pregnancy" SteadyHealth, n.d.

Section 44.3

Vancomycin-Intermediate/Resistance Staphylococcus aureus

This section includes text excerpted from "VISA/VRSA in Healthcare Settings," Centers for Disease Control and Prevention (CDC), November 24, 2010. Reviewed July 2019.

Vancomycin-intermediate *Staphylococcus aureus* (VISA) and vancomycin-resistant *Staphylococcus aureus* (VRSA) are specific types of antimicrobial-resistant bacteria. However, as of October 2010, all VISA and VRSA isolates have been susceptible to other U.S. Food and Drug Administration (FDA)-approved drugs. Persons who develop this type of staph infection may have underlying health conditions (such as diabetes and kidney disease), tubes going into their bodies (such as catheters), previous infections with methicillin-resistant *Staphylococcus aureus* (MRSA), and recent exposure to vancomycin and other antimicrobial agents.

What Is Staphylococcus aureus?

Staphylococcus aureus is a bacterium commonly found on the skin and in the nose of about 30 percent of individuals. Most of the time, staph does not cause any harm. These infections can look like pimples, boils, or other skin conditions, and most are able to be treated. Sometimes, staph bacteria can get into the bloodstream and cause serious infections which can be fatal, including:

- Bacteremia or sepsis when bacteria spread to the bloodstream, usually as a result of using catheters or having surgery

335

- Pneumonia, which predominantly affects people with underlying lung disease, including those on mechanical ventilators

- Endocarditis (infection of the heart valves), which can lead to heart failure.

- Osteomyelitis (bone infection), which can be caused by staph bacteria traveling in the bloodstream or put there by direct contact, such as following trauma (puncture wound of the foot or intravenous (IV) drug abuse)

Commonly Asked Questions about Vancomycin-Intermediate/Resistance Staphylococcus aureus

How Do Vancomycin-Intermediate Staphylococcus aureus and Vancomycin-Resistant Staphylococcus aureus Get Their Names?

Staph bacteria are classified as VISA or VRSA based on laboratory tests. Laboratories perform tests to determine if staph bacteria are resistant to antimicrobial agents that might be used for the treatment of infections. For vancomycin and other antimicrobial agents, laboratories determine how much of the agent it requires to inhibit the growth of the organism in a test tube. The result of the test is usually expressed as a minimum inhibitory concentration (MIC) or the minimum amount of antimicrobial agent that inhibits bacterial growth in the test tube. Therefore, staph bacteria are classified as VISA if the MIC for vancomycin is 4 to $8\mu g/ml$, and it is classified as VRSA if the vancomycin MIC is greater than $16\mu g/ml$.

Are Vancomycin-Intermediate Staphylococcus aureus and Vancomycin-Resistant Staphylococcus aureus Infections Treatable?

Yes. As of October 2010, all VISA and VRSA isolates have been susceptible to several FDA-approved drugs.

How Can the Spread of Vancomycin-Intermediate Staphylococcus aureus and Vancomycin-Resistant Staphylococcus aureus Be Prevented?

Use of appropriate infection control practices (such as wearing gloves before and after contact with infectious body substances and adherence to hand hygiene) by healthcare personnel can reduce the spread of VISA and VRSA.

What Should a Person Do If a Family Member or Close Friend Has Vancomycin-Intermediate Staphylococcus aureus or Vancomycin-Resistant Staphylococcus aureus?

VISA and VRSA are types of antibiotic-resistant staph bacteria. Therefore, as with all staph bacteria, spread occurs among people having close physical contact with infected patients or contaminated material, such as bandages. Persons having close physical contact with infected patients while they are outside of the healthcare setting should keep their hands clean by washing thoroughly with soap and water, and they should avoid contact with other people's wounds or material contaminated from wounds. If they go to the hospital to visit a friend or family member who is infected with VISA or VRSA, they must follow the hospital's recommended precautions.

What Is Centers for Disease Control and Prevention Doing to Address Vancomycin-Intermediate Staphylococcus aureus and Vancomycin-Resistant Staphylococcus aureus?

In addition to providing guidance for clinicians and infection control personnel, the Centers for Disease Control and Prevention (CDC) is also working with state and local health agencies, healthcare facilities, and clinical microbiology laboratories to ensure that laboratories are using proper methods to detect VISA and VRSA.

Chapter 45

Streptococcal Infections: Group A

Chapter Contents

Section 45.1—Strep Throat 340

Section 45.2—Scarlet Fever 344

Section 45.1

Strep Throat

This section includes text excerpted from "Strep Throat:
All You Need to Know," Centers for Disease Control
and Prevention (CDC), November 1, 2018.

Bacteria Cause Strep Throat

Viruses are the most common cause of a sore throat. However, strep throat is an infection in the throat and tonsils caused by bacteria called "group A *Streptococcus*" (group A strep).

How You Get Strep Throat

Group A strep live in the nose and throat, and it can easily spread to other people. It is important to know that all infected people do not have symptoms or seem sick. People who are infected spread the bacteria by coughing or sneezing, which creates small respiratory droplets that contain the bacteria.

People can get sick if they:

- Breathe in those droplets

- Touch something with droplets on it and then touch their mouth or nose

- Drink from the same glass or eat from the same plate as a sick person

- Touch sores on the skin caused by group A strep (impetigo)

Rarely, people can spread group A strep through food that is not handled properly. Experts do not believe pets or household items, such as toys, spread these bacteria.

Pain and Fever without a Cough Are Common Signs and Symptoms

In general, strep throat is a mild infection, but it can be very painful. The most common symptoms of strep throat include:

- Sore throat that can start very quickly

- Pain when swallowing

- Fever

- Red and swollen tonsils, sometimes with white patches or streaks of pus

- Tiny, red spots (petechiae) on the roof of the mouth (the soft or hard palate)

- Swollen lymph nodes in the front of the neck

Other symptoms may include a headache, stomach pain, nausea, or vomiting—especially in children. Someone with strep throat may also have a rash known as "scarlet fever" (also called "scarlatina").

The following symptoms suggest that a virus is the cause of the illness instead of strep throat:

- Cough

- Runny nose

- Hoarseness (changes in your voice that make it sound breathy, raspy, or strained)

- Conjunctivitis (also called "pink eye")

It usually takes two to five days for someone exposed to group A strep to become ill.

Children and Certain Adults Are at Increased Risk

Anyone can get strep throat, but there are some factors that can increase the risk of getting this common infection.

Strep throat is more common in children than adults. It is most common in children between the ages of 5 and 15. It is rare in children younger than 3 years of age. Adults who are at an increased risk for strep throat include:

- Parents of school-aged children

- Adults who are often in contact with children

Close contact with another person with strep throat is the most common risk factor for illness. For example, if someone has strep throat, it often spreads to other people in their household.

Infectious illnesses tend to spread wherever large groups of people gather together. Crowded conditions can increase the risk of getting a group A strep infection. These settings include:

341

- Schools
- Day care centers
- Military training facilities

A Simple Test Gives Fast Results

Only a rapid strep test or throat culture can determine if group A strep is the cause. A doctor cannot tell if someone has strep throat just by looking at her or his throat.

A rapid strep test involves swabbing the throat and running a test on the swab. The test quickly shows if group A strep is causing the illness. If the test is positive, doctors can prescribe antibiotics. If the test is negative but a doctor still suspects strep throat, then the doctor can take a throat culture swab. A throat culture takes time to see if group A strep bacteria grow from the swab. While it takes more time, a throat culture sometimes finds infections that the rapid strep test misses. Culture is important to use in children and teens since they can get a rheumatic fever from an untreated strep throat infection. For adults, it is usually not necessary to do a throat culture following a negative rapid strep test. Adults are generally not at risk of getting rheumatic fever following a strep throat infection.

Someone with strep throat should start feeling better in just a day or two after starting antibiotics. Call the doctor if you or your child are not feeling better after taking antibiotics for 48 hours.

Antibiotics Help You Get Well Fast

Doctors treat strep throat with antibiotics. Either penicillin or amoxicillin is recommended as the first choice for people who are not allergic to penicillin. Doctors can use other antibiotics to treat strep throat in people who are allergic to penicillin.

Benefits of antibiotics include:

- Decreasing how long someone is sick
- Decreasing symptoms (feeling better)
- Preventing the bacteria from spreading to others
- Preventing serious complications, such as rheumatic fever

Someone who tests positive for strep throat but has no symptoms (called a "carrier") usually does not need antibiotics. They are less likely to spread the bacteria to others and are very unlikely to get complications. If a carrier gets a sore throat illness caused by a virus, the rapid strep test can be positive. In these cases, it can be hard to know what is causing the sore throat. If someone keeps getting a sore throat after taking the right antibiotics, they may be a strep carrier and have a viral throat infection. Talk to a doctor if you think you or your child may be a strep carrier.

Serious Complications Are Not Common but Can Happen

Complications can occur after a strep throat infection. This can happen if the bacteria spread to other parts of the body. Complications can include:

- Abscesses (pockets of pus) around the tonsils
- Swollen lymph nodes in the neck
- Sinus infections
- Ear infections
- Rheumatic fever
- Poststreptococcal glomerulonephritis (a kidney disease)

Protect Yourself and Others

People can get strep throat more than once. Having strep throat does not protect someone from getting it again in the future. While there is no vaccine to prevent strep throat, there are things people can do to protect themselves and others.

Good Hygiene Helps Prevent Group A Strep Infections

The best way to keep from getting or spreading group A strep is to wash your hands often. This is especially important after coughing or sneezing and before preparing foods or eating. To practice good hygiene you should:

- Cover your mouth and nose with a tissue when you cough or sneeze.
- Put your used tissue in the wastebasket.
- Cough or sneeze into your upper sleeve or elbow, not your hands, if you do not have a tissue.

- Wash your hands often with soap and water for at least 20 seconds.

- Use an alcohol-based hand rub if soap and water are not available.

You should also wash glasses, utensils, and plates after someone who is sick uses them. These items are safe for others to use once washed.

People with strep throat should stay home from work, school, or day care until they:

- No longer have a fever

- Have taken antibiotics for at least 24 hours

Take the prescription exactly as the doctor says to. Do not stop taking the medicine, even if you or your child feel better unless the doctor says to stop.

Wash your hands often to help prevent germs from spreading.

Section 45.2

Scarlet Fever

This section includes text excerpted from "Scarlet Fever:
All You Need to Know," Centers for Disease Control
and Prevention (CDC), November 1, 2018.

Bacteria Cause Scarlet Fever

Bacteria called "group A *Streptococcus*" or "group A strep" cause scarlet fever. The bacteria sometimes make a poison (toxin), which causes a rash—the "scarlet" of scarlet fever.

How You Get Scarlet Fever

Group A strep live in the nose and throat, and it can easily spread to other people. It is important to know that all infected people do not have symptoms or seem sick. People who are infected spread the bacteria by coughing or sneezing, which creates small respiratory droplets that contain the bacteria.

People can get sick if they:

- Breathe in those droplets
- Touch something with droplets on it and then touch their mouth or nose
- Drink from the same glass or eat from the same plate as a sick person
- Touch sores on the skin caused by group A strep (impetigo)

Rarely, people can spread group A strep through food that is not handled properly. Experts do not believe pets or household items, such as toys, spread these bacteria.

Scarlet Fever: What to Expect

In general, scarlet fever is a mild infection. It usually takes two to five days for someone exposed to group A strep to become sick. The illness usually begins with a fever and sore throat. There may also be chills, vomiting, or abdominal pain. The tongue may have a whitish coating and appear swollen. It may also have a strawberry-like (red and bumpy) appearance. The throat and tonsils may be very red and sore, and swallowing may be painful.

One or two days after the illness begins, a red rash usually appears. However, the rash can appear before illness or up to seven days later. The rash may first appear on the neck, underarm, and groin (the area where your stomach meets your thighs). Over time, the rash spreads over the body. The rash usually begins as small, flat blotches that slowly become fine bumps that feel like sandpaper.

Although the cheeks might look flushed (rosy), there may be a pale area around the mouth. Underarm, elbow, and groin skin creases may become a brighter red than the rest of the rash. The rash from scarlet fever fades in about seven days. As the rash fades, the skin may peel around the fingertips, toes, and groin area. This peeling can last up to several weeks.

Children and Certain Adults Are at Increased Risk

Anyone can get scarlet fever, but there are some factors that can increase the risk of getting this infection.

Scarlet fever, like strep throat, is more common in children than adults. It is most common in children between the ages of 5 and 15. It is rare in children younger than 3 years of age. Adults who are at increased risk for scarlet fever include:

- Parents of school-aged children

- Adults who are often in contact with children

Close contact with another person with scarlet fever is the most common risk factor for illness. For example, if someone has scarlet fever, it often spreads to other people in their household.

Infectious illnesses tend to spread wherever large groups of people gather together. Crowded conditions can increase the risk of getting a group A strep infection. These settings include:

- Schools

- Day care centers

- Military training facilities

Doctors Can Test for and Treat Scarlet Fever

Many viruses and bacteria can cause an illness that includes a red rash and a sore throat. Only a rapid strep test or a throat culture can determine if group A strep is the cause.

A rapid strep test involves swabbing the throat and testing the swab. The test quickly shows if group A strep is causing the illness. If the test is positive, doctors can prescribe antibiotics. If the test is negative but a doctor still suspects scarlet fever, then the doctor can take a throat culture swab. A throat culture takes time to see if group A strep bacteria grow from the swab. While it takes more time, a throat culture sometimes finds infections that the rapid strep test misses. Culture is important to use in children and teens since they can get a rheumatic fever from an untreated scarlet fever infection. For adults, it is usually not necessary to do a throat culture following a negative rapid strep test. Adults are generally not at risk of getting rheumatic fever following scarlet fever.

Antibiotics Help You Get Well Fast

Doctors treat scarlet fever with antibiotics. Either penicillin or amoxicillin is recommended as the first choice for people who are not allergic to penicillin. Doctors can use other antibiotics to treat scarlet fever in people who are allergic to penicillin.

Benefits of antibiotics include:

- Decreasing how long someone is sick
- Decreasing symptoms (feeling better)
- Preventing the bacteria from spreading to others
- Preventing serious complications like rheumatic fever

Long-Term Health Problems Are Not Common but Can Happen

Complications are rare but can occur after having scarlet fever. This can happen if the bacteria spread to other parts of the body. Complications can include:

- Abscesses (pockets of pus) around the tonsils
- Swollen lymph nodes in the neck
- Ear, sinus, and skin infections
- Pneumonia (lung infection)
- Rheumatic fever (a heart disease)
- Poststreptococcal glomerulonephritis (a kidney disease)
- Arthritis (joint inflammation)

Treatment with antibiotics can prevent most of these health problems.

Protect Yourself and Others

People can get scarlet fever more than once. Having scarlet fever does not protect someone from getting it again in the future. While there is no vaccine to prevent scarlet fever, there are things people can do to protect themselves and others.

Good Hygiene Helps Prevent Group A Strep Infections

The best way to keep from getting or spreading group A strep is to wash your hands often. This is especially important after coughing or sneezing and before preparing foods or eating. To practice good hygiene you should:

- Cover your mouth and nose with a tissue when you cough or sneeze

- Put your used tissue in the wastebasket
- Cough or sneeze into your upper sleeve or elbow, not your hands, if you do not have a tissue
- Wash your hands often with soap and water for at least 20 seconds
- Use an alcohol-based hand rub if soap and water are not available

You should also wash glasses, utensils, and plates after someone who is sick uses them. These items are safe for others to use once washed.

Antibiotics Help Prevent Spreading the Infection to Others

People with scarlet fever should stay home from work, school, or day care until they:

- No longer have a fever
- Have taken antibiotics for at least 24 hours

Take the prescription exactly as the doctor says to. Do not stop taking the medicine, even if you or your child feel better unless the doctor says to stop.

Chapter 46

Streptococcal Infections: Group B

Chapter Contents

Section 46.1—*Streptococcus pneumoniae* 350

Section 46.2—Group B Strep in Pregnancy and
Newborns 356

Section 46.1

Streptococcus pneumoniae

This section includes text excerpted from "About Pneumococcal Disease," Centers for Disease Control and Prevention (CDC), September 6, 2017.

Pneumococcal disease is an infection caused by *Streptococcus pneumoniae* bacteria, sometimes referred to as "pneumococcus." Pneumococcus can cause many types of illnesses, including ear infections and meningitis. There are vaccines to prevent pneumococcal disease in children and adults.

Types of Infections

Streptococcus pneumoniae bacteria can cause many types of illnesses. Some of these illnesses can be life-threatening.

Pneumococcus is the most common cause of bloodstream infections, pneumonia, meningitis, and middle ear infections (otitis media) in young children.

You have probably heard of pneumonia, which is an infection of the lungs. Many different bacteria, viruses, and even fungi can cause pneumonia. Pneumococcus is one of the most common causes of severe pneumonia.

Besides pneumonia, pneumococcus can cause other types of infections too, such as:

• Ear infections

• Sinus infections

• Meningitis (infection of the tissue covering the brain and spinal cord)

• Bacteremia (bloodstream infection)

Doctors consider some of these infections "invasive." Invasive disease means that germs invade parts of the body that are normally free from germs. For example, pneumococcal bacteria can invade the bloodstream, causing bacteremia, and the tissues and fluids covering the brain and spinal cord, causing meningitis. When this happens, the disease is usually very severe, requiring treatment in a hospital and even causing death in some cases.

Risk Factors and Transmission

Anyone can get pneumococcal disease, but some people are at a greater risk for disease than others. Being a certain age or having some medical conditions can put you at an increased risk for pneumococcal disease.

Children at Risk for Pneumococcal Disease

Children at an increased risk for pneumococcal disease include those:

- Younger than two years of age

- Who have certain illnesses (sickle cell disease (SCD); human immunodeficiency virus (HIV) infection; diabetes; immunocompromising conditions; nephrotic syndrome; or chronic heart, lung, kidney, or liver disease)

- With cochlear implants or cerebrospinal fluid (CSF) leaks (escape of the fluid that surrounds the brain and spinal cord)

Adults at Risk for Pneumococcal Disease

If you are at an increased risk for pneumococcal disease, talk to your doctor about which pneumococcal vaccines you need and when.

Adults 65 years of age or older are at an increased risk for pneumococcal disease.

Some adults between the ages of 19 and 64 are also at an increased risk for pneumococcal disease, including those:

- With chronic illnesses (chronic heart, liver, kidney, or lung (including chronic obstructive lung disease, emphysema, and asthma) disease; diabetes; or alcoholism)

- With conditions that weaken the immune system (HIV/acquired immunodeficiency syndrome (AIDS), cancer, or a damaged/ absent spleen)

- With cochlear implants or CSF leaks (escape of the fluid that surrounds the brain and spinal cord)

- Who smoke cigarettes

Transmission

Pneumococcal bacteria spread from person-to-person by direct contact with respiratory secretions, such as saliva or mucus. Many people,

351

especially children, have the bacteria in their nose or throat at one time or another without being ill. Doctors call this "carriage" and do not know why it only rarely leads to sickness.

Symptoms and Complications

There are many types of pneumococcal disease. Symptoms and complications depend on the part of the body that is infected.

Symptoms

Pneumococcal pneumonia (lung infection) is the most common serious form of pneumococcal disease. Symptoms include:

- Fever and chills
- Cough
- Rapid breathing or difficulty breathing
- Chest pain

Older adults with pneumococcal pneumonia may experience confusion or low alertness rather than the more common symptoms listed above.

Pneumococcal meningitis is an infection of the tissue covering the brain and spinal cord. Symptoms include:

- Stiff neck
- Fever
- Headache
- Photophobia (eyes being more sensitive to light)
- Confusion

In babies, meningitis may cause poor eating and drinking, low alertness, and vomiting.

Pneumococcal bacteremia is a blood infection. Symptoms include:

- Fever
- Chills
- Low alertness

Sepsis is a complication caused by the body's overwhelming and life-threatening response to an infection, which can lead to tissue damage, organ failure, and death. Symptoms include:

- Confusion or disorientation

- Shortness of breath

- High heart rate

- Fever, shivering, or feeling very cold

- Extreme pain or discomfort

- Clammy or sweaty skin

Pneumococcus bacteria cause up to half of middle ear infections. Symptoms include:

- Ear pain

- A red, swollen eardrum

- Fever

- Sleepiness

Complications

Doctors consider some pneumococcal infections to be "invasive." Invasive disease means that germs invade parts of the body that are normally free from germs.

Most pneumococcal infections are mild. However, some can be deadly or result in long-term problems, such as brain damage or hearing loss.

Meningitis is the most severe type of invasive pneumococcal disease. Of children younger than 5 years of age who get pneumococcal meningitis, about 1 out of 15 dies of the infection. The chance of death from pneumococcal meningitis is higher among elderly patients. Others may have long-term problems, such as hearing loss or developmental delay.

Bacteremia is a type of invasive pneumococcal disease that infects the blood. About 1 out of 100 children younger than 5 years of age with this bloodstream infection die of it. The chance of death from pneumococcal bacteremia is higher among elderly patients.

Pneumonia is an infection of the lungs that can cause mild to severe illness in people of all ages. Complications of pneumococcal pneumonia include:

- Infection of the space between membranes that surround the lungs and chest cavity (empyema)

- Inflammation of the sac surrounding the heart (pericarditis)

- Blockage of the airway that allows air into the lungs (endobronchial obstruction), with a collapse within the lungs (atelectasis) and the collection of pus (abscess) in the lungs

About 5 out of 100 people with noninvasive pneumococcal pneumonia will die from it, but that rate may be higher among elderly patients. Doctors consider pneumococcal pneumonia noninvasive if there is not bacteremia or empyema occurring at the same time.

Sinus and ear infections are usually mild, and they are more common than the more severe forms of pneumococcal disease. However, some children develop repeated ear infections and may need ear tubes.

Diagnosis and Treatment

Early diagnosis and treatment are very important for invasive pneumococcal disease. It is important to know if it is pneumococcal disease because the treatment will change depending on the cause. In the case of pneumococcal disease, antibiotics can help prevent severe illness.

Diagnosis

If doctors suspect invasive pneumococcal disease, such as meningitis or bloodstream infections, they collect samples of cerebrospinal fluid or blood and send them to a laboratory for testing.

Identifying pneumococcus bacteria from the sample collected helps doctors confirm that pneumococcus is the cause of the illness. Additionally, growing the bacteria in a laboratory is important for identifying the specific type of bacteria that is causing the infection. It is also important for deciding which antibiotic will work best.

For noninvasive pneumococcal pneumonia in adults, there is also a urine test that can help make the diagnosis. For other pneumococcal infections, such as ear and sinus infections, healthcare professionals usually diagnose them based on the patient's medical history and physical exam findings that support pneumococcal infection.

Treatment

Antibiotics can treat pneumococcal disease. However, many types of pneumococcal bacteria have become resistant to some of the antibiotics used to treat these infections. Available data show that pneumococcal bacteria are resistant to one or more antibiotics in 3 out of every 10 cases.

Antibiotic treatment for invasive pneumococcal infections typically includes "broad-spectrum" antibiotics until results of antibiotic sensitivity testing are available. Broad-spectrum antibiotics work against a wide range of bacteria. Once the sensitivity of the bacteria is known, a more targeted (or "narrow-spectrum") antibiotic may be selected.

With the success of the pneumococcal conjugate vaccine, much less antibiotic-resistant pneumococcal infections are seen. In addition to the vaccine, appropriate use of antibiotics may also slow or reverse drug-resistant pneumococcal infections.

Prevention

The best way to prevent pneumococcal disease is to get the vaccine(s). Pneumococcal vaccines help protect against some of the more than 90 types of pneumococcal bacteria.

Vaccination

The pneumococcal conjugate vaccine (PCV13 or Prevnar 13®) protects against the 13 types of pneumococcal bacteria that cause most of the severe illness in children and adults. The vaccine can also help prevent some ear infections. The Centers for Disease Control and Prevention (CDC) recommends PCV13 for all children at 2, 4, 6, and 12 to 15 months old. The CDC also recommends PCV13 for adults 19 years of age or older with certain medical conditions and for all adults 65 years of age or older.

The pneumococcal polysaccharide vaccine (PPSV23 or Pneumovax 23®) protects against 23 types of pneumococcal bacteria. The CDC recommends this vaccine for all adults 65 years of age or older. It is also recommended for children and adults between 2 and 64 years of age who are at an increased risk for pneumococcal disease.

It is also important to get an influenza vaccine every year because having the flu increases your chances of getting pneumococcal disease.

Antibiotics

It is not common for people to develop pneumococcal disease after being exposed to someone with pneumococcal infection. Therefore, the CDC does not recommend prophylactic (preventative) antibiotics for contacts of patients with such infections.

Previous Infection

Because there are more than 90 known pneumococcal serotypes (strains or types) that cause disease, a previous pneumococcal infection will not protect you from future infection. Therefore, the CDC still recommends pneumococcal vaccines for children and adults who have had pneumococcal disease in the past.

Section 46.2

Group B Strep in Pregnancy and Newborns

This section includes text excerpted from "Group B Strep (GBS)," Centers for Disease Control and Prevention (CDC), June 25, 2019.

Group B *Streptococcus* (group B strep, GBS) are bacteria that come and go naturally in the body. Most of the time the bacteria are not harmful, but they can cause serious illness in people of all ages. In fact, group B strep disease is a common cause of severe infection in newborns. While GBS disease can be deadly, there are steps pregnant women can take to help protect their babies.

Causes

Bacteria called *"group B Streptococcus"* (group B strep, GBS) commonly live in people's gastrointestinal and genital tracts. The gastrointestinal tract is the part of the body that digests food and includes the stomach and intestines. The genital tract is the part of the body involved in reproduction and includes the vagina in women. Most of the time, the bacteria are not harmful and do not make people feel sick or have any symptoms. Sometimes, the bacteria invade the body and cause certain infections, which are known as "GBS disease."

Types of Infections

Group B strep bacteria can cause many types of infections:

- Bacteremia (bloodstream infection) and sepsis (the body's extreme response to an infection)
- Bone and joint infections
- Meningitis (infection of the tissue covering the brain and spinal cord)
- Pneumonia (lung infection)
- Skin and soft-tissue infections

Group B strep most commonly causes bacteremia, sepsis, pneumonia, and meningitis in newborns. It is very uncommon for GBS to cause meningitis in adults.

People at Increased Risk and How It Spreads

Anyone can get GBS disease, but some people are at a greater risk for disease than others. Being a certain age or having certain medical conditions can put you at an increased risk for GBS disease.

People at Increased Risk

Group B strep disease is most common in newborns. There are factors that can increase a pregnant woman's risk of having a baby who will develop GBS disease, including:

- Testing positive for GBS bacteria late in pregnancy
- Developing a fever during labor
- Having 18 hours or more pass between when their water breaks and when their baby is born

Talk to your doctor or midwife to learn more and find out if you are at risk.

How It Spreads

Group B strep bacteria commonly live in people's gastrointestinal and genital tracts.

The bacteria do not spread through food, water, or anything that people might have come into contact with. How people get these bacteria or spread them to others is generally unknown.

However, experts know that pregnant women can pass the bacteria to their babies during delivery. Most babies who get GBS disease in the first week of life (early-onset) are exposed to the bacteria this way. Babies who develop GBS disease from the first week through three months of life have late-onset disease. It can be hard to figure out how babies who develop late-onset GBS disease got the bacteria. The bacteria may have come from the mother during birth or from another source.

Other people that live with someone who has GBS bacteria, including other children, are not at risk of getting sick.

Signs and Symptoms

Symptoms of GBS disease are different in newborns when compared to people of other ages who get GBS disease.

In Newborns and Their Mothers

The symptoms of GBS disease can seem like other health problems in newborns and babies. Symptoms include:

- Fever
- Difficulty feeding
- Irritability or lethargy (limpness or hard to wake up the baby)
- Difficulty breathing
- Blue-ish color to skin

Most newborns with early-onset disease have symptoms on the day of birth. In contrast, babies who develop disease later can appear healthy at birth and during their first week of life.

Women who give birth to a baby who develops GBS disease usually do not feel sick or have any symptoms.

Diagnosis, Treatment, and Complications
Diagnosis

If doctors suspect someone has GBS disease, they will take samples of sterile body fluids. Examples of sterile body fluids are blood and spinal fluid. Doctors look to see if GBS bacteria grow from the samples (culture). It can take a few days to get these results since the bacteria need time to grow. Doctors may also order a chest X-ray to help determine if someone has GBS disease.

Sometimes, GBS bacteria can cause urinary tract infections (UTIs or bladder infections). Doctors use a sample of urine to diagnose UTIs.

Treatment

Doctors usually treat GBS disease with a type of antibiotic called "beta-lactams," which includes penicillin and ampicillin. Sometimes, people with soft tissue and bone infections may need additional treatment, such as surgery. Treatment will depend on the kind of infection caused by GBS bacteria. Patients should ask their or their child's doctor about specific treatment options.

Complications

Babies may have long-term problems, such as deafness and developmental disabilities, due to having GBS disease. Babies who had meningitis are especially at risk of having long-term problems. Care for sick babies has improved a lot in the United States. However, 2 to 3 in every 50 babies (4% to 6%) who develop GBS disease will die.

Group B strep bacteria may also cause some miscarriages, stillbirths, and preterm deliveries. However, many different factors can lead to stillbirth, preterm delivery, or miscarriage. Most of the time, the cause of these events is not known.

Serious GBS infections, such as bacteremia, sepsis, and pneumonia, can also be deadly for adults. On average, about 1 in 20 nonpregnant adults with serious GBS infections die. The risk of death is lower among younger adults and adults who do not have other medical conditions.

Prevention
Testing Pregnant Women

The American College of Obstetricians and Gynecologists (ACOG) and the American College of Nurse-Midwives (ACNM) recommend women get tested for GBS bacteria when they are 35 to 37 weeks pregnant. The test is simple and does not hurt. Clinicians use a sterile swab ("Q-tip") to collect a sample from the vagina and the rectum. They send the sample to a laboratory for testing.

Women who test positive for GBS are not sick. However, they are at an increased risk of passing the bacteria to their babies during birth.

Group B strep bacteria come and go naturally in people's bodies. A woman may test positive for the bacteria at some times and not others. That is why doctors test women late in their pregnancy, close to the time of delivery.

Antibiotics during Labor

Clinicians give antibiotics to women who are at an increased risk of having a baby who will develop GBS disease. The antibiotics help protect babies from infection, but only if they are given during labor. Doctors cannot give antibiotics before labor begins because the bacteria can grow back quickly.

Clinicians give the antibiotic by IV (through the vein). Clinicians most commonly prescribe beta-lactams. However, clinicians can also give other antibiotics to women who are severely allergic to these antibiotics. Antibiotics are very safe. For example, about 1 in 10 women have mild side effects from receiving penicillin. There is a rare chance (about 1 in 10,000 women) of having a severe allergic reaction that requires emergency treatment.

Vaccination

Currently, there is no vaccine to help pregnant women protect their newborns from GBS bacteria and disease. Researchers are working on developing a vaccine, which may become available in the future.

Strategies Proven Not to Work

The following strategies are not effective at preventing GBS disease in babies:

- Taking antibiotics by mouth

- Taking antibiotics before labor begins

- Using birth canal washes with the disinfectant chlorhexidine

Chapter 47

Syphilis

What Is Syphilis?

Syphilis is a sexually transmitted disease (STD) caused by the bacterium *Treponema pallidum*. Syphilis can cause serious health conditions if not adequately treated.

How Common Is Syphilis?

During 2017, there were 101,567 reported new diagnoses of syphilis (all stages), compared to 39,782 estimated new diagnoses of human immunodeficiency virus (HIV) infection in 2016 and 555,608 cases of gonorrhea in 2017. Of syphilis cases, 30,644 were primary and secondary (P&S) syphilis, the earliest and most transmissible stages of syphilis. In 2017, the majority of P&S syphilis cases occurred among gay, bisexual, and other men who have sex with men (MSM). In 2017, MSM accounted for 79.6 percent of all P&S syphilis cases among males in which sex of sex partner was known and 57.9 percent of all P&S syphilis cases overall.

Congenital syphilis (syphilis passed from pregnant women to their babies) continues to be a concern in the United States. During 2017, 918 cases of congenital syphilis were reported, compared to an estimated 99 cases of perinatal HIV infection during 2016. In 2017, congenital syphilis rates were 6.1 times and 3.5 times higher among

This chapter includes text excerpted from "Syphilis—CDC Fact Sheet (Detailed)," Centers for Disease Control and Prevention (CDC), January 30, 2017.

infants born to Black and Hispanic mothers (58.9 and 33.5 cases per 100,000 live births, respectively) when compared to White mothers (9.7 cases per 100,000 live births).

How Do People Get Syphilis?

Syphilis is transmitted from person to person by direct contact with a syphilitic sore, known as a "chancre." Chancres can occur on or around the external genitals, in the vagina, around the anus, or in the rectum, or in or around the mouth. Transmission of syphilis can occur during vaginal, anal, or oral sex. In addition, pregnant women with syphilis can transmit the infection to the fetus.

How Quickly Do Symptoms Appear after Infection?

The average time between acquisition of syphilis and the start of the first symptom is 21 days, but it can range from 10 to 90 days.

What Are the Signs and Symptoms in Adults?

Syphilis has been called "The Great Pretender," as its symptoms can look like many other diseases. However, syphilis typically follows a progression of stages that can last for weeks, months, or even years.

Primary Stage

The appearance of a single chancre marks the primary (first) stage of syphilis symptoms, but there may be multiple sores. The chancre is usually (but not always) firm, round, and painless. It appears at the location where syphilis entered the body. These painless chancres can occur in locations that make them difficult to notice (e.g., the vagina or anus). The chancre lasts three to six weeks and heals regardless of whether a person is treated or not. However, if the infected person does not receive adequate treatment, the infection progresses to the secondary stage.

Secondary Stage

Skin rashes and/or mucous membrane lesions (sores in the mouth, vagina, or anus) mark the second stage of symptoms. This stage typically starts with the development of a rash on one or more areas of the body. Rashes associated with secondary syphilis can appear when the primary chancre is healing or several weeks after the chancre has healed. The rash usually does not cause itching. The characteristic rash of secondary syphilis may appear as rough, red, or reddish brown spots both on the palms of the hands and the bottoms of the feet. However, rashes with a different appearance may occur on other parts of the body, sometimes resembling rashes caused by other diseases. Sometimes, rashes associated with secondary syphilis are so faint that they are not noticed. Large, raised, gray or white lesions, known as "condyloma lata," may develop in warm, moist areas, such as the mouth, underarm, or groin region. In addition to rashes, symptoms of secondary syphilis may include fever, swollen lymph glands, sore throat, patchy hair loss, headaches, weight loss, muscle aches, and fatigue. The symptoms of secondary syphilis will go away with or without treatment. However, without treatment, the infection will progress to the latent and possibly tertiary stage of the disease.

Latent Stage

The latent (hidden) stage of syphilis is a period of time when there are no visible signs or symptoms of syphilis. Without treatment, the infected person will continue to have syphilis in their body even though there are no signs or symptoms. Early latent syphilis is latent syphilis where infection occurred within the past 12 months. Late latent syphilis is latent syphilis where infection occurred more than 12 months ago. Latent syphilis can last for years.

Tertiary Syphilis

Tertiary syphilis is rare and develops in a subset of untreated syphilis infections; it can appear 10 to 30 years after infection was first acquired, and it can be fatal. Tertiary syphilis can affect multiple organ systems, including the brain, nerves, eyes, heart, blood vessels, liver, bones, and joints. Symptoms of tertiary syphilis vary depending on the organ system affected.

Neurosyphilis and Ocular Syphilis

Syphilis can invade the nervous system at any stage of infection and causes a wide range of symptoms, including headache, altered behavior, difficulty coordinating muscle movements, paralysis, sensory deficits, and dementia. This invasion of the nervous system is called "neurosyphilis."

Like neurosyphilis, ocular syphilis can occur at any stage of infection. Ocular syphilis can involve almost any eye structure, but posterior uveitis and panuveitis are the most common. Symptoms include vision changes, decreased visual acuity, and permanent blindness. Clinicians should be aware of ocular syphilis and screen for visual complaints in any patient at risk for syphilis (e.g., MSM, persons living with HIV, others with risk factors, and persons with multiple or anonymous partners).

How Does Syphilis Affect a Pregnant Woman and Her Baby?

When a pregnant woman has syphilis, the infection can be transmitted to the fetus. All pregnant women should be tested for syphilis at the first prenatal visit. For women who are at high risk for syphilis, live in areas of high syphilis morbidity, are previously untested, or had a positive screening test in the first trimester, the syphilis screening test should be repeated during the third trimester (28 to 32 weeks gestation) and again at delivery. Any woman who delivers a stillborn infant after 20 weeks gestation should also be tested for syphilis.

Depending on how long a pregnant woman has been infected, she may have a high risk of having a stillbirth or of giving birth to a baby who dies shortly after birth. Untreated syphilis in pregnant women results in infant death in up to 40 percent of cases.

An infected baby born alive may not have any signs or symptoms of the disease. However, if not treated immediately, the baby may develop serious problems within a few weeks. Untreated babies may become developmentally delayed, have seizures, or die. All babies born to mothers who test positive for syphilis during pregnancy should be screened for syphilis and examined thoroughly for evidence of congenital syphilis.

For pregnant women, only penicillin therapy can be used to treat syphilis and prevent passing the disease to the fetus; treatment with penicillin is extremely effective (success rate of 98%) in preventing mother-to-child transmission. Pregnant women who are allergic to penicillin should be referred to a specialist for desensitization to penicillin.

How Is Syphilis Diagnosed?

The definitive method for diagnosing syphilis is visualizing the *Treponema pallidum* bacterium via darkfield microscopy. Diagnoses are thus more commonly made using blood tests. There are two types of blood tests available for syphilis: nontreponemal tests and treponemal tests. Both types of tests are needed to confirm a diagnosis of syphilis.

Nontreponemal tests (e.g., venereal disease research laboratory (VDRL) and rapid plasma reagin (RPR)) are simple, inexpensive, and often used for screening. However, they are not specific for syphilis, can produce false-positive results, and, by themselves, are insufficient for diagnosis. VDRL and RPR should each have their antibody titer results reported quantitatively. Persons with a reactive nontreponemal test should always receive a treponemal test to confirm a syphilis diagnosis. This sequence of testing (nontreponemal, then treponemal test) is considered the "classical" testing algorithm.

Treponemal tests (e.g., fluorescent treponemal antibody absorption (FTA-ABS), *Treponema pallidum* particle agglutination (TP-PA), various enzyme-linked immunosorbent assays (EIAs), chemiluminescence immunoassays, immunoblots, and rapid treponemal assays) detect antibodies that are specific for syphilis. Treponemal antibodies appear earlier than nontreponemal antibodies and usually remain detectable for life, even after successful treatment. If a treponemal test is used for screening and the results are positive, a nontreponemal test with titer should be performed to confirm the diagnosis and guide patient management decisions. Based on the results, further treponemal testing may be indicated. This sequence of testing (treponemal, then nontreponemal, test) is considered the "reverse" sequence testing algorithm. Reverse sequence testing can be more convenient for laboratories, but its clinical interpretation is problematic, as this testing sequence can identify persons previously treated for syphilis, those with untreated or incompletely treated syphilis, and persons with false-positive results that can occur with a low likelihood of infection.

Special note: Because untreated syphilis in a pregnant woman can infect and possibly the fetus, every pregnant woman should have a blood test for syphilis. All women should be screened at their first prenatal visit. For patients who belong to communities and populations with high prevalence of syphilis and for patients at high risk, blood tests should also be performed during the third trimester (at 28 to 32 weeks) and at delivery.

All infants born to mothers who have reactive nontreponemal and treponemal test results should be evaluated for congenital syphilis. A quantitative nontreponemal test should be performed on infant serum and, if reactive, the infant should be examined thoroughly for evidence of congenital syphilis. Suspicious lesions, body fluids, or tissues (e.g., umbilical cord, placenta) should be examined by dark-field microscopy, polymerase chain reaction (PCR) testing, and/or special stains. Other recommended evaluations may include an analysis of cerebrospinal fluid by VDRL, cell count and protein, complete blood count (CBC) with differential and platelet count, and long-bone radiographs.

What Is the Link between Syphilis and Human Immunodeficiency Virus?

In the United States, approximately half of men who have sex with men with primary and secondary (P&S) syphilis were also living with HIV. In addition, MSM who are HIV-negative and diagnosed with P&S syphilis are more likely to be infected with HIV in the future. Genital sores caused by syphilis make it easier to transmit and acquire HIV infection sexually. There is an estimated two- to five-fold increased risk of acquiring HIV if exposed to that infection when syphilis is present. Furthermore, syphilis and certain other STDs might be indicators of ongoing behaviors and exposures that place a person at a greater risk for acquiring HIV.

What Is the Treatment for Syphilis?

The recommended treatment for adults and adolescents with primary, secondary, or early latent syphilis is benzathine penicillin G 2.4 million units administered intramuscularly in a single dose. The recommended treatment for adults and adolescents with late latent syphilis or latent syphilis of unknown duration is benzathine penicillin G 7.2 million units total, administered as 3 doses of 2.4 million units administered intramuscularly each at weekly intervals. The recommended treatment for neurosyphilis and ocular syphilis is 18 to 24 million units per day, administered as 3 to 4 million units intravenously every 4 hours or continuous infusion, for 10 to 14 days. Treatment will prevent disease progression, but it might not repair damage already done.

Selection of the appropriate penicillin preparation is important to properly treat and cure syphilis. Combinations of some penicillin preparations (e.g., Bicillin C-R, a combination of benzathine penicillin and procaine penicillin) are not appropriate replacements for benzathine penicillin as these combinations provide inadequate doses of penicillin.

Although data to support the use of alternatives to penicillin is limited, options for nonpregnant patients who are allergic to penicillin may include doxycycline, tetracycline, and for neurosyphilis, potentially ceftriaxone. These therapies should be used only in conjunction with close clinical and laboratory follow-up to ensure appropriate serological response and cure. Persons who receive syphilis treatment must abstain from sexual contact with new partners until the syphilis sores are completely healed. Persons with syphilis must notify their sex partners so that they also can be tested and receive treatment if necessary.

Who Should Be Tested for Syphilis?

Any person with signs or symptoms suggestive of syphilis should be tested for syphilis. Also, anyone with an oral, anal, or vaginal sex partner who has been recently diagnosed with syphilis should be tested for syphilis.

Some people should be tested for syphilis even if they do not have symptoms or know of a sex partner who has syphilis. Anyone who is sexually active should discuss her or his risk factors with a healthcare provider and ask whether she or he should be tested for syphilis or other STDs.

In addition, providers should routinely test for syphilis in persons who:

- Are pregnant

- Are sexually active MSM

- Are living with HIV and are sexually active

- Are taking pre-exposure prophylaxis (PrEP) for HIV prevention

Will Syphilis Recur?

After appropriate treatment, syphilis does not recur. However, having syphilis once does not protect a person from becoming infected again. Even following successful treatment, people can be reinfected. Patients with signs or symptoms that persist or recur, or those who have a sustained fourfold increase in nontreponemal test titer probably failed treatment or were reinfected. These patients should be retreated.

Because chancres can be hidden in the vagina, rectum, or mouth, it may not be obvious that a sex partner has syphilis. Unless a person knows that their sex partners have been tested and treated, they may be at risk of being reinfected by an untreated partner.

How Can Syphilis Be Prevented?

Correct and consistent use of latex condoms can reduce the risk of syphilis when the infected area or site of potential exposure is protected. However, a syphilis sore outside of the area covered by a latex condom can still allow transmission, so caution should be exercised even when using a condom.

The surest way to avoid transmission of STDs, including syphilis, is to abstain from sexual contact or to be in a long-term mutually monogamous relationship with a partner who has been tested and is known to be uninfected.

Partner-based interventions include partner notification—a critical component in preventing the spread of syphilis. Sexual partners of infected patients should be considered at risk and provided treatment per the 2015 STD Treatment Guidelines from the Centers for Disease Control and Prevention (CDC).

Chapter 48

Tuberculosis

Tuberculosis (TB) is caused by a bacterium called "*Mycobacterium tuberculosis*." The bacteria usually attack the lungs, but TB bacteria can attack any part of the body, such as the kidney, spine, and brain. Not everyone infected with TB bacteria becomes sick. As a result, two TB-related conditions exist: latent TB infection (LTBI) and TB disease. If not treated properly, TB disease can be fatal.

How Tuberculosis Spreads

Tuberculosis bacteria are spread through the air from one person to another. The TB bacteria are put into the air when a person with TB disease of the lungs or throat coughs, speaks, or sings. People nearby may breathe in these bacteria and become infected.

Tuberculosis is not spread by:

- Shaking someone's hand
- Sharing food or drink
- Touching bed linens or toilet seats
- Sharing toothbrushes
- Kissing

This chapter includes text excerpted from "Tuberculosis—Basic TB Facts," Centers for Disease Control and Prevention (CDC), March 20, 2016.

When a person breathes in TB bacteria, the bacteria can settle in the lungs and begin to grow. From there, they can move through the blood to other parts of the body, such as the kidney, spine, and brain.

Tuberculosis disease in the lungs or throat can be infectious. This means that the bacteria can be spread to other people. TB in other parts of the body, such as the kidney or spine, is usually not infectious.

People with TB disease are most likely to spread it to people they spend time with every day. This includes family members, friends, and coworkers or schoolmates.

Latent Tuberculosis Infection and Tuberculosis Disease

Not everyone infected with TB bacteria becomes sick. As a result, two TB-related conditions exist: latent TB infection and TB disease.

Latent Tuberculosis Infection

Tuberculosis bacteria can live in the body without making you sick. This is called "latent TB infection." In most people who breathe in TB bacteria and become infected, the body is able to fight the bacteria to stop them from growing. People with latent TB infection:

- Have no symptoms

- Do not feel sick

- Cannot spread TB bacteria to others

- Usually, have a positive TB skin test reaction or positive TB blood test

- May develop TB disease if they do not receive treatment for latent TB infection

Many people who have latent TB infection never develop TB disease. In these people, the TB bacteria remain inactive for a lifetime without causing disease. But in other people, especially people who have a weak immune system, the bacteria become active, multiply, and cause TB disease.

Tuberculosis Disease

Tuberculosis bacteria become active if the immune system cannot stop them from growing. When TB bacteria are active (multiplying

370

in your body), this is called "TB disease." People with TB disease are sick. They may also be able to spread the bacteria to people they spend time with every day.

Many people who have latent TB infection never develop TB disease. Some people develop TB disease soon after becoming infected (within weeks) before their immune system can fight the TB bacteria. Other people may get sick years later when their immune system becomes weak for another reason.

For people whose immune systems are weak, especially those with human immunodeficiency virus (HIV) infection, the risk of developing TB disease is much higher than for people with normal immune systems.

Signs and Symptoms of Tuberculosis

Symptoms of TB disease depend on where in the body the TB bacteria are growing. TB bacteria usually grow in the lungs (pulmonary TB). TB disease in the lungs may cause symptoms such as:

- A bad cough that lasts three weeks or longer

- Pain in the chest

- Coughing up blood or sputum (phlegm from deep inside the lungs)

Other symptoms of TB disease are:

- Weakness or fatigue

- Weight loss

- No appetite

- Chills

- Fever

- Sweating at night

Symptoms of TB disease in other parts of the body depend on the area affected.

People who have latent TB infection do not feel sick, do not have any symptoms, and cannot spread TB to others.

Risk Factors of Tuberculosis

Some people develop TB disease soon after becoming infected (within weeks) before their immune system can fight the TB bacteria.

Other people may get sick years later, when their immune system becomes weak for another reason.

Overall, about 5 to 10 percent of infected persons who do not receive treatment for latent TB infection will develop TB disease at some time in their lives. For persons whose immune systems are weak, especially those with HIV infection, the risk of developing TB disease is much higher than for persons with normal immune systems.

Generally, persons at a high risk for developing TB disease fall into two categories:

- Persons who have been recently infected with TB bacteria
- Persons with medical conditions that weaken the immune system

Persons Who Have Been Recently Infected with Tuberculosis Bacteria

This includes:

- Close contacts of a person with infectious TB disease
- Persons who have immigrated from areas of the world with high rates of TB
- Children less than five years of age who have a positive TB test
- Groups with high rates of TB transmission, such as homeless persons, injection drug users, and persons with HIV infection
- Persons who work or reside with people who are at a high risk for TB in facilities or institutions, such as hospitals, homeless shelters, correctional facilities, nursing homes, and residential homes for those with HIV

Persons with Medical Conditions That Weaken the Immune System

Babies and young children often have weak immune systems. Other people can have weak immune systems too, especially people with any of these conditions:

- HIV infection (the virus that causes acquired immunodeficiency syndrome (AIDS))
- Substance abuse
- Silicosis

- Diabetes mellitus

- Severe kidney disease

- Low body weight

- Organ transplants

- Head and neck cancer

- Medical treatments, such as corticosteroids or organ transplant

- Specialized treatment for rheumatoid arthritis (RA) or Crohn disease

Exposure to Tuberculosis
What to Do If You Have Been Exposed to Tuberculosis

You may have been exposed to TB bacteria if you spent time near someone with TB disease. The TB bacteria are put into the air when a person with active TB disease of the lungs or throat coughs, sneezes, speaks, or sings. You cannot get TB from:

- Clothes

- Drinking glasses

- Eating utensils

- Handshakes

- Toilets

- Other surfaces

If you think you have been exposed to someone with TB disease, you should contact your doctor or local health department about getting a TB skin test or a special TB blood test. Be sure to tell the doctor or nurse when you spent time with the person who has TB disease.

It is important to know that a person who is exposed to TB bacteria is not able to spread the bacteria to other people right away. Only persons with active TB disease can spread TB bacteria to others. Before you would be able to spread TB to others, you would have to breathe in TB bacteria and become infected. Then, the active bacteria would have to multiply in your body and cause active TB disease. At this point, you could possibly spread TB bacteria to others. People with TB disease are most likely to spread the bacteria to people they spend time with every day, such as family members, friends, coworkers, or schoolmates.

Many people with TB infection never develop TB disease.

Prevention of Tuberculosis
Preventing Latent Tuberculosis Infection from Progressing to Tuberculosis Disease

Many people who have latent TB infection never develop TB disease. But, some people who have latent TB infection are more likely to develop TB disease than others. Those at a high risk for developing TB disease include:

- People with HIV infection
- People who became infected with TB bacteria in the last two years
- Babies and young children
- People who inject illegal drugs
- People who are sick with other diseases that weaken the immune system
- Elderly people
- People who were not treated correctly for TB in the past

If you have latent TB infection and you are in one of these high-risk groups, you should take medicine to keep from developing TB disease. There are several treatment options for latent TB infection. You and your healthcare provider must decide which treatment is best for you. If you take your medicine as instructed, it can keep you from developing TB disease. Because there are less bacteria, treatment for latent TB infection is much easier than treatment for TB disease. A person with TB disease has a large amount of TB bacteria in the body. Several drugs are needed to treat TB disease.

Preventing Exposure to Tuberculosis Disease While Traveling Abroad

In many countries, TB is much more common than in the United States. Travelers should avoid close contact or prolonged time with known TB patients in crowded, enclosed environments (for example, clinics, hospitals, prisons, or homeless shelters).

Although multidrug-resistant (MDR) and extensively drug-resistant (XDR) TB are occurring globally, they are still rare. HIV-infected travelers are at greatest risk if they come in contact with a person with MDR or XDR TB.

Air travel itself carries a relatively low risk of infection with TB of any kind. Travelers who will be working in clinics, hospitals, or other health-care settings where TB patients are likely to be encountered should consult infection control or occupational health experts. They should ask about administrative and environmental procedures for preventing exposure to TB. Once those procedures are implemented, additional measures could include using personal respiratory protective devices.

Travelers who anticipate possible prolonged exposure to people with TB (for example, those who expect to come in contact routinely with clinic, hospital, prison, or homeless shelter populations) should have a TB skin test or a TB blood test before leaving the United States. If the test reaction is negative, they should have a repeat test 8 to 10 weeks after returning to the United States. Additionally, annual testing may be recommended for those who anticipate repeated or prolonged exposure or an extended stay over a period of years. Because people with HIV infection are more likely to have an impaired response to TB tests, travelers who are HIV-positive should tell their physicians about their HIV infection status.

Vaccines of Tuberculosis
Tuberculosis Vaccine

Bacille Calmette-Guérin (BCG) is a vaccine for tuberculosis (TB) disease. This vaccine is not widely used in the United States, but it is often given to infants and small children in other countries where TB is common. BCG does not always protect people from getting TB.

Bacille Calmette-Guérin Recommendations

In the United States, BCG should be considered for only very select people who meet specific criteria and in consultation with a TB expert. Healthcare providers who are considering BCG vaccination for their patients are encouraged to discuss this intervention with the TB control program in their area.

Children

Bacille Calmette-Guérin vaccination should only be considered for children who have a negative TB test and who are continually exposed, and they cannot be separated from adults who:

- Are untreated or ineffectively treated for TB disease, and the child cannot be given long-term primary preventive treatment for TB infection
- Have TB disease caused by strains resistant to isoniazid and rifampin

Healthcare Workers

Bacille Calmette-Guérin vaccination of healthcare workers should be considered on an individual basis in settings in which:

- A high percentage of TB patients are infected with TB strains resistant to both isoniazid and rifampin.
- There is an ongoing transmission of drug-resistant TB strains to healthcare workers, and subsequent infection is likely.
- Comprehensive TB infection-control precautions have been implemented but have not been successful.

Healthcare workers considered for BCG vaccination should be counseled regarding the risks and benefits associated with both BCG vaccination and treatment of latent TB infection.

Testing for Tuberculosis in Bacille Calmette-Guérin Vaccinated People

Many people born outside of the United States have been BCG-vaccinated.

People who were previously vaccinated with BCG may receive a TB skin test to test for TB infection. Vaccination with BCG may cause a positive reaction to a TB skin test. A positive reaction to a TB skin test may be due to the BCG vaccine itself or due to infection with TB bacteria.

Tuberculosis blood tests (interferon-gamma release assays (IGRAs)), unlike the TB skin test, are not affected by prior BCG vaccination and are not expected to give a false-positive result in people who have received BCG.

For children under the age of five, the TB skin test is preferred over TB blood tests.

A positive TB skin test or TB blood test only tells that a person has been infected with TB bacteria. It does not tell whether the person has latent TB infection or has progressed to TB disease. Other tests, such as a chest X-ray and a sample of sputum, are needed to see whether the person has TB disease.

Chapter 49

Typhoid Fever

What Is Typhoid Fever?

Typhoid fever is a serious disease spread by contaminated food and water. Symptoms of typhoid include lasting high fevers, weakness, stomach pains, headache, and a loss of appetite. Some patients have constipation, and some have a rash. Internal bleeding and death can occur, but both are rare.

Who Is at Risk?

Typhoid fever is common in most parts of the world except in industrialized regions, such as the United States, Canada, Western Europe, Australia, and Japan, so travelers to the developing world should consider taking precautions. Travelers to Asia, Africa, and Latin America are especially at risk, and the highest risk for typhoid is in South Asia.

About 300 people get typhoid fever in the United States each year, and most of these people have recently traveled. About 22 million cases of typhoid fever and 200,000 related deaths occur worldwide each year.

This chapter includes text excerpted from "Typhoid Fever," Centers for Disease Control and Prevention (CDC), March 10, 2013. Reviewed July 2019.

What Can Travelers Do to Prevent Typhoid Fever?
Get Vaccinated for Typhoid

- Ask your doctor or nurse about a typhoid vaccine. This could be pills or a shot, and your doctor will help you decide which one is best for you.
- Typhoid vaccine is only 50 to 80 percent effective, so you should still be careful about what you eat and drink.

Eat Safe Foods
Eat

- Food that is cooked and served hot
- Hard-cooked eggs
- Fruits and vegetables you have washed in clean water or peeled yourself
- Pasteurized dairy products

Do Not Eat

- Food served at room temperature
- Food from street vendors
- Raw or soft-cooked (runny) eggs
- Raw or undercooked (rare) meat or fish
- Unwashed or unpeeled raw fruits and vegetables
- Peelings from fruit or vegetables
- Condiments (such as salsa) made with fresh ingredients
- Salads
- Unpasteurized dairy products
- "Bushmeat" (monkeys, bats, or other wild game)

Drink Safe Beverages
Drink

- Bottled water that is sealed (carbonated is safer)
- Water that has been disinfected (boiled, filtered, treated)

- Ice made with bottled or disinfected water
- Bottled and sealed carbonated and sports drinks
- Hot coffee or tea
- Pasteurized milk

Do Not Drink

- Tap or well water
- Ice made with tap or well water
- Drinks made with tap or well water (such as reconstituted juice)
- Flavored ice and popsicles
- Unpasteurized milk
- Fountain drinks

Practice Hygiene and Cleanliness

- Wash your hands often.
- If soap and water are not available, clean your hands with hand sanitizer (containing at least 60% alcohol).
- Do not touch your eyes, nose, or mouth. If you need to touch your face, make sure your hands are clean.
- Try to avoid close contact, such as kissing, hugging, or sharing eating utensils or cups, with people who are sick.

Chapter 50

Vaginal and Reproductive Tract Infections

Understanding Bacterial Vaginosis
What Is Bacterial Vaginosis?

Bacterial vaginosis (BV) is a condition caused by changes in the number of certain types of bacteria in your vagina. BV is common, and any woman can get it. BV is easily treatable with medicine from your doctor or nurse. If left untreated, it can raise your risk for sexually transmitted infections (STIs) and cause problems during pregnancy.

Who Gets Bacterial Vaginosis

Bacterial vaginosis is the most common vaginal condition in women between the ages of 15 and 44. But women of any age can get it, even if they have never had sex.

This chapter contains text excerpted from the following sources: Text under the heading "Understanding Bacterial Vaginosis" is excerpted from "Bacterial Vaginosis," Office on Women's Health (OWH), U.S. Department of Health and Human Services (HHS), April 1, 2019; Text under the heading "Understanding Pelvic Inflammatory Disease" is excerpted from "Pelvic Inflammatory Disease," Office on Women's Health (OWH), U.S. Department of Health and Human Services (HHS), April 1, 2019; Text under the heading "Understanding Vaginal Yeast Infection" is excerpted from "Vaginal Yeast Infections," Office on Women's Health (OWH), U.S. Department of Health and Human Services (HHS), April 1, 2019.

You may be more at risk for BV if you:

- Have a new sex partner

- Have multiple sex partners

- Douche

- Do not use condoms or dental dams

- Are pregnant. BV is common during pregnancy. About one in four pregnant women get BV. The risk for BV is higher for pregnant women because of the hormonal changes that happen during pregnancy.

- Are African American. BV is twice as common in African American women as in White women.

- Have an intrauterine device (IUD), especially if you also have irregular bleeding

How Do You Get Bacterial Vaginosis?

Researchers are still studying how women get BV. You can get BV without having sex, but BV is more common in women who are sexually active. Having a new sex partner or multiple sex partners, as well as douching, can upset the balance of good and harmful bacteria in your vagina. This raises your risk of getting BV.

What Are the Symptoms of Bacterial Vaginosis?

Many women have no symptoms. If you do have symptoms, they may include:

- Unusual vaginal discharge. The discharge can be white (milky) or gray. It may also be foamy or watery. Some women report a strong fish-like odor, especially after sex.

- Burning when urinating

- Itching around the outside of the vagina

- Vaginal irritation

These symptoms may be similar to vaginal yeast infections and other health problems. Only your doctor or nurse can tell you for sure whether you have BV.

How Is Bacterial Vaginosis Treated?

Bacterial vaginosis is treated with antibiotics prescribed by your doctor.

If you get BV, your male sex partner would not need to be treated. But, if you are female and have a female sex partner, she might also have BV. If your current partner is female, she needs to see her doctor. She may also need treatment.

It is also possible to get BV again.

Bacterial vaginosis and vaginal yeast infections are treated differently. BV is treated with antibiotics prescribed by your doctor. Yeast infections can be treated with over-the-counter (OTC) medicines. But, you cannot treat BV with OTC yeast infection medicine.

What Should I Do If I Have Bacterial Vaginosis?

Bacterial vaginosis is easy to treat. If you think you have BV:

- See a doctor or nurse. Antibiotics will treat BV.

- Take all of your medicine. Even if symptoms go away, you need to finish all of the antibiotics.

- Tell your sex partner(s) if she is female so she can be treated.

- Avoid sexual contact until you finish your treatment.

- See your doctor or nurse again if you have symptoms that do not go away within a few days after finishing the antibiotic.

How Can I Lower My Risk of Bacterial Vaginosis?

Researchers do not know exactly how BV spreads. Steps that might lower your risk of BV include:

- **Keeping your vaginal bacteria balanced.** Use warm water only to clean the outside of your vagina. You do not need to use soap. Even mild soap can cause irritate your vagina. Always wipe front to back from your vagina to your anus. Keep the area cool by wearing cotton or cotton-lined underpants.

- **Not douching.** Douching upsets the balance of good and harmful bacteria in your vagina. This may raise your risk of BV. It may also make it easier to get BV again after treatment. Doctors do not recommend douching.

- **Not having sex.** Researchers are still studying how women get BV. You can get BV without having sex, but BV is more common in women who have sex.

- **Limiting your number of sex partners.** Researchers think that your risk of getting BV goes up with the number of partners you have.

Understanding Pelvic Inflammatory Disease
What Is Pelvic Inflammatory Disease?

Pelvic inflammatory disease is an infection of a woman's reproductive organs. The reproductive organs include the uterus (womb), fallopian tubes, ovaries, and cervix.

PID can be caused by many different types of bacteria. Usually, PID is caused by bacteria from STIs. Sometimes, PID is caused by normal bacteria found in the vagina.

Who Gets Pelvic Inflammatory Disease

Pelvic inflammatory disease affects about 5 percent of women in the United States. Your risk for PID is higher if you:

- Have had an STI

- Have had PID before

- Are younger than 25 years of age and have sex. PID is most common in women between 15 and 24 years of age.

- Have more than one sex partner or have a partner who has multiple sexual partners

- Douche. Douching can push bacteria into the reproductive organs and cause PID. Douching can also hide the signs of PID.

- Recently had an IUD inserted. The risk of PID is higher for the first few weeks only after the insertion of an IUD, but PID is rare after that. Getting tested for STIs before the IUD is inserted lowers your risk for PID.

What Are the Signs and Symptoms of Pelvic Inflammatory Disease?

Many women do not know they have PID because they do not have any signs or symptoms.

When symptoms do happen, they can be mild or more serious. Signs and symptoms include:

- Pain in the lower abdomen (this is the most common symptom)
- Fever (100.4°F or higher)
- Vaginal discharge that may smell foul
- Painful sex
- Pain when urinating
- Irregular menstrual periods
- Pain in the upper right abdomen (this is rare)

Pelvic inflammatory disease can come on fast, with extreme pain and fever, especially if it is caused by gonorrhea.

How Is Pelvic Inflammatory Disease Diagnosed?

To diagnose PID, doctors usually do a physical exam to check for signs of PID and test for STIs. If you think that you may have PID, see a doctor or nurse as soon as possible.

If you have pain in your lower abdomen, your doctor or nurse will check for:

- Unusual discharge from your vagina or cervix
- An abscess (collection of pus) near your ovaries or fallopian tubes
- Tenderness or pain in your reproductive organs

Your doctor may do tests to find out whether you have PID or a different problem that looks like PID. These can include:

- Tests for STIs, especially gonorrhea and chlamydia. These infections can cause PID.
- A test for a urinary tract infection (UTI) or other conditions that can cause pelvic pain
- Ultrasound or another imaging test so your doctor can look at your internal organs for signs of PID

How Is Pelvic Inflammatory Disease Treated?

Your doctor or nurse will give you antibiotics to treat PID. Most of the time, at least two antibiotics have been used that work against many different types of bacteria. You must take all of your antibiotics, even if your symptoms go away. This helps to make sure the infection is fully cured. See your doctor or nurse again two to three days after starting the antibiotics to make sure they are working.

Your doctor or nurse may suggest going into the hospital to treat your PID if:

- You are very sick.

- You are pregnant.

- Your symptoms do not go away after taking the antibiotics or if you cannot swallow pills. If this is the case, you will need IV antibiotics.

- You have an abscess in a fallopian tube or ovary.

If you still have symptoms or if the abscess does not go away after treatment, you may need surgery. Problems caused by PID, such as chronic pelvic pain and scarring, are often hard to treat. But sometimes they get better after surgery.

How Can I Prevent Pelvic Inflammatory Disease?

You may not be able to prevent PID. It is not always caused by an STI. Sometimes, normal bacteria in your vagina can travel up to your reproductive organs and cause PID.

But, you can lower your risk of PID by not douching. You can also prevent STIs by not having vaginal, oral, or anal sex.

If you do have sex, lower your risk of getting an STI with the following steps:

- **Use condoms.** Condoms are the best way to prevent STIs when you have sex. Because a man does not need to ejaculate to give or get STIs, make sure to put the condom on before the penis touches the vagina, mouth, or anus. Other methods of birth control, such as birth control pills, shots, implants, or diaphragms, will not protect you from STIs.

- **Get tested.** Be sure you and your partner are tested for STIs. Talk to each other about the test results before you have sex.

- **Be monogamous.** Having sex with just one partner can lower your risk for STIs. After being tested for STIs, be faithful to each other. That means that you have sex only with each other and no one else.

- **Limit your number of sex partners.** Your risk of getting STIs goes up with the number of partners you have.

- **Do not douche.** Douching removes some of the normal bacteria in the vagina that protect you from infection. Douching may also raise your risk for PID by helping bacteria travel to other areas, such as your uterus, ovaries, and fallopian tubes.

- **Do not abuse alcohol or drugs.** Drinking too much alcohol or using drugs increases risky behavior and may put you at risk of sexual assault and possible exposure to STIs.

- **The steps work best when used together.** No single step can protect you from every single type of STI.

Understanding Vaginal Yeast Infection

What Is a Vaginal Yeast Infection?

A vaginal yeast infection is an infection of the vagina that causes itching and burning of the vulva, the area around the vagina. Vaginal yeast infections are caused by an overgrowth of the fungus *Candida*.

Who Gets Vaginal Yeast Infections

Women and girls of all ages can get vaginal yeast infections. Three out of four women will have a yeast infection at some point in their lives. Almost half of women have two or more infections.

Vaginal yeast infections are rare before puberty and after menopause.

Are Some Women More at Risk for Yeast Infections?

Yes. Your risk for yeast infections is higher if:

- You are pregnant.

- You have diabetes and your blood sugar is not under the control.

- You use a type of hormonal birth control that has higher doses of estrogen.

- You douche or use vaginal sprays.

- You recently took antibiotics, such as amoxicillin, or steroid medicines.

- You have a weakened immune system, such as from HIV.

What Are the Symptoms of Vaginal Yeast Infections?

The most common symptom of a vaginal yeast infection is extreme itchiness in and around the vagina.

Other signs and symptoms include:

- Burning, redness, and swelling of the vagina and the vulva

- Pain when urinating

- Pain during sex

- Soreness

- A thick, white vaginal discharge that looks like cottage cheese and does not have a bad smell

You may have only a few of these symptoms. They may be mild or severe.

How Is a Yeast Infection Diagnosed?

Your doctor will do a pelvic exam to look for swelling and discharge. Your doctor may also use a cotton swab to take a sample of the discharge from your vagina. A lab technician will look at the sample under a microscope to see whether there is an overgrowth of the fungus *Candida* that causes a yeast infection.

How Is a Yeast Infection Treated?

Yeast infections are usually treated with antifungal medicine. See your doctor or nurse to make sure that you have a vaginal yeast infection and not another type of infection.

You can then buy antifungal medicine for yeast infections at a store without a prescription. Antifungal medicines come in the form of creams, tablets, ointments, or suppositories that you insert into your vagina. You can apply treatment in one dose or daily for up to seven days, depending on the brand you choose.

Your doctor or nurse can also give you a single dose of antifungal medicine taken by mouth, such as fluconazole. If you get more than four vaginal yeast infections a year, or if your yeast infection does not go away after using over-the-counter (OTC) treatment, you may need to take regular doses of antifungal medicine for up to six months.

How Can I Prevent a Yeast Infection?

You can take steps to lower your risk of getting yeast infections:

- Do not douche. Douching removes some of the normal bacteria in the vagina that protects you from infection.

- Do not use scented feminine products, including bubble bath, sprays, pads, and tampons.

- Change tampons, pads, and panty liners often.

- Do not wear tight underwear, pantyhose, pants, or jeans. These can increase body heat and moisture in your genital area.

- Wear underwear with a cotton crotch. Cotton underwear helps keep you dry and does not hold in warmth and moisture.

- Change out of wet swimsuits and workout clothes as soon as you can.

- After using the bathroom, always wipe from front to back.

- Avoid hot tubs and very hot baths.

- If you have diabetes, be sure your blood sugar is under control.

Chapter 51

Vancomycin-Resistant Enterococci

What Is Vancomycin-Resistant Enterococci?

Enterococci are bacteria that are normally present in the human intestines and in the female genital tract, and they are often found in the environment. These bacteria can sometimes cause infections. Vancomycin is an antibiotic that is used to treat some drug-resistant infections caused by enterococci. In some instances, enterococci have become resistant to this drug and thus are called "vancomycin-resistant enterococci." Most VRE infections occur in hospitals.

What Types of Infections Does Vancomycin-Resistant Enterococci Cause?

Vancomycin-resistant enterococci can live in the human intestines and female genital tract without causing disease (often called "colonization"). However, sometimes it can cause infections of the urinary tract, the bloodstream, or of wounds associated with catheters or surgical procedures.

This chapter includes text excerpted from "VRE in Healthcare Settings," Centers for Disease Control and Prevention (CDC), November 24, 2010. Reviewed July 2019.

Are Certain People at Risk of Getting Vancomycin-Resistant Enterococci?

The following persons are at an increased risk of becoming infected with VRE:

- People who have been previously treated with the antibiotic vancomycin or other antibiotics for long periods of time

- People who are hospitalized, particularly when they receive antibiotic treatment for long periods of time

- People with weakened immune systems, such as patients in intensive care units (ICUs) or in cancer or transplant wards

- People who have undergone surgical procedures, such as abdominal or chest surgery

- People with medical devices that stay in for some time, such as urinary catheters or central intravenous (IV) catheters

- People who are colonized with VRE

What Is the Treatment for Vancomycin-Resistant Enterococci?

People with colonized VRE do not need treatment. Most VRE infections can be treated with antibiotics other than vancomycin. Laboratory testing of the VRE can determine which antibiotics will work. For people who get VRE infections in their bladder and have urinary catheters, removal of the catheter when it is no longer needed can also help get rid of the infection.

How Is Vancomycin-Resistant Enterococci Spread?

Vancomycin-resistant enterococci is often passed from person to person by the contaminated hands of caregivers. VRE can get onto a caregiver's hands after they have contact with other people with VRE or after contact with contaminated surfaces. VRE can also be spread directly to people after they touch surfaces that are contaminated with VRE. VRE is not spread through the air by coughing or sneezing.

How Can Patients Prevent the Spread of Vancomycin-Resistant Enterococci?

If a patient or someone in their household has VRE, the following are some things they can do to prevent the spread of VRE:

- Keep their hands clean. Always wash their hands thoroughly after using the bathroom and before preparing food. Clean their hands after contact with persons who have VRE. Wash with soap and water (particularly when visibly soiled), or use alcohol-based hand rubs.

- Frequently clean areas of the home, such as bathrooms, that may become contaminated with VRE.

- Wear gloves if hands may come in contact with body fluids that may contain VRE, such as stool or bandages from infected wounds. Always wash their hands after removing gloves.

- If someone has VRE, be sure to tell healthcare providers so that they are aware of the infection. Healthcare facilities use special precautions to help prevent the spread of VRE to others.

What Should Patients Do If They Think They Have Vancomycin-Resistant Enterococci?

Anyone who thinks they have VRE must talk with their healthcare provider.

Monitoring Vancomycin-Resistant Enterococci

The Centers for Disease Control and Prevention's (CDC) National Healthcare Safety Network (NHSN) (www.cdc.gov/nhsn/index.html) Patient Safety Component, an online training module, includes surveillance methods to identify and track device-associated infections, such as central-line associated bloodstream infections.

Chapter 52

Whooping Cough

Pertussis, also known as "whooping cough," is a highly contagious respiratory disease. It is caused by the bacterium *Bordetella pertussis*.

Pertussis is known for uncontrollable, violent coughing which often makes it hard to breathe. After cough fits, someone with pertussis often needs to take deep breaths, which result in a "whooping" sound. Pertussis can affect people of all ages, but it can be very serious, even deadly, for babies less than one year of age.

The best way to protect against pertussis is by getting vaccinated.

Causes of Whooping Cough

Bordetella pertussis attach to the cilia (tiny, hair-like extensions) that line part of the upper respiratory system. The bacteria release toxins (poisons), which damage the cilia and cause airways to swell.

Transmission of Whooping Cough

Pertussis is a very contagious disease only found in humans. Pertussis spreads from person to person. People with pertussis usually spread the disease to another person by coughing or sneezing, or when spending a lot of time near one another where you share breathing space. Many babies who get pertussis are infected by older siblings, parents, or caregivers who might not even know they have the disease.

This chapter includes text excerpted from "Pertussis (Whooping Cough)," Centers for Disease Control and Prevention (CDC), August 7, 2017.

Infected people are most contagious up to about two weeks after the cough begins. Antibiotics (medications that can help treat diseases caused by bacteria) may shorten the amount of time someone is contagious.

While pertussis vaccines are the most effective tool to prevent this disease, no vaccine is 100 percent effective. When pertussis circulates in the community, there is a chance that a fully vaccinated person of any age can catch this disease. If you have gotten the pertussis vaccine but still get sick, the infection is usually not as bad.

Signs and Symptoms of Whooping Cough

Pertussis can cause serious illness in babies, children, teens, and adults. Symptoms of pertussis usually develop within 5 to 10 days after you are exposed. Sometimes, pertussis symptoms do not develop for as long as 3 weeks.

Early Symptoms

The disease usually starts with cold-like symptoms and maybe a mild cough or fever. In babies, the cough can be minimal or not even there. Babies may have a symptom known as "apnea." Apnea is a pause in the child's breathing pattern. Pertussis is most dangerous for babies. About half of babies younger than one year of age who get the disease need care in the hospital.

Early symptoms can last for one to two weeks and usually include:

- Runny nose

- Low-grade fever (generally minimal throughout the course of the disease)

- Mild, occasional cough

- Apnea (in babies)

Pertussis in its early stages appears to be nothing more than the common cold. Therefore, healthcare professionals often do not suspect or diagnose it until more severe symptoms appear.

Later-Stage Symptoms

After one to two weeks and as the disease progresses, the traditional symptoms of pertussis may appear and include:

- Paroxysms (fits) of many, rapid coughs followed by a high-pitched "whoop" sound

- Vomiting (throwing up) during or after coughing fits

- Exhaustion (very tired) after coughing fits

Pertussis can cause violent and rapid coughing, over and over, until the air is gone from your lungs. When there is no more air in the lungs, you are forced to inhale with a loud "whooping" sound. This extreme coughing can cause you to throw up and be very tired. Although you are often exhausted after a coughing fit, you usually appear fairly well in-between. Coughing fits generally become more common and severe as the illness continues, and they can occur more often at night. The coughing fits can go on for up to 10 weeks or more. In China, pertussis is known as the "100-day cough."

The "whoop" is often not there if you have a milder (less serious) disease. The infection is generally milder in teens and adults, especially those who have gotten the pertussis vaccine.

Recovery

Recovery from pertussis can happen slowly. The cough becomes milder and less common. However, coughing fits can return with other respiratory infections for many months after the pertussis infection started.

Complications of Whooping Cough
Babies and Children

Pertussis can cause serious and sometimes deadly complications in babies and young children, especially those who have not received all recommended pertussis vaccines.

About half of babies younger than one year of age who get pertussis need care in the hospital. The younger the baby, the more likely they will need treatment in the hospital. Of those babies who are treated in the hospital with pertussis about:

- 1 out of 4 (23%) get pneumonia (lung infection)

- 1 out of 100 (1.1%) will have convulsions (violent, uncontrolled shaking)

- 3 out of 5 (61%) will have apnea

- 1 out of 300 (0.3%) will have encephalopathy (disease of the brain)
- 1 out of 100 (1%) will die

Teens and Adults

Teens and adults can also get complications from pertussis. They are usually less serious in this older age group, especially in those who have been vaccinated with a pertussis vaccine. The cough itself often causes complications in teens and adults. For example, you may pass out or break (fracture) a rib during violent coughing fits.

In one study, less than 1 out of 20 (5%) teens and adults with pertussis needed care in the hospital. Healthcare professionals diagnosed pneumonia in 1 out of 50 (2%) of those patients. The most common complications in another study were:

- Weight loss in 1 out of 3 (33%) adults
- Loss of bladder control in 1 out of 3 (28%) adults
- Passing out in 3 out of 50 (6%) adults
- Rib fractures from severe coughing in 1 out of 25 (4%) adults

Diagnosis of Whooping Cough

Healthcare providers diagnose pertussis by considering if you have been exposed to pertussis and by doing a:

- History of typical signs and symptoms
- Physical examination
- Laboratory test which involves taking a sample of mucus (with a swab or syringe filled with saline) from the back of the throat through the nose
- Blood test

Treatment of Whooping Cough

Healthcare providers generally treat pertussis with antibiotics, and early treatment is very important. Treatment may make your infection less serious if you start it early before coughing fits begin. Treatment can also help prevent spreading the disease to close contacts (people who have spent a lot of time around the infected person). Treatment after three weeks of illness is unlikely to help. The bacteria are gone from your body by then, even though you usually will still have symptoms. This is because the bacteria have already done damage to your body.

There are several antibiotics available to treat pertussis. If a healthcare professional diagnoses you or your child with pertussis, they will explain how to treat the infection.

Pertussis can sometimes be very serious, requiring treatment in the hospital. Babies are at greatest risk for serious complications from pertussis.

If Your Child Gets Treatment for Pertussis at Home

Do not give cough medications unless instructed by your doctor. Giving cough medicine probably will not help and is often not recommended for kids younger than four years of age.

Manage pertussis and reduce the risk of spreading it to others by:

- Following the schedule for giving antibiotics exactly as your child's doctor prescribed

- Keeping your home free from irritants—as much as possible—that can trigger coughing, such as smoke, dust, and chemical fumes

- Using a clean, cool mist vaporizer to help loosen mucus and soothe the cough

- Practicing good hand washing

- Encouraging your child to drink plenty of fluids, including water, juices, and soups, and eating fruits to prevent dehydration (lack of fluids). Report any signs of dehydration to your doctor immediately. These include dry, sticky mouth; sleepiness or tiredness; or thirst. They also include decreased urination or fewer wet diapers, few or no tears when crying, muscle weakness, headache, dizziness, or light-headedness.

- Encouraging your child to eat small meals every few hours to help prevent vomiting from occurring

If Your Child Gets Treatment for Pertussis in the Hospital

Your child may need help keeping breathing passages clear, which may require suctioning (drawing out) of mucus. Doctors monitor breathing and give oxygen if needed. Children might need intravenous (IV, through the vein) fluids if they show signs of dehydration or have difficulty eating. You should take precautions, such as practicing good hand hygiene and keeping surfaces clean.

Prevention of Whooping Cough
Vaccines

The best way to prevent pertussis among babies, children, teens, and adults is to get vaccinated. Also, keep babies and other people at a high risk for pertussis complications away from infected people.

In the United States, the recommended pertussis vaccine for babies and children is called "DTaP." This is a combination vaccine that helps protect against three diseases: diphtheria, tetanus, and pertussis.

Vaccine protection for these 3 diseases fades with time. Before 2005, the only booster (called "tetanus and diphtheria" (Td)) available contained protection against tetanus and diphtheria. This vaccine was recommended for teens and adults every 10 years. There is a booster (Tdap) for preteens, teens, and adults that contains protection against tetanus, diphtheria, and pertussis.

Infection

If your doctor confirms that you have pertussis, your body will have a natural defense (immunity) to future pertussis infections. Some observational studies suggest that pertussis infection can provide immunity for 4 to 20 years. Since this immunity fades and does not offer lifelong protection, The Centers for Disease Control and Prevention (CDC) still recommends the pertussis vaccination.

Antibiotics

If you or a member of your household has been diagnosed with pertussis, your doctor or local health department may recommend preventive antibiotics to other members of the household to help prevent the spread of disease. Additionally, they may recommend preventive antibiotics to some other people outside the household who have been exposed to a person with pertussis, including:

- People at risk for serious disease

- People who have routine contact with someone that is considered at high risk of serious disease

Babies younger than one year of age are most at risk for serious complications from pertussis. Pregnant women are not at an increased risk for serious disease. However, experts consider those in their third trimester to be at an increased risk since they could in turn expose their newborn to pertussis. You should discuss whether or not you need preventative antibiotics with your doctor. This is especially important if there is a baby or pregnant woman in your household. It is also important if you plan to have contact with a baby or pregnant woman.

Hygiene

As with many respiratory illnesses, pertussis spreads by coughing and sneezing while in close contact with others who then breathe in the bacteria. The CDC recommends practicing good hygiene to prevent the spread of respiratory illnesses. To practice good hygiene you should:

- Cover your mouth and nose with a tissue when you cough or sneeze.
- Put your used tissue in the wastebasket.
- Cough or sneeze into your upper sleeve or elbow, not your hands, if you do not have a tissue.
- Wash your hands often with soap and water for at least 20 seconds.
- Use an alcohol-based hand rub if soap and water are not available.

Part Four

Parasitic and Fungal Contagious Diseases

Chapter 53

Amebiasis

What Is Amebiasis?

Amebiasis is a disease caused by a one-celled parasite called *"Entamoeba histolytica"* (*E. histolytica*).

Who Is at Risk for Amebiasis?

Although anyone can have this disease, it is more common in people who live in tropical areas with poor sanitary conditions. In the United States, amebiasis is most common in:

- People who have traveled to tropical places that have poor sanitary conditions

- Immigrants from tropical countries that have poor sanitary conditions

- People who live in institutions that have poor sanitary conditions

- Men who have sex with men

This chapter includes text excerpted from "Amebiasis—General Information," Centers for Disease Control and Prevention (CDC), July 20, 2015. Reviewed July 2019.

How Can I Become Infected with Entamoeba histolytica?

E. histolytica infection can occur when a person:

- Puts anything into their mouth that has touched the feces of a person who is infected with *E. histolytica*

- Swallows something, such as water or food, that is contaminated with *E. histolytica*

- Swallows *E. histolytica* cysts (eggs) picked up from contaminated surfaces or fingers

What Are the Symptoms of Amebiasis?

Only about 10 to 20 percent of people who are infected with *E. histolytica* become sick from the infection. The symptoms are often quite mild and can include loose feces, stomach pain, and stomach cramping. Amebic dysentery is a severe form of amebiasis associated with stomach pain, bloody stools, and fever. Rarely, *E. histolytica* invades the liver and forms an abscess (a collection of pus). In a small number of instances, it has been shown to spread to other parts of the body, such as the lungs or brain, but this is very uncommon.

If I Swallowed Entamoeba histolytica, How Quickly Would I Become Sick?

Only about 10 to 20 percent of people who are infected with *E. histolytica* become sick from the infection. Those people who do become sick usually develop symptoms within 2 to 4 weeks, though it can sometimes take longer.

How Is Amebiasis Diagnosed?

Your healthcare provider will ask you to submit fecal samples. Because *E. histolytica* is not always found in every stool sample, you may be asked to submit several stool samples from several different days.

The diagnosis of amebiasis can be very difficult. One problem is that other parasites and cells can look very similar to *E. histolytica* when seen under a microscope. Therefore, people are sometimes told that they are infected with *E. histolytica* even though they are not.

Entamoeba histolytica and another ameba, *Entamoeba dispar*, which is about 10 times more common, look the same when seen under a microscope. Unlike infection with *E. histolytica*, which sometimes makes people sick, infection with *E. dispar* does not make people sick and, therefore, does not need to be treated.

If you have been told that you are infected with *E. histolytica* but you are feeling fine, you might be infected with *E. dispar* instead. Unfortunately, most laboratories do not yet have the tests that can tell whether a person is infected with *E. histolytica* or with *E. dispar*. Until these tests become more widely available, it usually is best to assume that the parasite is *E. histolytica*.

A blood test is also available but is only recommended when your healthcare provider thinks that your infection may have spread beyond the intestine (gut) to some other organ of your body, such as the liver. However, this blood test may not be helpful in diagnosing your current illness because the test can be positive if you had amebiasis in the past, even if you are not infected now.

How Is Amebiasis Treated?

Several antibiotics are available to treat amebiasis. Treatment must be prescribed by a physician. You will be treated with only one antibiotic if your *E. histolytica* infection has not made you sick. You probably will be treated with two antibiotics (first one and then the other) if your infection has made you sick.

I Am Going to Travel to a Country That Has Poor Sanitary Conditions. What Should I Eat and Drink There so I Will Not Become Infected with Entamoeba histolytica or Other Such Germs?

The following items are safe to drink:

- Bottled water with an unbroken seal

- Tap water that has been boiled for at least one minute

- Carbonated (bubbly) water from sealed cans or bottles

- Carbonated (bubbly) drinks (such as soda) from sealed cans or bottles

You can also make tap water safe for drinking by filtering it through an absolute one micron or less filter and dissolving the chlorine, chlorine dioxide, or iodine tablets in the filtered water. Absolute one-micron filters can be found in camping/outdoor supply stores.

The following items may not be safe to drink or eat:

- Fountain drinks or any drinks with ice cubes

- Fresh fruit or vegetables that you did not peel yourself

- Milk, cheese, or dairy products that may not have been pasteurized

- Food or drinks sold by street vendors

Should I Be Concerned about Spreading the Infection to Others?

Yes, but the risk of spreading infection is low if the infected person is treated with antibiotics and practices good personal hygiene. This includes thorough handwashing with soap and water after using the toilet, after changing diapers, and before handling or preparing food.

Chapter 54

Cryptosporidiosis

What Is Cryptosporidiosis?

Cryptosporidiosis is a disease that causes watery diarrhea. It is caused by microscopic germs—parasites called *"Cryptosporidium."* *Cryptosporidium*, or "Crypto" for short, can be found in water, food, soil or on surfaces, or dirty hands that have been contaminated with the feces of humans, or animals infected with the parasite. From 2001 to 2010, Crypto was the leading cause of waterborne disease outbreaks, linked to recreational water in the United States. The parasite is found in every region of the United States and throughout the world.

How Is Cryptosporidiosis Spread?

Crypto lives in the gut of infected humans or animals. An infected person or animal sheds Crypto parasites in their feces. An infected person can shed 10,000,000 to 100,000,000 Crypto germs in a single bowel movement. The shedding of Crypto in feces begins when symptoms such as diarrhea begin, and it can last for weeks after symptoms stop. Swallowing as few as 10 Crypto germs can cause infection.

This chapter includes text excerpted from "Cryptosporidium—General Information for the Public," Centers for Disease Control and Prevention (CDC), August 16, 2017.

Crypto can be spread by:

- Swallowing recreational water (for example, the water in swimming pools, fountains, lakes, rivers) contaminated with Crypto

  - Crypto's high tolerance to chlorine enables the parasite to survive for long periods of time in chlorinated drinking and swimming pool water.

- Drinking untreated water from a lake or river that is contaminated with Crypto

- Swallowing water, ice, or beverages contaminated with feces from infected humans or animals

- Eating undercooked food or drinking unpasteurized/raw apple cider or milk that gets contaminated with Crypto

- Touching your mouth with contaminated hands

  - Hands can become contaminated through a variety of activities, such as touching surfaces or objects (e.g., toys, bathroom fixtures, changing tables, diaper pails, etc.) that have been contaminated by feces from an infected person, changing diapers, caring for an infected person, and touching an infected animal.

- Exposure to feces from an infected person through oral-anal sexual contact

Crypto is not spread through contact with blood.

What Are the Symptoms of Cryptosporidiosis, When Do They Begin, and How Long Do They Last?

Symptoms of Crypto generally begin 2 to 10 days (average 7 days) after becoming infected with the parasite. Symptoms include:

- Watery diarrhea
- Stomach cramps or pain
- Dehydration
- Nausea
- Vomiting

- Fever

- Weight loss

Symptoms usually last about one to two weeks (with a range of a few days to four or more weeks) in people with healthy immune systems.

The most common symptom of cryptosporidiosis is watery diarrhea. Some people with Crypto will have no symptoms at all.

Who Is Most at Risk of Cryptosporidiosis?

People who are most likely to become infected with *Cryptosporidium* include:

- Children who attend child care centers, including diaper-aged children

- Child care workers

- Parents of infected children

- Older adults (75 years of age and older)

- People who take care of other people with Crypto

- International travelers

- Backpackers, hikers, and campers who drink unfiltered, untreated water

- People who drink from untreated shallow, unprotected wells

- People, including swimmers, who swallow water from contaminated sources

- People who handle infected calves or other ruminants such as sheep

- People exposed to human feces through sexual contact

Contaminated water might include water that has not been boiled or filtered, as well as contaminated recreational water sources (e.g., swimming pools, lakes, rivers, ponds, and streams). Several community-wide outbreaks have been linked to drinking tap water or recreational water contaminated with *Cryptosporidium*. Crypto's high tolerance to chlorine enables the parasite to survive for long periods of time in chlorinated drinking and swimming pool water. This means anyone swallowing contaminated water could get ill.

411

What Should I Do If I Think I Might Have Cryptosporidiosis?

For diarrhea whose cause has not been determined, the following actions may help relieve symptoms:

- Drink plenty of fluids to remain well hydrated and avoid dehydration. Serious health problems can occur if the body does not maintain proper fluid levels. For some people, diarrhea can be severe and result in hospitalization due to dehydration.

- Maintain a well-balanced diet. Doing so may help speed recovery.

- Avoid beverages that contain caffeine, such as tea, coffee, and many soft drinks.

- Avoid alcohol, as it can lead to dehydration.

How Is Cryptosporidiosis Diagnosed?

Cryptosporidiosis is a diarrheal disease that is spread through contact with the stool of an infected person or animal. The disease is diagnosed by examining stool samples. People infected with Crypto can shed the parasite irregularly in their feces (for example, one day they shed parasite, the next day they do not, the third day they do), so patients may need to give three samples collected on three different days to help make sure that a negative test result is accurate and really means that they do not have Crypto. Healthcare providers should specifically request testing for Crypto. Routine ova and parasite testing does not normally include Crypto testing.

What Is the Treatment of Cryptosporidiosis?

Most people with healthy immune systems will recover from cryptosporidiosis without treatment. The following actions may help relieve symptoms:

- Drink plenty of fluids to remain well-hydrated and to avoid dehydration. Serious health problems can occur if the body does not maintain proper fluid levels. For some people, diarrhea can be severe and result in hospitalization due to dehydration.

- Maintain a well-balanced diet. Doing so may help speed recovery.

- Avoid beverages that contain caffeine, such as tea, coffee, and many soft drinks.

- Avoid alcohol, as it can lead to dehydration.

Over-the-counter (OTC) antidiarrheal medicine might help slow down diarrhea, but a healthcare provider should be consulted before such medicine is taken.

A drug called "nitazoxanide" has been approved by the U.S. Food and Drug Administration (FDA) for treatment of diarrhea caused by *Cryptosporidium* in people with healthy immune systems and is available by prescription. Consult with your healthcare provider for more information about potential advantages and disadvantages of taking nitazoxanide.

Individuals who have health concerns should talk to their healthcare provider.

How Should I Clean My House to Help Prevent Spread of Cryptosporidiosis?

No cleaning method is guaranteed to be completely effective against Crypto. However, you can lower the chance of spreading Crypto by taking the following precautions:

- Wash linens, clothing, dishwasher or dryer-safe soft toys, etc. soiled with feces or vomit as soon as possible.
  - Flush excess vomit or feces on clothes or objects down the toilet.
  - Use laundry detergent, and wash in hot water: 113°F or hotter for at least 20 minutes or at 122°F or hotter for at least 5 minutes.
  - Machine dry on the highest heat setting.
- For other household object and surfaces (for example, diaper-change areas):
  - Remove all visible feces.
  - Clean with soap and water.
  - Let dry completely for at least four hours.
    - If possible, expose to direct sunlight during the four hours.
- Wash your hands with soap and water after cleaning objects or surfaces that could be contaminated with Crypto.

How Can I Protect Myself and Others from Getting Cryptosporidiosis?

The following recommendations are intended to help prevent and control cryptosporidiosis in members of the general public.

Practice Good Hygiene
Everywhere

Wet hands with clean, running water and apply soap. Lather all surfaces of hands and scrub for at least 20 seconds. Rinse with clean, running water and dry with a clean towel or air:

- Before preparing or eating food

- After using the toilet

- After changing diapers or cleaning up a child who has used the toilet

- Before and after caring for someone who is ill with diarrhea

- After handling an animal, particularly young livestock, or its stool

- After gardening, even if wearing gloves

At Child care Facilities

Exclude children who are ill with diarrhea from child care settings until diarrhea has stopped.

Information about preventing cryptosporidiosis and controlling cryptosporidiosis outbreaks at child care facilities is available on the Centers for Disease Control and Prevention's (CDC) child care facilities page.

At the Pool

- Protect others by not swimming if ill with diarrhea.

- If cryptosporidiosis is diagnosed, do not swim for at least two weeks after diarrhea stops.

- Do not swallow the water.

- Take young children on bathroom breaks every 60 minutes, or check their diapers every 30 to 60 minutes.

Avoid Water That Might Be Contaminated

- Do not drink untreated water from lakes, rivers, springs, ponds, streams, or shallow wells.

- Follow the advice given during local drinking water advisories.

- If the safety of drinking water is in doubt (e.g., during an outbreak or if water treatment is unknown) use at least one of the following:

  - Commercially bottled water

  - Water that has been previously boiled for 1 minute and left to cool. At elevations above 6,500 feet (1,981 meters), boil for 3 minutes.

  - Use a filter designed to remove Cryptosporidium.

    - The label might read "NSF 53" or "NSF 58."

    - Filter labels that read "absolute pore size of 1 micron or smaller" are also effective.

- If the safety of drinking water is in doubt, (e.g., during an outbreak or if water treatment is unknown), use bottled, boiled, or filtered water to wash fruits and vegetables that will be eaten raw.

Practice Extra Caution while Traveling

- Do not use or drink inadequately treated water or use ice when traveling in countries where the water might be unsafe.

- Avoid eating uncooked foods when traveling in countries where the food supply might be unsafe.

Prevent Contact and Contamination with Feces during Sex

- Use barriers (e.g., condoms, natural rubber latex sheets, dental dams, or cut-open nonlubricated condoms) between the mouth and a partner's genitals or rectum.

- Wash hands immediately after handling a condom or other barrier used during anal sex and after touching the anus or rectal area.

Chapter 55

Lice

Chapter Contents

Section 55.1—Body Lice 418

Section 55.2—Head Lice 420

Section 55.3—Pubic Lice 425

Section 55.1

Body Lice

This section includes text excerpted from "Body Lice—Frequently
Asked Questions (FAQs)," Centers for Disease Control and
Prevention (CDC), November 5, 2018.

What Are Body Lice?

Body lice are parasitic insects that live on clothing and bedding
used by infected persons. Body lice frequently lay their eggs on or
near the seams of clothing. Body lice must feed on blood and usually
only move to the skin to feed. Body lice exist worldwide and infect
people of all races. Body lice infestations can spread rapidly under
crowded living conditions where hygiene is poor (the homeless, refu-
gees, victims of war, or natural disasters). In the United States, body
lice infestations are found only in homeless transient populations who
do not have access to bathing and regular changes of clean clothes.
Infestation is unlikely to persist on anyone who bathes regularly
and who has at least weekly access to freshly laundered clothing
and bedding.

What Do Body Lice Look Like?

Body lice have three forms: the egg (also called a "nit"), the nymph,
and the adult.

Nit: Nits are lice eggs. They are generally easy to see in the seams
of an infected person's clothing, particularly around the waistline and
under armpits. Body lice nits occasionally also may be attached to body
hair. They are oval and usually yellow to white in color. Body lice nits
may take one to two weeks to hatch.

Nymph: A nymph is an immature louse that hatches from the nit.
A nymph looks like an adult body louse, but it is smaller. Nymphs
mature into adults about 9 to 12 days after hatching. To live, the
nymph must feed on blood.

Adult: The adult body louse is about the size of a sesame seed, has
six legs, and is tan to greyish-white. Females lay eggs. To live, lice
must feed on blood. If a louse falls off of a person, it dies within about
five to seven days at room temperature.

Where Are Body Lice Found?

Body lice generally are found on clothing and bedding used by infected people. Sometimes body lice are be seen on the body when they feed. Body lice eggs usually are seen in the seams of clothing or on bedding. Occasionally eggs are attached to body hair.

Lice found on the head and scalp are not body lice; they are head lice.

What Are the Signs and Symptoms of Body Lice?

Intense itching ("pruritus") and rash caused by an allergic reaction to the louse bites are common symptoms of body lice infestation. When body lice infestation has been present for a long time, heavily bitten areas of the skin can become thickened and discolored, particularly around the midsection of the body (the waist, groin, and upper thighs); this condition is called "vagabond's disease."

As with other lice infestations, intense itching can lead to scratching, which can cause sores on the body; these sores sometimes can become infected with bacteria or fungi.

Can Body Lice Transmit Disease?

Yes. Body lice can spread epidemic typhus, trench fever, and louse-borne relapsing fever. Although louse-borne typhus is no longer widespread, outbreaks of this disease still occur during times of war, civil unrest, natural or human-made disasters, and in prisons where people live together in unsanitary conditions. Louse-borne typhus still exists in places where climate, chronic poverty, and social customs or war and social upheaval prevent regular changes and laundering of clothing.

How Are Body Lice Spread?

Body lice are spread through direct physical contact with a person who has body lice or through contact with articles, such as clothing, beds, bed linens, or towels, that have been in contact with an infected person. In the United States, actual infestation with body lice tends to occur only in persons, such as homeless, transient persons, who do not have access to regular (at least weekly) bathing and changes of clean clothes, such as homeless, transient persons.

How Are the Body Lice Infestations Diagnosed?

Body lice infestation is diagnosed by finding eggs and crawling lice in the seams of clothing. Sometimes, a body louse can be seen on the skin crawling or feeding. Although body lice and nits can be large enough to be seen with the naked eye, sometimes a magnifying lens may be necessary to find lice or nits. A diagnosis should be made by a healthcare provider if you are unsure about an infestation.

How Are Body Lice Treated?

A body lice infestation is treated by improving the personal hygiene of the infected person, including ensuring a regular (at least weekly) change of clean clothes. Clothing, bedding, and towels used by the infected person should be laundered using hot water (at least 130°F) and machine dried using the hot cycle.

Sometimes, the infected person also is treated with a pediculicide, a medicine that can kill lice; however, a pediculicide generally is not necessary if hygiene is maintained and items are laundered appropriately at least once a week. A pediculicide should be applied exactly as directed on the bottle or by your physician.

If you choose to treat body lice, guidelines for the choice of the pediculicide are the same as for head lice.

Section 55.2

Head Lice

This section includes text excerpted from "Head Lice—Frequently Asked Questions (FAQs)," Centers for Disease Control and Prevention (CDC), August 28, 2015. Reviewed July 2019.

What Are Head Lice?

The head louse, or *Pediculus humanus capitis*, is a parasitic insect that can be found on the head, eyebrows, and eyelashes of people. Head lice feed on human blood several times a day and live close to the human scalp. Head lice are not known to spread disease.

Who Is at Risk for Getting Head Lice?

Head lice are found worldwide. In the United States, infestation with head lice is most common among preschool children attending child care, elementary-school children, and the household members of infected children. Although reliable data on how many people in the United States get head lice each year are not available, an estimated 6 million to 12 million infestations occur each year in the United States among children between the ages of 3 and 11. In the United States, infestation with head lice is much less common among African Americans than among persons of other races, possibly because the claws of the head louse found most frequently in the United States are better adapted for grasping the shape and width of the hair shaft of other races.

Head lice move by crawling; they cannot hop or fly. Head lice are spread by direct contact with the hair of an infected person. Anyone who comes in head-to-head contact with someone who already has head lice is at greatest risk. Spread by contact with clothing (such as hats, scarves, or coats) or other personal items (such as combs, brushes, or towels) used by an infected person is uncommon. Personal hygiene or cleanliness in the home or school has nothing to do with getting head lice.

What Do Head Lice Look Like?

Head lice have three forms: the egg (also called a "nit"), the nymph, and the adult.

Egg/nit: Nits are lice eggs laid by the adult female head louse at the base of the hair shaft nearest the scalp. Nits are firmly attached to the hair shaft and are oval-shaped and very small (about the size of a knot in thread), making them hard to see. Nits often appear yellow or white; although, live nits sometimes appear to be the same color as the hair of the infected person. Nits are often confused with dandruff, scabs, or hair-spray droplets. Head lice nits usually take about 8 to 9 days to hatch. Eggs that are likely to hatch are usually located no more than ¼ inch from the base of the hair shaft. Nits located further than ¼ inch from the base of hair shaft may very well be already hatched, nonviable nits, or empty nits or casings. This is difficult to distinguish with the naked eye.

Nymph: A nymph is an immature louse that hatches from the nit. A nymph looks like an adult head louse, but it is smaller. To live, a nymph must feed on blood. Nymphs mature into adults about 9 to 12 days after hatching from the nit.

Adult: The fully grown and developed adult louse is about the size of a sesame seed, has 6 legs, and is tan to grayish-white in color. Adult head lice may look darker in persons with dark hair than in persons with light hair. To survive, adult head lice must feed on blood. An adult head louse can live about 30 days on a person's head but will die within 1 or 2 days if it falls off a person. Adult female head lice are usually larger than males and can lay about 6 eggs each day.

Where Are Head Lice Most Commonly Found?

Head lice and head lice nits are found almost exclusively on the scalp, particularly around and behind the ears and near the neckline at the back of the head. Head lice or head lice nits sometimes are found on the eyelashes or eyebrows, but this is uncommon. Head lice hold tightly to hair with hook-like claws at the end of each of their six legs. Head lice nits are cemented firmly to the hair shaft, and they can be difficult to remove even after the nymphs hatch and empty casings remain.

What Are the Signs and Symptoms of Head Lice Infestation?

- Tickling feeling of something moving in the hair
- Itching, caused by an allergic reaction to the bites of the head louse
- Irritability and difficulty sleeping; head lice are most active in the dark
- Sores on the head caused by scratching. These sores can sometimes become infected with bacteria found on the person's skin

How Did My Child Get Head Lice?

Head-to-head contact with an already infected person is the most common way to get head lice. Head-to-head contact is common during play at school, at home, and elsewhere (sports activities, playgrounds, slumber parties, camp, etc.).

Although uncommon, head lice can be spread by sharing clothing or belongings. This happens when lice crawl, or when nits attached to shed hair hatch, and get on the shared clothing or belongings. Examples include:

- Sharing clothing (hats, scarves, coats, sports uniforms, etc.) or articles (hair ribbons, barrettes, combs, brushes, towels, stuffed animals, etc.) recently worn or used by an infected person

- Lying on a bed, couch, pillow, or carpet that has recently been in contact with an infected person

Dogs, cats, and other pets do not play a role in the spread of head lice.

How Is Head Lice Infestation Diagnosed?

The diagnosis of a head lice infestation is best made by finding a live nymph or adult louse on the scalp or hair of a person. Because nymphs and adult lice are very small, move quickly, and avoid light, they can be difficult to find. A magnifying lens and a fine-toothed comb may be helpful to find live lice. If crawling lice are not seen, finding nits firmly attached within a ¼ inch of the base of the hair shafts strongly suggests, but does not confirm, that a person is infected and should be treated. Nits that are attached more than ¼ inch from the base of the hair shaft are almost always dead or already hatched. Nits are often confused with other things found in the hair, such as dandruff, hair-spray droplets, and dirt particles. If no live nymphs or adult lice are seen, and the only nits found are more than ¼ inch from the scalp, the infestation is probably old and no longer active, and it does not need to be treated.

If you are not sure if a person has head lice, the diagnosis should be made by their healthcare provider, local health department, or other person trained to identify live head lice.

Is Infestation with Head Lice Reportable to Health Departments?

Most health departments do not require reporting of head lice infestation. However, it may be beneficial for the sake of others to share information with school nurses, parents of classmates, and others about contact with head lice.

I Do Not like My School "No-Nit" Policy; Can the Centers for Disease Control and Prevention Do Something?

No. The Centers for Disease Control and Prevention (CDC) is not a regulatory agency. School head lice policies often are determined by local school boards. Local health departments may have guidelines that address school head lice policies; check with your local and state health departments to see if they have such recommendations.

Do Head Lice Spread Disease?

Head lice should not be considered as a medical or public-health hazard. Head lice are not known to spread disease. Head lice can be an annoyance because their presence may cause itching and loss of sleep. Sometimes, the itching can lead to excessive scratching that can sometimes increase the chance of a secondary skin infection.

Can Head Lice Be Spread by Sharing Sports Helmets or Headphones?

Head lice are spread most commonly by direct contact with the hair of an infected person. Spread by contact with inanimate objects and personal belongings may occur but is very uncommon. Head lice feet are specially adapted for holding onto human hair. Head lice would have difficulty attaching firmly to smooth or slippery surfaces such as plastic, metal, polished synthetic leathers, and other similar materials.

Can Wigs or Hairpieces Spread Lice?

Head lice and their eggs soon perish if separated from their human host. Adult head lice can live only a day or so off the human head without blood for feeding. Nymphs (young head lice) can live only for several hours without feeding on a human. Nits generally die within a week away from their human host, and they cannot hatch at a temperature lower than that close to the human scalp. For these reasons, the risk of transmission of head lice from a wig or other hairpiece is extremely small, particularly if the wig or hairpiece has not been worn within the preceding 48 hours by someone who is actively infected with live head lice.

Can Swimming Spread Lice?

Data show that head lice can survive underwater for several hours but are unlikely to be spread by the water in a swimming pool. Head lice have been seen to hold tightly to human hair and not let go when submerged under water. Chlorine levels found in pool water do not kill head lice.

Head lice may be spread by sharing towels or other items that have been in contact with an infected person's hair, although such spread is uncommon. Children should be taught not to share towels, hair brushes, and similar items either at the poolside or in the changing room.

Swimming or washing the hair within one to two days after treatment with some head lice medicines might make some treatments less effective. Seek the advice of your healthcare provider or health department if you have questions.

Section 55.3

Pubic Lice

This section includes text excerpted from "Pubic "Crab" Lice—Frequently Asked Questions (FAQs)," Centers for Disease Control and Prevention (CDC), November 5, 2018.

What Are the Pubic Lice?

Also called "crab lice" or "crabs," pubic lice are parasitic insects found primarily in the pubic or genital area of humans. Pubic lice infestation is found worldwide and occurs in all races, ethnic groups, and levels of society.

What Do Pubic Lice Look Like?

Pubic lice have three forms: the egg (also called a "nit"), the nymph, and the adult.

Nit: Nits are lice eggs. They can be hard to see and are found firmly attached to the hair shaft. They are oval and usually yellow to white in color. Pubic lice nits take about 6 to 10 days to hatch.

Nymph: The nymph is an immature louse that hatches from the nit (egg). A nymph looks like an adult pubic louse, but it is smaller. Pubic lice nymphs take about two to three weeks after hatching to mature into adults capable of reproducing. To live, a nymph must feed on blood.

Adult: The adult pubic louse resembles a miniature crab when viewed through a strong magnifying glass. Pubic lice have six legs; their two front legs are very large and look like the pincher claws of a crab. This is how they got the nickname "crabs." Pubic lice are tan to grayish-white in color. Females lay nits and are usually larger than males. To live, lice must feed on blood. If the louse falls off a person, it dies within one to two days.

Where Are the Pubic Lice Found?

Pubic lice usually are found in the genital area on pubic hair; but, they may occasionally be found on other coarse body hair, such as hair on the legs, armpits, mustache, beard, eyebrows, or eyelashes. Pubic lice on the eyebrows or eyelashes of children may be a sign of sexual exposure or abuse. Lice found on the head generally are head lice, not pubic lice.

Animals do not get or spread pubic lice.

What Are the Signs and Symptoms of Pubic Lice?

Signs and symptoms of pubic lice include:

* Itching in the genital area

* Visible nits or crawling lice

How Did I Get Pubic Lice?

Pubic lice usually are spread through sexual contact and are most common in adults. Pubic lice found on children may be a sign of sexual exposure or abuse. Occasionally, pubic lice may be spread by close personal contact or contact with articles, such as clothing, bed linens, or towels, that have been used by an infected person. A common misconception is that pubic lice are spread easily by sitting on a toilet seat. This would be extremely rare because lice cannot live long away from a warm human body, and they do not have feet designed to hold onto or walk on smooth surfaces, such as toilet seats.

Persons infected with pubic lice should be examined for the presence of other sexually transmitted diseases (STDs).

How Is a Pubic Infestation Diagnosed?

A pubic lice infestation is diagnosed by finding a "crab" louse or egg on hair in the pubic region or, less commonly, elsewhere on the body (eyebrows, eyelashes, beard, mustache, armpit, perianal area, groin, trunk, or scalp). Pubic lice may be difficult to find because there may be only a few. Pubic lice often attach themselves to more than one hair and generally do not crawl as quickly as head and body lice. If crawling lice are not seen, finding nits in the pubic area strongly suggests that a person is infected and should be treated. If you are unsure about infestation or if treatment is not successful, see a healthcare provider for a diagnosis. Persons infected with pubic lice should be investigated for the presence of other STDs.

Although pubic lice and nits can be large enough to be seen with the naked eye, a magnifying lens may be necessary to find lice or eggs.

How Is a Pubic Infestation Treated?

A lice-killing lotion containing one percent permethrin or a mousse containing pyrethrins and piperonyl butoxide can be used to treat pubic ("crab") lice. These products are available over-the-counter (OTC) without a prescription at a local drug store or pharmacy. These medications are safe and effective when used exactly according to the instructions in the package or on the label.

Lindane shampoo is a prescription medication that can kill lice and lice eggs. However, lindane is not recommended as first-line therapy. Lindane can be toxic to the brain and other parts of the nervous system; its use should be restricted to patients who have failed treatment with or cannot tolerate other medications that pose less risk. Lindane should not be used to treat premature infants, persons with a seizure disorder, women who are pregnant or breastfeeding, persons who have very irritated skin or sores where the lindane will be applied, infants, children, the elderly, and persons who weigh less than 110 pounds.

Malathion lotion 0.5 (Ovide) is a prescription medication that can kill lice and some lice eggs; however, malathion lotion currently has not been approved by the U.S. Food and Drug Administration (FDA) for treatment of pubic lice.

Both topical and oral ivermectin have been used successfully to treat lice; however, only topical ivermectin lotion currently is approved by the FDA for treatment of lice. Oral ivermectin is not FDA-approved for the treatment of lice.

How to treat pubic lice infestations: (Warning: See special instructions for the treatment of lice and nits on eyebrows or eyelashes. The lice medications described in this section should not be used near the eyes.)

- Wash the infested area; towel dry.

- Carefully follow the instructions in the package or on the label. Thoroughly saturate the pubic hair and other infested areas with lice medication. Leave the medication on hair for the time recommended in the instructions. After waiting the recommended time, remove the medication by carefully following the instructions on the label or in the box.

- Following treatment, most nits will still be attached to hair shafts. Nits may be removed with fingernails or by using a fine-toothed comb.

- Put on clean underwear and clothing after treatment.

- To kill any lice or nits remaining on clothing, towels, or bedding, machine-wash and machine-dry those items that the infected person used during the 2 to 3 days before treatment. Use hot water (at least 130°F) and the hot dryer cycle.

- Items that cannot be laundered can be dry-cleaned or stored in a sealed plastic bag for two weeks.

- All sex partners from within the previous month should be informed that they are at risk for infestation and should be treated.

- Persons should avoid sexual contact with their sex partner(s) until both they and their partners have been successfully treated and reevaluated to rule out persistent infestation.

- Repeat treatment in 9 to 10 days if live lice are still found.

- Persons with pubic lice should be evaluated for other STDs.

Special instructions for the treatment of lice and nits found on eyebrows or eyelashes:

- If only a few live lice and nits are present, it may be possible to remove these with fingernails or a nit comb.

- If additional treatment is needed for lice or nits on the eyelashes, careful application of ophthalmic-grade petrolatum ointment (only available by prescription) to the eyelid margins 2 to 4 times a day for 10 days is effective. Regular petrolatum (e.g., Vaseline) should not be used because it can irritate the eyes if applied.

Chapter 56

Parasitic, Amebic, and Fungal Meningitis

Understanding Parasitic Meningitis

Various parasites can cause meningitis or can affect the brain or nervous system in other ways. Overall, parasitic meningitis is much less common than viral and bacterial meningitis.

Causes of Parasitic Meningitis

Some parasites can cause a rare form of meningitis called "eosinophilic meningitis," eosinophilic meningoencephalitis (EM), with increased levels of eosinophils (a type of white blood cell) in the cerebrospinal fluid. EM also can be caused by other types of infections (not just by parasites) and can have noninfectious causes, such as medications.

The three main parasites that cause EM in some infected people are:

- *Angiostrongylus cantonensis (neurologic angiostrongyliasis)*

- *Baylisascaris procyonis (baylisascariasis; neural larva migrans)*

- *Gnathostoma spinigerum (neurognathostomiasis)*

This chapter includes text excerpted from "Meningitis," Centers for Disease Control and Prevention (CDC), March 13, 2019.

How These Parasites Spread

These parasites normally infect animals not people, and they are not spread from one person to another. People get infected by ingesting something that has the infectious form or stage of the parasite:

- People can get infected with A. *cantonensis* in various ways, such as by ingesting raw or undercooked snails or slugs or by eating contaminated produce.

- People get infected with B. *procyonis* by accidentally ingesting infectious parasite eggs in raccoon feces or in something (such as dirt) contaminated with raccoon feces.

- People can get infected with G. *spinigerum* in various ways, such as by eating raw or undercooked freshwater fish or eels, frogs, poultry, or snakes.

People at Risk

Some people may have increased risk for infection because of where they live or travel:

- People in many parts of the world have gotten infected with A. *cantonensis*—especially, but not only, in parts of Asia and the Pacific Islands, including in Hawaii.

- B. *procyonis* is found in raccoons in parts of the United States, especially in the mid-Atlantic, northeastern, and midwestern regions, as well as parts of California. People in these areas, particularly young children, who put dirt or animal waste in their mouth or who spend time around raccoons are at an increased risk for *Baylisascaris infection*.

- The neurologic form of G. *spinigerum* infection is most common in Southeast Asia, particularly in Thailand.

Signs and Symptoms of Parasitic Meningitis

If you think that you or your child might have meningitis, see a healthcare provider right away, for the appropriate testing and clinical management.

As with meningitis caused by other infections, people who develop symptomatic EM from these parasites can have headache, stiff neck, nausea, vomiting, photophobia, and/or altered mental status (confusion). Other symptoms/signs can be noted. For example, people with

EM caused by A. *cantonensis* often have tingling or painful feelings in their skin and may have a low-grade fever.

All three of these parasites sometimes infect the eye(s). All three parasites, but most commonly *Baylisascaris*, can cause severe illness, such as those with a loss of coordination and muscle control, weakness/paralysis, coma, permanent disability, or death.

Diagnosis of Parasitic Meningitis

If meningitis is suspected, samples of blood and CSF are collected and sent for laboratory testing, to look for evidence of infection with these parasites and to rule out other causes. It often is hard to find these parasites in the CSF or in other parts of the body. But the person's travel/exposure history may provide helpful clues, along with the findings of clinical examinations, laboratory testing, and scans (such as brain scans).

Treatment of Parasitic Meningitis

The most common types of treatment for EM caused by these parasites are for the symptoms—such as pain medication for headache or medications to reduce the body's reaction to the parasite—rather than for the infection itself. However, treatment for the infection might help some people.

Understanding Amebic Meningitis

Primary amebic meningoencephalitis (PAM) is a very rare form of parasitic meningitis that causes a brain infection that is usually fatal.

Causes of Amebic Meningitis

Primary amebic meningoencephalitis is caused by the microscopic ameba (a single-celled living organism) *Naegleria fowleri* when water containing the ameba enters the body through the nose.

Risk Factors of Amebic Meningitis

Naegleria fowleri is found around the world. In the United States, the majority of infections have been linked to swimming in warm freshwater located in southern-tier states, such as Florida and Texas. The ameba can be found in:

- Bodies of warm freshwaters, such as lakes and rivers

- Geothermal (naturally hot) water, such as hot springs

- Warm water discharge from industrial plants

- Untreated geothermal (naturally hot) drinking water sources

- Swimming pools that are poorly maintained, minimally-chlorinated, and/or un-chlorinated

- Water heaters. *Naegleria fowleri* grows best at higher temperatures up to 115°F (46°C) and can survive for short periods at higher temperatures.

- Soil

Naegleria fowleri is not found in salt water, such as the ocean.

How It Spreads

Naegleria fowleri infects people by entering the body through the nose. This typically occurs when people go swimming or diving in warm freshwater places, such as lakes and rivers. The *Naegleria fowleri* ameba travels up the nose to the brain, where it destroys the brain tissue.

You cannot be infected with *Naegleria fowleri* by drinking contaminated water. In very rare instances, *Naegleria* infections may also occur when contaminated water from other sources (such as inadequately chlorinated swimming pool water or contaminated tap water) enters the nose, for example when people submerge their heads or cleanse their noses during religious practices, and when people irrigate their sinuses (nose) using contaminated tap water.

Naegleria fowleri infections are rare. In the 10 years from 2006 to 2015, 37 infections were reported in the United States and there were two survivors.

Primary amebic meningoencephalitis cannot be spread from one person to another.

Signs and Symptoms of Amebic Meningitis

Naegleria fowleri causes the disease PAM. In its early stages, symptoms of PAM are similar to symptoms of bacterial meningitis.

Initial symptoms of PAM start 1 to 7 days after infection. The initial symptoms include headache, fever, nausea, vomiting, and stiff neck. Later symptoms include confusion, lack of attention to people and surroundings, loss of balance, seizures, and hallucinations. After the start of symptoms, the disease progresses rapidly and usually causes death within about 5 days (range 1 to 12 days).

Diagnosis of Amebic Meningitis

Primary amebic meningoencephalitis is rare, with no more than eight cases reported each year in the United States. The early symptoms of PAM are more likely to be caused by other more common illnesses, such as bacterial or viral meningitis. People should seek medical care immediately whenever they develop a sudden onset of fever, headache, stiff neck, and vomiting, particularly if they have been in warm freshwater recently.

Treatment of Amebic Meningitis

Several drugs are effective against *Naegleria fowleri* in the laboratory. However, their effectiveness is unclear since almost all infections have been fatal, even when people were treated.

Prevention of Amebic Meningitis

Naegleria fowleri infects people when water containing the ameba enters the body through the nose. Infection is rare and typically occurs when people go swimming or diving in warm freshwater places, such as lakes and rivers. Very rarely, infections have been reported when people submerge their heads, cleanse their noses during religious practices, or irrigate their sinuses (nose) using contaminated tap or faucet water. *Naegleria fowleri* can grow in pipes, hot water heaters, and water systems, including treated public drinking water systems.

Personal actions to reduce the risk of *Naegleria fowleri* infection should focus on limiting the amount of water going up the nose and lowering the chances that *Naegleria fowleri* may be in the water.

Understanding Fungal Meningitis

Fungal meningitis is rare and usually caused by fungus spreading through blood to the spinal cord. Although anyone can get fungal meningitis, people with weakened immune systems, such as those with a human immunodeficiency virus (HIV) infection or cancer, are at an increased risk.

Causes of Fungal Meningitis

The most common cause of fungal meningitis for people with weak immune systems is *Cryptococcus*. This disease is one of the most common causes of adult meningitis in Africa.

How It Spreads

Fungal meningitis is not spread from person to person. Fungal meningitis can develop after a fungus spreads through the bloodstream from somewhere else in the body to the brain or spinal cord or from an infection next to the brain or spinal cord.

You may also get fungal meningitis after taking medications that weaken your immune system. Examples of these medications include steroids, such as prednisone; medications given after organ transplantation; or anti-Arboviruses medications, sometimes given for the treatment of rheumatoid arthritis or other autoimmune conditions.

Different types of fungus are transmitted in several ways.

- *Cryptococcus* is thought to be acquired through inhaling soil contaminated with bird droppings.
- *Histoplasma* is found in environments with heavy contamination of bird or bat droppings, particularly in the Midwest near the Ohio and Mississippi Rivers.
- *Blastomyces* is thought to exist in soil rich in decaying organic matter in the Midwest United States, particularly the northern Midwest.
- *Coccidioides* is found in the soil of endemic areas (Southwestern U.S. and parts of Central and South America).

When these environments are disturbed, the fungal spores (small pieces of fungus) can be inhaled. Meningitis results from the fungal infection spreading from the lungs to the spinal cord. Unlike the fungi above, Candida, which can also cause meningitis, is usually acquired in a hospital setting.

Risk Factors of Fungal Meningitis

Certain diseases, medications, and surgical procedures may weaken the immune system and increase your risk of getting a fungal infection, which can lead to fungal meningitis. Premature babies with very low birth weights are also at an increased risk of getting *Candida* blood-stream infection, which may spread to the brain.

Living in certain areas of the United States may increase your risk for fungal lung infections, which can also cause meningitis. For example, bird and bat droppings in the Midwestern United States may contain *Histoplasma*, and soil in the Southwestern United States may contain *Coccidioides*.

African Americans, Filipinos, pregnant women in the third trimester, and people with weakened immune systems are more likely to get *Coccidiodes* infection, which is also called "valley fever."

Signs and Symptoms of Fungal Meningitis

Signs and symptoms of fungal meningitis may include the following:

- Fever

- Headache

- Stiff neck

- Nausea and vomiting

- Photophobia (sensitivity to light)

- Altered mental status (confusion)

Diagnosis of Fungal Meningitis

If meningitis is suspected, samples of blood or cerebrospinal fluid are collected and sent to a laboratory for testing. Knowing the specific cause of meningitis is important because the severity of illness and the treatment depend on the cause.

To confirm fungal meningitis, specific lab tests can be performed, depending on the type of fungus suspected.

Treatment of Fungal Meningitis

Fungal meningitis is treated with long courses of high dose anti-fungal medications, usually given through an IV in the hospital. The length of treatment depends on how strong the immune system is and the type of fungus that caused the infection. For people with weak immune systems, such as those with acquired immunodeficiency syndrome (AIDS), diabetes, or cancer, treatment is often longer.

Prevention of Fungal Meningitis

No specific activities are known to cause fungal meningitis. Avoid soil and other environments that are likely to contain fungus. People with weak immune systems, such as those with HIV infection or cancer, should try to avoid bird droppings and avoid digging and dusty activities—particularly if they live in a geographic region where fungi, such as *Histoplasma*, *Coccidioides*, or *Blastomyces*, exist. HIV-infected people cannot completely avoid exposure.

Chapter 57

Pinworms

Pinworm infection is caused by a small, thin, white roundworm called *"Enterobius vermicularis."* Although pinworm infection can affect all people, it most commonly occurs among children, institutionalized persons, and household members of persons with pinworm infection. Pinworm infection is treatable with over-the-counter (OTC) or prescription medication, but reinfection, which occurs easily, should be prevented.

Risk Factors

The people most likely to be infected with pinworm are children under 18 years of age, people who take care of infected children, and people who are institutionalized. In these groups, the prevalence can reach 50 percent.

Pinworm is the most common worm infection in the United States. Humans are the only species that can transfer this parasite. Household pets, such as dogs and cats, cannot become infected with human pinworms. Pinworm eggs can survive in the indoor environment for two to three weeks.

This chapter includes text excerpted from "Parasites—Enterobiasis (Also Known as Pinworm Infection)," Centers for Disease Control and Prevention (CDC), January 10, 2013. Reviewed July 2019.

Epidemiology

Pinworm infections are more common within families with school-aged children, in primary caregivers of infected children, and in institutionalized children.

A person is infected with pinworms by ingesting pinworm eggs either directly or indirectly. These eggs are deposited around the anus by the worm and can be carried to common surfaces, such as hands, toys, bedding, clothing, and toilet seats. By putting anyone's contaminated hands (including one's own) around the mouth area or putting one's mouth on common contaminated surfaces, a person can ingest pinworm eggs and become infected with the pinworm parasite. Since pinworm eggs are so small, it is possible to ingest them while breathing.

Once someone has ingested pinworm eggs, there is an incubation period of one to two months or longer for the adult gravid female to mature in the small intestine. Once mature, the adult female worm migrates to the colon and lays eggs around the anus at night, when many of their hosts are asleep. People who are infected with pinworm can transfer the parasite to others for as long as there is a female pinworm depositing eggs on the perianal skin. A person can also reinfect themselves or be reinfected by eggs from another person.

Symptoms

The most common clinical manifestation of a pinworm infection is an itchy anal region. When the infection is heavy, there can be a secondary bacterial infection due to the irritation and scratching of the anal area. Often, the patient will complain of teeth grinding and insomnia due to disturbed sleep, or even abdominal pain or appendicitis. Infection of the female genital tract has been well reported.

Diagnosis

A person infected with pinworm is often asymptomatic, but itching around the anus is a common symptom. Diagnosis of pinworm can be reached from three simple techniques. The first option is to look for the worms in the perianal region two to three hours after the infected person is asleep. The second option is to touch the perianal skin with transparent tape to collect possible pinworm eggs around the anus first thing in the morning. If a person is infected, the eggs on the tape will be visible under a microscope. The tape method should be conducted on three consecutive mornings right after the infected person wakes up and before she or he does any washing. Since anal itching is a common symptom of pinworm, the third option for diagnosis is analyzing samples from under fingernails under a microscope. An infected person who has scratched the anal area may have picked up some pinworm eggs under the nails that could be used for diagnosis.

Since pinworm eggs and worms are often sparse in stool, examining stool samples is not recommended. Serologic tests are not available for diagnosing pinworm infections.

Treatment

The medications used for the treatment of pinworm are either mebendazole, pyrantel pamoate, or albendazole. Any of these drugs are given in one dose initially and then another single dose of the same drug two weeks later. Pyrantel pamoate is available without a prescription. The medication does not reliably kill pinworm eggs. Therefore, the second dose is to prevent reinfection by adult worms that hatch from any eggs not killed by the first treatment. Health practitioners and parents should weigh the health risks and benefits of these drugs for patients under two years of age.

Repeated infections should be treated by the same method as the first infection. In households where more than one member is infected or where repeated, symptomatic infections occur, it is recommended that all household members be treated at the same time. In institutions, mass and simultaneous treatment that is repeated within two weeks can be effective.

Prevention and Control

Washing your hands with soap and warm water after using the toilet, changing diapers, and before handling food is the most successful way to prevent pinworm infection. In order to stop the spread of pinworm and possible reinfection, people who are infected should bathe every morning to help remove a large amount of the eggs on the skin. Showering is a better method than taking a bath because showering avoids potentially contaminating the bath water with pinworm eggs. Infected people should not co-bathe with others during their time of infection.

Also, infected people should comply with good hygiene practices, such as washing their hands with soap and warm water after using the toilet, changing diapers, and before handling food. They should also cut their fingernails regularly, and avoid biting the nails and scratching around the anus. Frequent changing of underclothes and bed linens first thing in the morning is a great way to prevent the possible transmission of eggs in the environment and risk of reinfection. These items should not be shaken, and they should be carefully placed into a washer and laundered in hot water followed by a hot dryer to kill any eggs that may be there.

In institutions, day care centers, and schools, control of pinworm can be difficult, but mass drug administration during an outbreak can be successful. Teach children the importance of washing their hands to prevent infection.

Chapter 58

Scabies

What Is Scabies?

Scabies is an infestation of the skin by the human itch mite (*Sarcoptes scabiei* var. *hominis*). The microscopic scabies mite burrows into the upper layer of the skin where it lives and lays its eggs. The most common symptoms of scabies are intense itching and a pimple-like skin rash. The scabies mite usually is spread by direct, prolonged, skin-to-skin contact with a person who has scabies.

Scabies is found worldwide and affects people of all races and social classes. Scabies can spread rapidly under crowded conditions where close body and skin contact is frequent. Institutions, such as nursing homes, extended care facilities, and prisons, are often sites of scabies outbreaks. Child care facilities also are a common site of scabies infestations.

What Is Crusted Scabies?

Crusted scabies is a severe form of scabies that can occur in some persons who are immunocompromised (have a weak immune system), elderly, disabled, or debilitated. It is also called "Norwegian scabies." Persons with crusted scabies have thick crusts of skin that contain large numbers of scabies mites and eggs. Persons with crusted scabies are very contagious to other persons and can spread the infestation

This chapter includes text excerpted from "Scabies Frequently Asked Questions (FAQs)," Centers for Disease Control and Prevention (CDC), October 24, 2018.

easily both by direct skin-to-skin contact and by contamination of items (fomites), such as their clothing, bedding, and furniture. Persons with crusted scabies may not show the usual signs and symptoms of scabies, such as the characteristic rash or itching (pruritus). Persons with crusted scabies should receive quick and aggressive medical treatment for their infestation to prevent outbreaks of scabies.

How Soon after Infestation Do Symptoms of Scabies Begin?

If a person has never had scabies before, symptoms may take as long as four to six weeks to begin. It is important to remember that an infected person can spread scabies during this time, even if she or he does not have symptoms yet.

In a person who has had scabies before, symptoms usually appear much sooner (one to four days) after exposure.

What Are the Signs and Symptoms of Scabies Infestation?

The most common signs and symptoms of scabies are intense itching, especially at night, and a pimple-like (papular) itchy rash. The itching and rash each may affect much of the body or be limited to common sites, such as the wrist, elbow, armpit, webbing between the fingers, nipple, penis, waist, beltline, and buttocks. The rash also can include tiny blisters (vesicles) and scales. Scratching the rash can cause skin sores; sometimes, these sores become infected by bacteria.

Tiny burrows sometimes are seen on the skin; these are caused by the female scabies mite tunneling just beneath the surface of the skin. These burrows appear as tiny raised and crooked (serpiginous) grayish-white or skin-colored lines on the skin surface. Because mites are often few in number (only 10 to 15 mites per person), these burrows may be difficult to find. They are found most often in the webbing between the fingers; in the skin folds on the wrist, elbow, or knee; and on the penis, breast, or shoulder blades.

The head, face, neck, palms, and soles often are involved in infants and very young children, but usually not adults and older children.

Persons with crusted scabies may not show the usual signs and symptoms of scabies, such as the characteristic rash or itching.

How Did You Get Scabies?

Scabies usually is spread by direct, prolonged, skin-to-skin contact with a person who has scabies. Contact generally must be prolonged; a quick handshake or hug usually will not spread scabies. Scabies is spread easily to sexual partners and household members. Scabies in adults frequently is sexually acquired. Scabies sometimes is spread indirectly by sharing articles, such as clothing, towels, or bedding used by an infested person; however, such indirect spread can occur much more easily when the infested person has crusted scabies.

How Is Scabies Infestation Diagnosed?

Diagnosis of a scabies infestation usually is made based on the customary appearance and distribution of the rash and the presence of burrows. Whenever possible, the diagnosis of scabies should be confirmed by identifying the mite, mite eggs, or mite fecal matter (scybala). This can be done by carefully removing a mite from the end of its burrow using the tip of a needle or by obtaining skin scraping to examine under a microscope for mites, eggs, or mite fecal matter. It is important to remember that a person can still be infected even if mites, eggs, or fecal matter cannot be found; typically, fewer than 10 to 15 mites can be present on the entire body of an infected person who is otherwise healthy. However, persons with crusted scabies can be infested with thousands of mites and should be considered highly contagious.

How Long Can Scabies Mites Live?

On a person, scabies mites can live for as long as 1 to 2 months. Off a person, scabies mites usually do not survive more than 48 to 72 hours. Scabies mites will die if exposed to a temperature of 50°C (122°F) for 10 minutes.

Can Scabies Be Treated?

Yes. Products used to treat scabies are called "scabicides" because they kill scabies mites; some also kill eggs. Scabicides to treat human scabies are available only with a doctor's prescription; no over-the-counter (OTC) products have been tested and approved for humans.

Always carefully follow the instructions provided by the doctor and pharmacist, as well as those contained in the box or printed on the label. When treating adults and older children, scabicide cream or lotion is applied to all areas of the body from the neck down to the feet and toes; when treating infants and young children, the cream or lotion also is applied to the head and neck. The medication should be left on the body for the recommended time before it is washed off. Clean clothes should be worn after treatment.

In addition to the infected person, the treatment also is recommended for household members and sexual contacts, particularly those who have had prolonged skin-to-skin contact with the infected person. All persons should be treated at the same time in order to prevent reinfestation. Retreatment may be necessary if itching continues more than two to four weeks after treatment or if new burrows or rash continue to appear.

Never use a scabicide intended for veterinary or agricultural use to treat humans.

Who Should Be Treated for Scabies?

Anyone who is diagnosed with scabies, as well as her or his sexual partners and other contacts who have had prolonged skin-to-skin contact with the infested person, should be treated. Treatment is recommended for members of the same household as the person with scabies, particularly those persons who have had prolonged skin-to-skin contact with the infected person. All persons should be treated at the same time to prevent reinfestation.

Retreatment may be necessary if itching continues more than two to four weeks after treatment or if new burrows or rash continue to appear.

How Soon after Treatment Will You Feel Better?

If itching continues more than two to four weeks after initial treatment or if new burrows or rash continue to appear (if initial treatment includes more than one application or dose, then the two to four time period begins after the last application or dose), retreatment with scabicide may be necessary; seek the advice of a physician.

Did You Get Scabies from Your Pet?

No. Animals do not spread human scabies. Pets can become infected with a different kind of scabies mite that does not survive or reproduce on humans but causes "mange" in animals. If an animal with "mange" has close contact with a person, the animal mite can get under the person's skin and cause temporary itching and skin irritation. However, the animal mite cannot reproduce on a person and will die on its own in a couple of days. Although the person does not need to be treated, the animal should be treated because its mites can continue to burrow into the person's skin and cause symptoms until the animal has been treated successfully.

Can Scabies Be Spread by Swimming in a Public Pool?

Scabies is spread by prolonged skin-to-skin contact with a person who has scabies. Scabies sometimes also can be spread by contact with items, such as clothing, bedding, or towels that have been used by a person with scabies, but such spread is very uncommon unless the infested person has crusted scabies.

Scabies is very unlikely to be spread by the water in a swimming pool. Except for a person with crusted scabies, only about 10 to 15 scabies mites are present on an infested person; it is extremely unlikely that any would emerge from under wet skin.

Although uncommon, scabies can be spread by sharing a towel or item of clothing that has been used by a person with scabies.

How Can You Remove Scabies Mites from Your House or Carpet?

Scabies mites do not survive more than 2 to 3 days away from human skin. Items such as bedding, clothing, and towels used by a person with scabies can be decontaminated by machine-washing in hot water and drying using the hot cycle or by dry-cleaning. Items that cannot be washed or dry-cleaned can be decontaminated by removing from any body contact for at least 72 hours.

Because persons with crusted scabies are considered very infectious, careful vacuuming of furniture and carpets in rooms used by these persons is recommended.

Fumigation of living areas is unnecessary.

How Can You Remove Scabies Mites from Your Clothes?

Scabies mites do not survive more than 2 to 3 days away from human skin. Items, such as bedding, clothing, and towels used by a person with scabies can be decontaminated by machine-washing in hot water and drying using the hot cycle or by dry-cleaning. Items that cannot be washed or dry-cleaned can be decontaminated by removing from any body contact for at least 72 hours.

Your Spouse and You Were Diagnosed with Scabies. After Several Treatments, She or He Still Has Symptoms while You Are Cured. Why?

The rash and itching of scabies can persist for several weeks to a month after treatment, even if the treatment was successful and all the mites and eggs have been killed. Your healthcare provider may prescribe additional medication to relieve itching if it is severe. Symptoms that persist for longer than two weeks after treatment can be due to a number of reasons, including:

- Incorrect diagnosis of scabies. Many drug reactions can mimic the symptoms of scabies and cause a skin rash and itching; the diagnosis of scabies should be confirmed by a skin scraping that includes observing the mite, eggs, or scybala under a microscope. If you are sleeping in the same bed with your spouse and have not become reinfested, and you have not retreated yourself for at least 30 days, then it is unlikely that your spouse has scabies.

- Reinfestation with scabies from a family member or other infested person if all patients and their contacts are not treated at the same time; infested persons and their contacts must be treated at the same time to prevent reinfestation.

- Treatment failure caused by resistance to medication, by faulty application of topical scabicides, or by failure to do a second application when necessary; no new burrows should appear 24 to 48 hours after effective treatment.

- Treatment failure of crusted scabies because of poor penetration of scabicide into thick scaly skin containing large numbers of scabies mites; repeated treatment with a combination of both topical and oral medication may be necessary to treat crusted scabies successfully.

- Reinfestation from fomites, such as clothing, bedding, or towels that were not appropriately washed or dry-cleaned (this is mainly of concern for items used by persons with crusted scabies); potentially contaminated items should be machine washed in hot water and dried using the hot temperature cycle, dry-cleaned, or removed from skin contact for at least 72 hours.

- An allergic skin rash (dermatitis)

- Exposure to household mites that cause symptoms to persist because of cross-reactivity between mite antigens

If itching continues more than two to four weeks or if new burrows or rash continue to appear, seek the advice of a physician; retreatment with the same or a different scabicide may be necessary.

If You Come in Contact with a Person Who Has Scabies, Should You Treat Yourself?

No. Animals do not spread human scabies. Pets can become infected with a different kind of scabies mite that does not survive or reproduce on humans but causes "mange" in animals. If an animal with "mange" has close contact with a person, the animal mite can get under the person's skin and cause temporary itching and skin irritation. However, the animal mite cannot reproduce on a person and will die on its own in a couple of days. Although the person does not need to be treated, the animal should be treated because its mites can continue to burrow into the person's skin and cause symptoms until the animal has been treated successfully.

Chapter 59

Tinea Infections

Ringworm is a common infection of the skin and nails that is caused by fungus. The infection is called "ringworm" because it can cause an itchy, red, circular rash. Ringworm is also called "tinea" or "dermato-phytosis." The different types of ringworm are usually named for the location of the infection on the body.

Areas of the body that can be affected by ringworm include:

- Feet (tinea pedis, commonly called "athlete's foot")

- Groin, inner thighs, or buttocks (tinea cruris, commonly called "jock itch")

- Scalp (tinea capitis)

- Beard (tinea barbae)

- Hands (tinea manuum)

- Toenails or fingernails (tinea unguium, also called "onychomycosis")

- Other parts of the body, such as arms or legs (tinea corporis)

This chapter contains text excerpted from the following sources: Text in this chapter begins with excerpts from "About Ringworm," Centers for Disease Control and Prevention (CDC), August 6, 2018; Text under the heading *"Tinea Pedis"* is excerpted from "Hygiene-Related Diseases," Centers for Disease Control and Prevention (CDC), February 6, 2017.

Approximately 40 different species of fungi can cause ringworm; the scientific names for the types of fungi that cause ringworm are *"Trichophyton," "Microsporum," and "Epidermophyton."*

Symptoms of Ringworm Infections

Ringworm can affect the skin on almost any part of the body, as well as fingernails and toenails. The symptoms of ringworm often depend on which part of the body is infected, but they generally include:

- Itchy skin

- Ring-shaped rash

- Red, scaly, cracked skin

- Hair loss

Symptoms typically appear between 4 and 14 days after the skin comes in contact with the fungi that cause ringworm.

Symptoms of ringworm by its location on the body are as follows:

- **Tinea pedis or "athlete's foot":** The symptoms of ringworm on the feet include red, swollen, peeling, itchy skin between the toes (especially between the pinky toe and the one next to it). The sole and heel of the foot may also be affected. In severe cases, the skin on the feet can blister.

- **Tinea capitis:** Ringworm on the scalp usually looks like a scaly, itchy, red, circular bald spot. The bald spot can grow in size and multiple spots might develop if the infection spreads. Ringworm on the scalp is more common in children than it is in adults.

- **Tinea cruris or "jock itch":** Ringworm on the groin looks like scaly, itchy, red spots, usually on the inner sides of the skin folds of the thigh.

- **Tinea barbae:** Symptoms of ringworm on the beard include scaly, itchy, red spots on the cheeks, chin, and upper neck. The spots might become crusted over or filled with pus, and the affected hair might fall out.

Ringworm Risk and Prevention
Who Gets Ringworm

Ringworm is very common. Anyone can get ringworm, but people who have weakened immune systems may be especially at risk for infection and may have problems fighting off a ringworm infection. People who use public showers or locker rooms, athletes (particularly those who are involved in contact sports, such as wrestling), people who wear tight shoes and have excessive sweating, and people who have close contact with animals may also be more likely to come in contact with the fungi that cause ringworm.

How Can I Prevent Ringworm?

- Keep your skin clean and dry.
- Wear shoes that allow air to circulate freely around your feet.
- Do not walk barefoot in areas, such as locker rooms or public showers.
- Clip your fingernails and toenails short and keep them clean.
- Change your socks and underwear at least once a day.
- Do not share clothing, towels, sheets, or other personal items with someone who has ringworm.
- Wash your hands with soap and running water after playing with pets. If you suspect that your pet has ringworm, take it to see a veterinarian. If your pet has ringworm, follow the steps below to prevent spreading the infection.
- If you are an athlete involved in close contact sports, shower immediately after your practice session or match, and keep all of your sports gear and uniform clean. Do not share sports gear (helmet, etc.) with other players.

My Pet Has Ringworm and I Am Worried about Ringworm in My House. What Should I Do?

Ringworm can easily transfer from animals to humans. You can take the following steps to protect yourself and your pet:

For People

Do:

- Wash your hands with soap and running water after playing with or petting your pet.
- Wear gloves and long sleeves if you must handle animals with ringworm, and always wash your hands after handling the animal.

453

- Vacuum the areas of the home that the infected pet commonly visits. This will help to remove infected fur or flakes of skin.

- Disinfect areas the pet has spent time in, including surfaces and bedding.

  - The spores of this fungus can be killed with common disinfectants, such as diluted chlorine bleach (¼ cup per 1 gallon of water), benzalkonium chloride, or strong detergents.

  - Never mix cleaning products. This may cause harmful gases.

Do not handle animals with ringworm if your immune system is weak in any way (if you have human immunodeficiency virus/acquired immunodeficiency syndrome (HIV/AIDS), are undergoing cancer treatment, or are taking medications that suppress the immune system, for example).

For Pets
Protect Your Pet's Health

- If you suspect that your pet has ringworm, make sure it is seen by a veterinarian so treatment can be started.

- If one of your pets has ringworm, make sure you have every pet in the household checked.

There Is a Ringworm Outbreak in My Child's School / Day Care Center. What Should I Do?

- Contact your local health department for more information.

- Tell your child not to share personal items, such as clothing, hairbrushes, and hats, with other people.

- Take your child to see a pediatrician if she or he develops ringworm symptoms.

- Check with your child's school or day care to see if she or he can still attend classes or participate in athletics.

Sources of Infection

The fungi that cause ringworm can live on the skin and in the environment. There are three main ways that ringworm can spread:

From a Person Who Has Ringworm

People can get ringworm after contact with someone who has the infection. To avoid spreading the infection, people with ringworm should not share clothing, towels, combs, or other personal items with other people.

From an Animal That Has Ringworm

People can get ringworm after touching an animal that has ringworm. Many different kinds of animals can spread ringworm to people, including dogs and cats, especially kittens and puppies. Other animals, such as cows, goats, pigs, and horses, can also spread ringworm to people.

From the Environment

The fungi that cause ringworm can live on surfaces, particularly in damp areas, such as locker rooms and public showers. For that reason, it is a good idea not to walk barefoot in these places.

How Is Ringworm Diagnosed?

Your healthcare provider can usually diagnose ringworm by looking at the affected skin and asking questions about your symptoms. She or he may also take a small skin scraping to be examined under a microscope or sent to a laboratory for a fungal culture.

Treatment for Ringworm

The treatment for ringworm depends on its location on the body and how serious the infection is. Some forms of ringworm can be treated with nonprescription (over-the-counter (OTC)) medications, but other forms of ringworm need treatment with prescription antifungal medication.

- Ringworm on the skin, such as athlete's foot and jock itch can usually be treated with nonprescription antifungal creams, lotions, or powders applied to the skin for two to four weeks. There are many nonprescription products available to treat ringworm, including:

  - Clotrimazole (Lotrimin, Mycelex)

  - Miconazole (Aloe Vesta Antifungal, Azolen, Baza Antifungal, Carrington Antifungal, Critic-Aid Clear, Cruex Prescription

Strength, DermaFungal, Desenex, Fungoid Tincture, Micaderm, Micatin, Micro-Guard, Miranel, Mitrazol, Podactin, Remedy Antifungal, Secura Antifungal)

- Terbinafine (Lamisil)

- Ketoconazole (Xolegel)

For nonprescription creams, lotions, or powders, follow the directions on the package label. Contact your healthcare provider if your infection does not go away or gets worse.

- Tinea capitis usually needs to be treated with prescription antifungal medication taken by mouth for one to three months. Creams, lotions, or powders do not work for ringworm on the scalp. Prescription antifungal medications used to treat ringworm on the scalp include:

  - Griseofulvin (Grifulvin V, Gris-PEG)

  - Terbinafine

  - Itraconazole (Onmel, Sporanox)

  - Fluconazole (Diflucan)

You should contact your healthcare provider if:

- Your infection gets worse or does not go away after using nonprescription medications.

- You or your child has ringworm on the scalp. Ringworm on the scalp needs to be treated with prescription antifungal medication.

Tinea Pedis

Tinea pedis is an infection of the skin and feet that can be caused by a variety of different fungi. Although tinea pedis can affect any portion of the foot, the infection most often affects the space between the toes. Athlete's foot is typically characterized by skin fissures or scales that can be red and itchy.

Tinea pedis is spread through contact with infected skin scales or contact with fungi in damp areas (for example, showers, locker rooms, swimming pools). Tinea pedis can be a chronic infection that recurs frequently. Treatment may include topical creams (applied to the surface of the skin) or oral medications.

Appropriate hygiene techniques may help to prevent or control tinea pedis. The following hygiene techniques should be followed:

Prevention of athlete's foot:

- Nails should be clipped short and kept clean. Nails can house and spread the infection.

- Avoid walking barefoot in locker rooms or public showers (wear sandals).

For control of athlete's foot infection, persons with active tinea pedis infection should:

- Keep their feet clean, dry, and cool.

- Avoid using swimming pools, public showers, or foot baths.

- Wear sandals when possible or air shoes out by alternating them every two to three days.

- Avoid wearing closed shoes and wearing socks made from fabric that does not dry easily (for example, nylon).

- Treat the infection with recommended medication.

Chapter 60

Trichomoniasis

What Is Trichomoniasis?

Trichomoniasis or "trich" is a sexually transmitted infection (STI) caused by a parasite. The parasite is spread most often through vaginal, oral, or anal sex. It is one of the most common STIs in the United States and affects more women than men. It is treated easily with antibiotics, but many women do not have symptoms. If left untreated, trichomoniasis can raise your risk of getting the human immunodeficiency virus (HIV).

Who Gets Trichomoniasis

Trichomoniasis is more common in women than men. It affects more than 2 million women between the ages of 14 and 49 in the United States.

Trichomoniasis affects more African American women than White and Hispanic women. The risk for African American women increases with age and lifetime number of sex partners.

This chapter includes text excerpted from "Trichomoniasis," Office on Women's Health (OWH), U.S. Department of Health and Human Services (HHS), April 1, 2019.

How Do You Get Trichomoniasis?

Trichomoniasis is spread through:

- **Vaginal, oral, or anal sex.** Trichomoniasis can be spread even if there are no symptoms. This means you can get trichomoniasis from someone who has no signs or symptoms.

- **Genital touching.** A man does not need to ejaculate for trichomoniasis to spread. Trichomoniasis can also be passed between women who have sex with women (WSW).

What Are the Symptoms of Trichomoniasis?

Most infected women have no symptoms. If you do get symptoms, they might appear 5 to 28 days after exposure and can include:

- Irritation and itching in the genital area

- Thin or frothy discharge with an unusual foul odor that can be clear, white, yellowish, or greenish

- Discomfort during sex and when urinating

- Lower abdominal pain (this is rare)

If you think you may have trichomoniasis, you and your sex partner(s) need to see a doctor or nurse as soon as possible.

How Is Trichomoniasis Diagnosed?

To find out whether you have trichomoniasis, your doctor or nurse may:

- Do a pelvic exam

- Use a cotton swab to take a fluid sample from your vagina to look for the parasite under a microscope

- Do a lab test, such as a deoxyribonucleic acid (DNA) test or a fluid culture. A culture test uses urine or a swab from your vagina. The parasite then grows in a lab. It takes up to a week for the parasite to grow enough to be seen.

A Papanicolaou (Pap) test is not used to detect trichomoniasis.
If you have trichomoniasis, you need to be tested for other STIs too.

How Is Trichomoniasis Treated?

Trichomoniasis is easily cured with one of two antibiotics:

- Metronidazole
- Tinidazole

These antibiotics are usually a pill you swallow in a single dose.

If you are treated for trichomoniasis, your sex partner(s) needs to be treated too. Do not have sex until you and your sex partner(s) finish taking all of the antibiotics and have no symptoms.

What Can Happen If Trichomoniasis Is Not Treated?

Most people with trichomoniasis have no symptoms and never know they have it. Even without symptoms, it can be passed to others.

If you have trichomoniasis, you are at a higher risk of getting HIV (the virus that causes acquired immunodeficiency virus (AIDS)) if you are exposed to HIV. If you are HIV-positive, having trichomoniasis also raises your risk of passing HIV to your sex partner(s). The Centers for Disease Control and Prevention (CDC) recommends that women with HIV get screened for trichomoniasis at least once a year.

What Should I Do If I Have Trichomoniasis?

Trichomoniasis is easy to treat. But, you need to be tested and treated as soon as possible.

If you have trichomoniasis:

- See a doctor or nurse as soon as possible. Antibiotics will treat trichomoniasis.

- Take all of your medicine. Even if symptoms go away, you need to finish all of the antibiotics.

- Tell your sex partner(s) so they can be tested and treated.

- Avoid sexual contact until you and your partner(s) have been treated and cured. Even after you finish your antibiotics, you can get trichomoniasis again if you have sex with someone who has trichomoniasis.

- See your doctor or nurse again if you have symptoms that do not go away within a few days after finishing the antibiotics.

461

How Does Trichomoniasis Affect Pregnancy?

Pregnant women with trichomoniasis are at a higher risk of a premature birth (babies born before 37 weeks of pregnancy) or having a low-birth-weight (LBW) baby (less than 5½ pounds). A premature birth and a low birth weight raise the risk of health and developmental problems at birth and later in life.

The antibiotic metronidazole can be used to treat trichomoniasis during any stage of pregnancy. Talk to your doctor about the benefits and risks of taking any medicine during pregnancy.

Can I Take Medicine for Trichomoniasis If I Am Breastfeeding?

You can take the antibiotic metronidazole if you are breastfeeding. Your doctor may suggest waiting 12 to 24 hours after taking metronidazole before breastfeeding. Do not take tinidazole if you are breastfeeding.

How Can I Prevent Trichomoniasis?

The best way to prevent trichomoniasis or any STI is to not have vaginal, oral, or anal sex.

If you do have sex, lower your risk of getting an STI with the following steps:

- **Use condoms.** Condoms are the best way to prevent STIs when you have sex. Because a man does not need to ejaculate to give or get trichomoniasis, make sure to put the condom on before the penis touches the vagina, mouth, or anus. Other methods of birth control, such as birth control pills, shots, implants, or diaphragms, will not protect you from STIs.

- **Get tested.** Be sure you and your partner are tested for STIs. Talk to each other about the test results before you have sex.

- **Be monogamous.** Having sex with just one partner can lower your risk for STIs. After being tested for STIs, be faithful to each other. That means that you have sex only with each other and no one else.

- **Limit your number of sex partners.** Your risk of getting STIs goes up with the number of partners you have.

- **Do not douche.** Douching removes some of the normal bacteria in the vagina that protects you from infection. This may increase your risk of getting STIs.

- **Do not abuse alcohol or drugs.** Drinking too much alcohol or using drugs increases risky behavior and may put you at risk of sexual assault and possible exposure to STIs.

The steps work best when used together. No single step can protect you from every single type of STI.

Can Women Who Have Sex with Women Get Trichomoniasis?

Yes. It is possible to get trichomoniasis, or any other STI, if you are a woman who has sex only with women.

Talk to your partner about her sexual history before having sex, and ask your doctor about getting tested if you have signs or symptoms of trichomoniasis.

Part Five

Self-Treatment for Contagious Diseases

Chapter 61

Self-Care for Colds or Flu

Chapter Contents

Section 61.1—What to Do for Colds and Flu.............................. 468

Section 61.2—Cold, Flu, or Allergy? Know the
             Difference... 471

Section 61.3—Antibiotics Do Not Work for a Cold
             or the Flu 473

Section 61.4—Healthy Habits to Help Prevent Flu.................. 474

Section 61.5—Taking Care of Yourself When You
             Have Seasonal Flu 476

Section 61.1

What to Do for Colds and Flu

This section includes text excerpted from "Is It a
Cold or the Flu? Prevention, Symptoms, Treatments,"
U.S. Food and Drug Administration (FDA), March 15, 2018.

Most viral respiratory infections, such as the common cold, come
and go within a few days, with no lasting effects. But, the flu can cause
serious health problems and can result in hospitalization or death.

You can fight back by adopting healthy habits and by using medicines and vaccines approved by the U.S. Food and Drug Administration
(FDA) to combat and help prevent the flu.

If you are generally healthy, here is how to tell if you have a cold
or the flu and when to seek medical care.

Symptoms of Colds and Flu

Flu and cold viruses spread mainly by respiratory droplets, when
infected people cough, sneeze, or talk. You also can get infected by
touching a surface or object that has viruses on it. Flu season in the
United States may begin as early as October and can last as late as
May, and generally peaks between December and February.

Colds. Symptoms of colds usually are a stuffy or runny nose and
sneezing. Other symptoms include coughing, a scratchy throat, and
watery eyes. There is no vaccine to prevent colds, which come on grad-
ually and often spread through everyday contact.

Flu. Symptoms of the flu come on suddenly and can include
fever, headache, chills, dry cough, sore throat, body or muscle aches,
tiredness, and feeling generally miserable. As with the viruses that
cause a cold, flu viruses can cause a stuffy or runny nose, sneezing,
and watery eyes. Young children also may experience nausea and
vomiting.

Check with your healthcare provider promptly if you are at a high
risk for flu-related complications and you have flu symptoms—or
if you have flu symptoms that do not improve. People at high risk
include:

- Children younger than five years of age, but especially those
  younger than the age of two

- Pregnant women

- People with certain chronic health conditions (such as asthma, diabetes, or heart and lung disease)

- People 65 years of age or older

Rapid Flu Tests Are Available

Some healthcare providers can give you an FDA-approved rapid flu test. There are 13 rapid flu tests on the market with updated performance criteria that the FDA created to provide reasonable assurance that the test is accurate, reliable, and clinically valid.

But know that, according to the Centers for Disease Control and Prevention's (CDC) flu testing guidelines, you do not need testing—or to await test results—before your healthcare provider can prescribe antiviral medication. Your healthcare provider will decide what to prescribe based on the signs and symptoms you have.

What to Do If You Are Already Sick

Colds usually run their course. When you are sick, limit exposing yourself to other people. Cover your mouth and nose when you cough or sneeze. Also, stay hydrated and rested; avoid alcohol and caffeinated products.

There are FDA-approved prescription medications—called "antivirals"—for treating flu. Also, a cold or flu may lead to a bacterial infection (such as bronchitis, sinusitis, ear infections, and pneumonia) that could require antibiotics.

Rest assured, most people with the flu who are not at a high risk have mild illness and do not need medical care or antiviral drugs. Still, your symptoms may last up to two weeks.

How to Safely Take Over-the-Counter Medicines for Cold or Flu Symptoms

Read medicine labels carefully, and follow the directions. People with certain health conditions, such as high blood pressure or diabetes, should check with a doctor or pharmacist before taking a new cough or cold medicine.

Choose the right over-the-counter (OTC) medicines for your symptoms.

- Nasal decongestants help unclog a stuffy nose.

- Cough suppressants help relieve coughs.

469

- Expectorants help loosen mucus.

- Antihistamines help stop a runny nose and sneezing.

- Pain relievers can help ease fever, headaches, and minor aches.

Check the medicine's side effects. Medications can cause drowsiness and interact with food, alcohol, dietary supplements, and other medicines. Tell your doctor and pharmacist about every medical product and supplement you are taking.

Check with a healthcare professional before giving medicine to children.

Prevention Tips

Get vaccinated against the flu. The best way to prevent the flu is by getting vaccinated every year. That is because flu viruses can change from year to year, so the vaccines may need to be updated to protect against new strains. Also, the protection provided by the previous year's vaccine will diminish over time and may be too low to provide protection into the next year.

With rare exceptions, everyone six months of age and older should be vaccinated against flu. The vaccine is an important step for reducing flu illnesses and preventing flu-related hospitalizations and deaths.

Annual vaccination is especially important for people at a high risk of developing serious complications from flu. People who use tobacco or who are exposed to secondhand smoke, healthcare workers, and anyone who lives with or cares for people at high risk for serious flu-related complications should also get vaccinated.

Babies younger than six months of age are too young to get a flu vaccine. So, the CDC recommends that pregnant women and parents of infants should get a flu shot to help protect themselves and their babies during those early months. Also, all the baby's caregivers and close contacts should be vaccinated.

Wash your hands often. Teach children to do the same. Both colds and flu can be passed through contaminated surfaces, including the hands. Wash your hands with warm water and soap for at least 20 seconds.

Limit exposure to infected people. Keep infants away from crowds for the first few months of life.

Section 61.2

Cold, Flu, or Allergy? Know the Difference

This section includes text excerpted from "Cold, Flu, or Allergy?" *NIH News in Health*, National Institutes of Health (NIH), October 2014. Reviewed July 2019.

You are feeling pretty lousy. You have got sniffles, sneezing, and a sore throat. Is it a cold, flu, or allergies? It can be hard to tell them apart because they share so many symptoms. But, understanding the differences will help you choose the best treatment.

"If you know what you have, you would not take medications that you do not need, that are not effective, or that might even make your symptoms worse," says the National Institutes of Health's (NIH) Dr. Teresa Hauguel, an expert on infectious diseases that affect breathing.

The cold, flu, and allergies all affect your respiratory system, which can make it hard to breathe. Each condition has key symptoms that set them apart.

Colds and flu are caused by different viruses. "As a rule of thumb, the symptoms associated with the flu are more severe," says Hauguel. Both illnesses can lead to a runny, stuffy nose; congestion; cough; and sore throat. But the flu can also cause high fever that lasts for three to four days, along with a headache, fatigue, and general aches and pain. These symptoms are less common when you have a cold.

"Allergies are a little different because they are not caused by a virus," Hauguel explains. "Instead, it is your body's immune system reacting to a trigger, or allergen, which is something you are allergic to." If you have allergies and breathe in things such as pollen or pet dander, the immune cells in your nose and airways may overreact to these harmless substances. Your delicate respiratory tissues may then swell, and your nose may become stuffed up or runny.

"Allergies can also cause itchy, watery eyes, which you do not normally have with a cold or flu," Hauguel adds.

Allergy symptoms usually last as long as you are exposed to the allergen, which may be about six weeks during pollen seasons in the Spring, Summer, or Fall. Colds and flu rarely last beyond two weeks.

Most people with a cold or flu recover on their own without medical care. But, check with a healthcare provider if symptoms last beyond 10 days or if symptoms are not relieved by over-the-counter (OTC) medicines.

Table 61.1. Symptoms of Cold, Flu, and Airborne Allergy

Symptoms	Cold	Flu	Airborne Allergy
Fever	Rare	Usual, high (100–102°F), sometimes higher, especially in young children); lasts 3–4 days	Never
Headache	Uncommon	Common	Uncommon
General Aches, Pains	Slight	Usual; often severe	Never
Fatigue, Weakness	Sometimes	Usual, can last up to 3 weeks	Sometimes
Extreme Exhaustion	Never	Usual, at the beginning of the illness	Never
Stuffy, Runny Nose	Common	Sometimes	Common
Sneezing	Usual	Sometimes	Usual
Sore Throat	Common	Sometimes	Sometimes
Cough	Common	Common, can become severe	Sometimes
Chest Discomfort	Mild to moderate	Common	Rare, except for those with allergic asthma
Treatment	Get plenty of rest. Stay hydrated. (Drink plenty of fluids.) Decongestants. Aspirin (ages 18 and up), acetaminophen, or ibuprofen for aches and pains	Get plenty of rest. Stay hydrated. Aspirin (ages 18 and up), acetaminophen, or ibuprofen for aches, pains, and fever Antiviral medicines (see your doctor)	Avoid allergens (things that you are allergic to) Antihistamines Nasal steroids Decongestants
Prevention	Wash your hands often. Avoid close contact with anyone who has a cold.	Get the flu vaccine each year. Wash your hands often. Avoid close contact with anyone who has the flu.	Avoid allergens, such as pollen, house dust mites, mold, pet dander, cockroaches.
Complications	Sinus infection middle ear infection, asthma	Bronchitis, pneumonia; can be life-threatening	Sinus infection, middle ear infection, asthma

To treat colds or flu, get plenty of rest and drink lots of fluids. If you have the flu, pain relievers such as aspirin, acetaminophen, or ibuprofen can reduce fever or aches. Allergies can be treated with antihistamines or decongestants.

Be careful to avoid "drug overlap" when taking medicines that list two or more active ingredients on the label. For example, if you take two different drugs that contain acetaminophen—one for a stuffy nose and the other for headache—you may be getting too much acetaminophen.

"Read medicine labels carefully—the warnings, side effects, dosages. If you have questions, talk to your doctor or pharmacist, especially if you have children who are sick," Hauguel says. "You do not want to overmedicate, and you do not want to risk taking a medication that may interact with another."

Section 61.3

Antibiotics Do Not Work for a Cold or the Flu

This section includes text excerpted from "Sniffle or Sneeze? No Antibiotics Please," Centers for Disease Control and Prevention (CDC), November 3, 2003. Reviewed July 2019.

What Not to Do If You Are Already Sick

The problem is, taking antibiotics when they are not needed can do more harm than good. Widespread inappropriate use of antibiotics is fueling an increase in drug-resistant bacteria. And sick individuals are not the only people who can suffer the consequences. Families and entire communities feel the impact when disease-causing germs become resistant to antibiotics.

The most obvious consequence of inappropriate antibiotic use is its effect on the sick patient. When antibiotics are incorrectly used to treat children or adults with viral infections, such as colds and flu, they are not getting the best care for their condition. A course of antibiotics would not fight the virus, make the patient feel better, yield a quicker recovery or keep others from getting sick.

A less obvious consequence of antibiotic overuse is the boost it gives to drug-resistant disease-causing bacteria. Almost every type of bacteria has become stronger and less responsive to antibiotic treatment when it really is needed. These antibiotic-resistant bacteria can quickly spread to family members, schoolmates, and coworkers—threatening the community with a new strain of infectious disease that is more difficult to cure and more expensive to treat.

According to the Centers for Disease Control and Prevention (CDC), antibiotic resistance is one of the world's most pressing public health problems. Americans of all ages can lower this risk by talking to their doctors and using antibiotics appropriately during this cold and flu season.

Section 61.4

Healthy Habits to Help Prevent Flu

This section includes text excerpted from "Healthy Habits to Help Prevent Flu," Centers for Disease Control and Prevention (CDC), July 20, 2018.

The single best way to prevent seasonal flu is to get vaccinated each year, but good health habits, such as covering your cough and washing your hands often, can help stop the spread of germs and prevent respiratory illnesses like the flu. There also are flu antiviral drugs that can be used to treat and prevent flu. The tips and resources below will help you learn about steps you can take to protect yourself and others from flu and help stop the spread of germs.

1. **Avoid close contact.**

   Avoid close contact with people who are sick. When you are sick, keep your distance from others to protect them from getting sick too.

2. **Stay home when you are sick.**

   If possible, stay home from work, school, and errands when you are sick. This will help prevent spreading your illness to others.

3. Cover your mouth and nose.

Cover your mouth and nose with a tissue when coughing or sneezing. It may prevent those around you from getting sick. Flu and other serious respiratory illnesses, such as respiratory syncytial virus (RSV), whooping cough, and severe acute respiratory syndrome (SARS), are spread by cough, sneezing, or unclean hands.

4. Clean your hands.

Washing your hands often will help protect you from germs. If soap and water are not available, use an alcohol-based hand rub.

5. Avoid touching your eyes, nose or mouth.

Germs are often spread when a person touches something that is contaminated with germs and then touches his or her eyes, nose, or mouth.

6. Practice other good health habits.

Clean and disinfect frequently touched surfaces at home, work, or school, especially when someone is ill. Get plenty of sleep, be physically active, manage your stress, drink plenty of fluids, and eat nutritious food.

Preventing Flu at Work and School
At School

• Find out about plans your child's school, child care program, or college has if an outbreak of flu or another illness occurs and whether flu vaccinations are offered on-site.

• Make sure your child's school, child care program, or college routinely cleans frequently touched objects and surfaces, and that they have a good supply of tissues, soap, paper towels, alcohol-based hand rubs, and disposable wipes on-site.

• Ask how sick students and staff are separated from others and who will care for them until they can go home.

At Work

• Find out about your employer's plans if an outbreak of flu or another illness occurs and whether flu vaccinations are offered on-site.

- Routinely clean frequently touched objects and surfaces, including doorknobs, keyboards, and phones, to help remove germs.

- Make sure your workplace has an adequate supply of tissues, soap, paper towels, alcohol-based hand rubs, and disposable wipes.

- Train others on how to do your job so they can cover for you in case you or a family member gets sick and you have to stay home.

- If you begin to feel sick while at work, go home as soon as possible.

Section 61.5

Taking Care of Yourself When You Have Seasonal Flu

This section includes text excerpted from "Flu: What to Do If You Get Sick," Centers for Disease Control and Prevention (CDC), February 28, 2019.

What Should I Do If I Get Sick?

Most people with the flu have mild illness and do not need medical care or antiviral drugs. If you get sick with flu symptoms, in most cases, you should stay home and avoid contact with other people except to get medical care.

If, however, you have symptoms of flu and are in a high-risk group, or you are very sick or worried about your illness, contact your health-care provider (doctor, physician assistant, etc.).

Certain people are at a high risk of serious flu-related complications (including young children, people 65 years of age and older, pregnant women, and people with certain medical conditions). This is true both for seasonal flu and novel flu virus infections. If you are in a high-risk group and develop flu symptoms, it is best for you to contact your doctor early in your illness. Remind them about your high-risk status for flu.

The Centers for Disease Control and Prevention (CDC) recommends that people at a high risk for complications should get antiviral treatment as early as possible, because benefit is greatest if treatment is started within two days after illness onset.

Do I Need to Go the Emergency Room If I Am Only a Little Sick?

No. The emergency room should be used for people who are very sick. You should not go to the emergency room if you are only mildly ill.

If you have the emergency warning signs of flu sickness, you should go to the emergency room. If you get sick with flu symptoms and are at a high risk of flu complications or you are concerned about your illness, call your healthcare provider for advice. If you go to the emergency room and you are not sick with the flu, you may catch it from people who do have it.

Are There Medicines to Treat the Flu?

Yes. There are drugs your doctor may prescribe for treating the flu called "antivirals." These drugs can make you better faster and may also prevent serious complications.

How Long Should I Stay Home If I Am Sick?

The CDC recommends that you stay home for at least 24 hours after your fever is gone except to get medical care or other necessities. Your fever should be gone without the need to use a fever-reducing medicine, such as Tylenol®. Until then, you should stay home from work, school, travel, shopping, social events, and public gatherings.

The CDC also recommends that children and teenagers (anyone 18 years of age and younger) who have flu or are suspected to have flu should not be given Aspirin (acetylsalicylic acid) or any salicylate-containing products (e.g., Pepto Bismol); this can cause a rare, very serious complication called "Reye syndrome."

What Should I Do While I Am Sick?

Stay away from others as much as possible to keep from infecting them. If you must leave home, for example, to get medical care, wear a facemask if you have one or cover coughs and sneezes with a tissue. Wash your hands often to keep from spreading flu to others.

Chapter 62

Sore Throat Care

Most sore throats will go away on their own without antibiotics. In some cases (like for strep throat), a lab test will need to be done to see if you or your child need antibiotics.

Causes of Sore Throat

Most sore throats are caused by viruses, such as the ones that cause a cold or the flu, and do not need antibiotic treatment.

Some sore throats are caused by bacteria, such as group A *Streptococcus* (group A strep). Sore throats caused by these bacteria are known as "strep throat." In children, 20 to 30 out of every 100 sore throats are strep throat. In adults, only 5 to 15 out of every 100 sore throats is strep throat.

Other common causes of sore throats include:

- Allergies

- Dry air

- Pollution (airborne chemicals or irritants)

- Smoking or exposure to secondhand smoke

This chapter includes text excerpted from "Sore Throat," Centers for Disease Control and Prevention (CDC), April 17, 2015. Reviewed July 2019.

Risk Factors of Sore Throat

There are many things that can increase your risk for a sore throat, including:

- Age. Children and teens between 5 and 15 years of age are most likely to get a sore throat.

- Exposure to someone with a sore throat or strep throat

- Time of the year. Winter and early Spring are common times for strep throat.

- Weather. Cold air can irritate your throat.

- Irregularly shaped or large tonsils

- Pollution or smoke exposure

- A weak immune system or taking drugs that weaken the immune system

- Postnasal drip or allergies

- Acid reflux disease

Signs and Symptoms of Sore Throat

A sore throat can make it painful to swallow. A sore throat can also feel dry and scratchy, and it may be a symptom of the common cold or other upper respiratory tract infection.

The following symptoms are often associated with sore throats caused by a viral infection or due to allergies:

- Sneezing

- Coughing

- Watery eyes

- Mild headache or body aches

- Runny nose

- Low fever (less than 101°F)

Symptoms more commonly associated with strep throat include:

- Red and swollen tonsils, sometimes with white patches or streaks of pus

- Tiny red spots (petechiae) on the soft or hard palate (the roof of the mouth)

- High fever (101°F or above)
- Nausea
- Vomiting
- Swollen lymph nodes in the neck
- Severe headache or body aches
- Rash

When to Seek Medical Care

See a healthcare professional if you or your child has any of the following:

- Sore throat that lasts longer than one week
- Difficulty swallowing or breathing
- Excessive drooling (young children)
- Temperature higher than 100.4°F
- Pus on the back of the throat
- Rash
- Joint pain
- Hoarseness lasting longer than two weeks
- Blood in saliva or phlegm
- Dehydration (symptoms include a dry, sticky mouth; sleepiness or tiredness; thirst; decreased urination or fewer wet diapers; few or no tears when crying; muscle weakness; headache; and dizziness or light-headedness)
- Recurring sore throats

If your child is younger than three months of age and has a fever, it is important to always call your healthcare professional right away.

Diagnosis and Treatment of Sore Throat

Antibiotics are not needed to treat most sore throats, which usually improve on their own within one to two weeks. Antibiotics will not help if a sore throat is caused by a virus or irritation from the air. Antibiotic treatment in these cases may cause harm in both children and adults.

Your healthcare professional may prescribe other medicine or give you tips to help with other symptoms, such as fever and coughing.

Antibiotics are needed if a healthcare professional diagnoses you or your child with strep throat, which is caused by bacteria. This diagnosis can be done using a quick swab of the throat. Strep throat cannot be diagnosed by looking in the throat—a lab test must be done.

Antibiotics are prescribed for strep throat to prevent rheumatic fever. If diagnosed with strep throat, an infected patient should stay home from work, school, or day care until 24 hours after starting an antibiotic.

Prevention of Sore Throat

There are steps you can take to help prevent getting a sore throat, including:

- Practice good hand hygiene.

- Avoid close contact with people who have sore throats, colds, or other upper respiratory infections.

- Avoid smoking and exposure to secondhand smoke.

Chapter 63

Fever: What You Can Do

What Is a Fever?

A fever—also called high temperature or pyrexia—is a temporary rise in the body's temperature. It is not an illness itself but a natural defense against bacteria or viruses that thrive best at normal body temperature, around 98.6°F.

Hyperthermia is a form of fever in which the body's temperature rises far above normal and can be caused, for example, by side effects of illicit drugs or certain medications, stroke, or by temperature-related conditions like heat stroke. Usually, a fever is not considered life-threatening, but hyperthermia can lead to a critical elevation of the body's temperature.

An adult is considered to have a fever if the body temperature is above 99°F to 99.5°F (37.2°C to 37.5°C), depending on the time of the day. (Body temperature is usually highest in late afternoon.) A child is considered to have a fever if the temperature is at or above:

- 100.4°F (38°C) rectally

- 99.5°F (37.5°C) orally

- 99°F (37.2°C) axillary (measured under the arm)

"Fever: What You Can Do," © 2017 Omnigraphics. Reviewed July 2019.

What Causes Fever

The hypothalamus, a region in the brain that helps the body main its normal temperature, may cause temperature to fluctuate in response to a number of factors, such as eating, heavy clothing, high humidity, medications, physical activity, room temperature, strong emotions, and menstrual cycles in women. The hypothalamus may also cause an increase in the body temperature as a response to an infection or illness.

Although the most frequent causes of fever are common infections, such as colds, other possibilities include:

- Appendicitis

- Autoimmune or inflammatory conditions

- Blood clots or thrombophlebitis

- Bone infections (osteomyelitis)

- Cancer, particularly leukemia, Hodgkin disease, and non-Hodgkin lymphoma

- Reaction to medications, such as certain antibiotics, antihistamines, and seizure medicines

- Hormone disorders, such as hyperthyroidism

- Immunization, in some children

- Infections of the bladder or kidney

- Meningitis

- Respiratory infections, such as flu, sinus infections, mononucleosis, bronchitis, pneumonia, and tuberculosis

- Side effects of drugs like amphetamines and cocaine

- Skin infections or cellulitis

- Teething

Signs and Symptoms of Fever

In addition to an elevated body temperature, other symptoms of fever, depending on its underlying cause, can include headache, sweating, chills, muscle ache, weakness, and dehydration.

In children, symptoms may also include fussiness, lethargy, poor appetite, stiff neck, rashes, earache, sore throat, cough, vomiting, diarrhea, and a weakened immune system.

How Is a Fever Diagnosed?

Once a fever is measured with a thermometer, a physician will attempt to determine its cause by a physical examination (including thorough examination of the skin, eyes, ears, nose, throat, neck, chest, and abdomen) and by asking about recent behavior and interactions, including travel to regions that are known to be sources of infections. For instance, conditions like Lyme disease and Rocky Mountain spotted fever (RMSF) are endemic to certain parts of the United States, while such conditions as malaria are more common in sub-Saharan Africa and southern Asia. In certain cases, a person might be diagnosed with a "fever of unknown origin," one in which the cause is not attributable to an obvious condition.

To diagnose fever, the doctor may order tests that include:

- Blood tests (such as a complete blood count or blood differential)
- Chest X-ray
- Urinalysis

How Is Fever Treated?

A fever is treated based on its duration and cause, along with other symptoms that may accompany the elevated temperature. Typically, medications for fever include over-the-counter drugs, such as acetaminophen (Tylenol®), and nonsteroidal anti-inflammatory medicines, such as naproxen (Aleve) and ibuprofen (Advil, Motrin). If the fever is the result of a bacterial infection, such as strep throat, antibiotics would be prescribed. Aspirin may be taken by adults but is not recommended for children and teens, as it is associated with Reye syndrome, which can cause damage to the brain and liver.

Home Care

Fever is not necessarily a symptom of a serious problem. While a simple cold can lead to body temperatures as high as 104°F (40°C), some serious conditions may cause no fever at all.

A mild fever does not generally require treatment; enough rest and proper fluid consumption will usually suffice. The condition is most likely not serious if the patient:

- Is alert and active
- Continues to eat and drink well

- Has a normal skin color

- Looks well when the body temperature returns to normal

If a person with high body temperature is uncomfortable and experiences vomiting, dehydration, or inadequate sleep, follow these steps reduce the fever:

- Make the room comfortable. It should neither be too hot nor too cool.

- Remove excess clothing from the person. A single layer of lightweight clothing will be sufficient. If the patient has chills, do not bundle him/her up excessively.

- Cool the person with a lukewarm bath or sponge bath. This may be particularly effective after medication is given.

- Avoid cold baths, ice, or alcohol rubs, as they worsen the situation by making the person shiver, which can increase the core body temperature.

When Taking Medicine to Lower a Fever

- Always consult a doctor before giving medicines to a child three months of age or younger.

- In adults and children, acetaminophen and ibuprofen help reduce fever. A doctor may recommend the use of either type of medicine, although ibuprofen is not generally recommended for children under the age of six months.

- Aspirin is highly effective for treating fever but is recommended only for adults unless prescribed for a child by a doctor.

- The correct dose of medicine should be given to a child based on the child's weight and per the instructions on the package.

Eating and Drinking

It is important for adults, and even more so for children, to drink plenty of fluids to keep the body hydrated. Water, soup, popsicles, and gelatin are good choices. Consumption of fruit juice should be limited, and sports drinks should be avoided in young children. Eating is fine; however, food should not be forced.

When to Contact a Medical Professional

Call a doctor immediately if the fever:

- Is 100.4°F (38°C) or higher in a child 3 months or younger.

- Is 102.2°F (39°C) or higher in children between 3 and 12 months old.

- Is 105°F (40.5°C) or higher and does not come down readily when treated, and the person is not comfortable.

- Lasts longer than 24 to 48 hours in children 2 years or younger.

- Lasts longer than 48 to 72 hours in those older than 2 years.

Medical assistance will also be required if the patient:

- Has a fever that stays at 103°F or keeps rising.

- Has symptoms (such as a sore throat, cough, or earache) that are usually associated with other illnesses.

- Has had recurrent mild fevers for a week or more.

- Has bruises or a new rash.

- Has been vaccinated recently.

- Has pain when urinating.

- Traveled to another region or country recently.

- Is suffering from a serious medical condition, such as diabetes, heart disease, sickle cell anemia, chronic obstructive pulmonary disease (COPD), other chronic lung problems, or cystic fibrosis.

- Has problems with the immune system (such as one caused by a bone marrow or organ transplant, cancer treatment, chronic steroid therapy, HIV, or spleen removal).

If an infant three months old or younger has a temperature above 100.4°F, or any child has a temperature above 104°F, you should call a doctor or visit an emergency room immediately, since this could be a sign of potentially life-threatening condition. Febrile seizure can occur in some children with such high body temperatures, although this generally does not cause any permanent damage. But brain damage can occur if the fever is above 107.6°F (42°C).

References

1. Kaneshiro, Neil K. "Fever," MedlinePlus, National Institutes of Health (NIH), August 30, 2014.

2. Blahd, William. "Fever Facts," WebMD, LLC, April 16, 2015.

Chapter 64

Mouth Sores: Causes and Care

Mouth sores are common ailments that appear on the soft tissues of your mouth, including the cheeks, lips, tongue, gums, and roof and floor of the mouth. There is also a possibility of developing mouth sores in your esophagus—a muscular tube that carries food and liquids from your mouth to the stomach.

There are many types of mouth sores; however, the most common types are cold sores and canker sores. Cold sores, sometimes called "fever blisters," form around your lips.

Canker sores, also called "aphthous ulcers," are shallow, small lesions that develop on the soft tissues in the mouth or at the base of your gums.

Causes of Mouth Sores

Mostly, mouth sores occur as a result of irritation from:

- Biting your cheek, tongue, or lip
- Burning your mouth from hot drinks or foods
- Chewing tobacco
- A sharp or broken tooth
- Braces

"Mouth Sores: Causes and Care," © 2019 Omnigraphics. Reviewed July 2019.

In other cases, mouth sores can develop due to the following reasons:

- High acidic foods
- Stress
- Hormonal changes during pregnancy
- Vitamin and folate deficiencies

The sores can spread from person to person by close contact (such as kissing).

Cold sores are caused by the herpes simplex virus (HSV) and are contagious. Unlike cold sores, canker sores do not occur on the surface of the lips and are not contagious. The cause of the canker sores remains unclear, but it may be related to:

- Virus
- Irritation
- Minor injury during dental operations
- Overzealous brushing
- Mouth rinses and toothpastes containing lauryl sulfate
- Diet lacking in vitamin B_{12}, zinc, folate, or iron
- Hormonal changes during menstruation

Rarely, mouth sores can be a sign of a tumor or illness. In such cases, they may form in response to:

- Mouth cancer
- Infection (such as hand-foot-mouth syndrome)
- Bleeding disorders
- Weakened immune system
- Autoimmune disorders

Certain drugs and medications, such as aspirin, penicillin, phenytoin, streptomycin, chemotherapeutic agents, and sulfa drugs. tend to cause mouth sores.

Signs and Symptoms of Mouth Sores
Cold Sores

Cold sores are tiny, fluid-filled blisters that occur around your lips. These blisters are often grouped together in patches. The symptoms of cold sores are:

- Blisters, lesions, or ulcers in the mouth
- Pain in the mouth or tongue
- Lip swelling
- Sore throat
- Difficulty swallowing
- Swollen glands
- Fever
- Headache

The signs and symptoms may vary depending on whether this is a recurrence or the first outbreak.

Canker Sores

Canker sores appear either as a single pale or yellow ulcer with a red outer ring or as a cluster of sores. The major symptoms of canker sores are:

- Severe pain
- Fever
- Extreme difficulty eating and drinking

How to Take Care of Your Mouth Sores

Mouth sores can last from 10 to 14 days. Usually, mouth sores do not need any treatment, but persistent, large, and painful sores often do need medical attention. Follow these steps to make yourself feel better:

- Gargle with salt or cold water.
- Apply cool compression.
- Avoid hot beverages.
- Avoid eating spicy and salty foods.
- Avoid citrus fruits.
- Avoid alcohol.
- Take pain relievers, such as acetaminophen.

For canker sores:

- Apply a thin paste of water and baking soda to the sore.

- For severe cases, anti-inflammatory amlexanox paste (Aphthasol) or fluocinonide gel (Lidex) is recommended.

Over-the-counter (OTC) medicines (such as creams, pastes, gels, or liquids) can help relieve the pain caused by mouth sores and to speed up the healing process.

When to See the Doctor

You must consult the doctor, if:

- You have large patches on the tongue or roof of the mouth

- The sore begins after starting new medication

- The sore lasts more than two weeks

- You have other symptoms, such as a skin rash, drooling, fever, or difficulty swallowing

What to Expect during a Doctor's Visit

The doctor will perform a physical examination of your tongue and mouth and review your medical history and symptoms.

The treatment will consist of the following:

- Antiviral medication to treat the sores that are caused by the HSV virus

- Medicine to numb the area that is causing extreme pain; this medicine may be prescribed as an ointment, such as lidocaine (which must not be used for children)

- Steroid gel to apply to the mouth sore

- A paste that stops swelling and inflammation (Aphthasol)

The doctor will prescribe a mouthwash, such as chlorhexidine gluconate (Peridex), or a solution to use to rinse the mouth. This will help you to heal and prevent further infections. The doctor may recommend a nutritional supplement, such as folate, zinc, or vitamin B_{12}, if you are low on nutrients.

Prevention of Mouth Sores

Mouth sores are common and can be prevented from spreading. The following steps can be followed to prevent mouth sores from spreading:

- Avoid close contact with people who have sores. The virus spreads more quickly when the sores secrete moisture from blisters.

- Avoid sharing items. Towels, utensils, and lip balms can spread the virus when blisters are present.

- Keep your hands clean.

References

1. "Cold Sore," Mayo Clinic, December 20, 2018.

2. "Canker Sore," Mayo Clinic, April 3, 2018.

3. Fletcher, Jenna. "Mouth Sores: Everything You Need to Know," Medical News Today, March 12, 2019.

4. Nordqvist, Christian. "Everything You Need to Know about Cold Sores," Medical News Today, May 19, 2017.

Chapter 65

Over-the-Counter Medications

Chapter Contents

Section 65.1—Over-the-Counter Medications and
How They Work 496

Section 65.2—Kids Are Not Just Small Adults:
Tips on Giving Over-the-Counter
Medicine to Children 499

Section 65.3—Over-the-Counter Cough and Cold
Products for Children 502

Section 65.1

Over-the-Counter Medications and How They Work

This section includes text excerpted from "Over-the-Counter Medicines," National Institute on Drug Abuse (NIDA), December 2017.

What Are Over-the-Counter Medicines?

Over-the-counter (OTC) medicines are those that can be sold directly to people without a prescription. OTC medicines treat a variety of illnesses and their symptoms including pain, coughs and colds, diarrhea, constipation, acne, and others. Some OTC medicines have active ingredients with the potential for misuse at higher-than-recommended dosages.

How Do People Misuse Over-the-Counter Medicines?

Misuse of an OTC medicine means:

- Taking medicine in a way or dose other than directed on the package

- Taking medicine for the effect it causes—for example, to get high

- Mixing OTC medicines together to create new products

What Are Some of the Commonly Misused Over-the-Counter Medicines?

There are two OTC medicines that are most commonly misused.

Dextromethorphan (DXM) is a cough suppressant found in many OTC cold medicines. The most common sources of abused DXM are extra strength cough syrup, tablets, and gel capsules. OTC medications that contain DXM often also contain antihistamines and decongestants. DXM may be swallowed in its original form or may be mixed with soda for flavor, called "robotripping" or "skittling." Users sometimes inject it. These medicines are often misused in combination with other drugs, such as alcohol and marijuana.

Loperamide is an antidiarrheal that is available in tablet, capsule, or liquid form. When misusing loperamide, people swallow large quantities of medicine. It is unclear how often this drug is misused.

How Do These Over-the-Counter Medicines Affect the Brain?

DXM is an opioid without effects on pain reduction and does not act on the opioid receptors. When taken in large doses, DXM causes a depressant effect and sometimes a hallucinogenic effect, similar to phencyclidine (PCP) and ketamine. Repeatedly seeking to experience that feeling can lead to addiction—a chronic relapsing brain condition characterized by an inability to stop using a drug despite damaging consequences to a person's life and health.

Loperamide is an opioid designed not to enter the brain. However, when taken in large amounts and combined with other substances, it may cause the drug to act in a similar way to other opioids. Other opioids, such as certain prescription pain relievers and heroin, bind to and activate opioid receptors in many areas of the brain, especially those involved in feelings of pain and pleasure. Opioid receptors are also located in the brainstem, which controls important processes, such as blood pressure, arousal, and breathing.

What Are the Health Effects of These Over-the-Counter Medicines?
Dextromethorphan

Short-term effects of DXM misuse can range from mild stimulation to alcohol- or marijuana-like intoxication. At high doses, a person may have hallucinations or feelings of physical distortion, extreme panic, paranoia, anxiety, and aggression.

Other health effects from DXM misuse can include the following:

- Hyperexcitability
- Poor motor control
- Lack of energy
- Stomach pain
- Vision changes
- Slurred speech

- Increased blood pressure
- Sweating

Misuse of DXM products containing acetaminophen can cause liver damage.

Loperamide

In the short term, loperamide is sometimes misused to lessen cravings and withdrawal symptoms; however, it can cause euphoria, similar to other opioids.

Loperamide misuse can also lead to fainting, stomach pain, constipation, eye changes, and loss of consciousness. It can cause the heart to beat erratically or rapidly, or it can cause kidney problems. These effects may increase if taken with other medicines that interact with loperamide. Other effects have not been well studied and reports are mixed, but the physical consequences of loperamide misuse can be severe.

Can a Person Overdose on These Over-the-Counter Medicines?

Yes, a person can overdose on cold medicines containing DXM or loperamide. An overdose occurs when a person uses enough of the drug to produce a life-threatening reaction or death.

As with other opioids, when people overdose on DXM or loperamide, their breathing often slows or stops. This can decrease the amount of oxygen that reaches the brain, a condition called "hypoxia." Hypoxia can have short- and long-term mental effects and effects on the nervous system, including coma and permanent brain damage and death.

How Can These Over-the-Counter Medicine Overdoses Be Treated?

A person who has overdosed needs immediate medical attention. Call 911. If the person has stopped breathing or if breathing is weak, begin cardiopulmonary resuscitation (CPR). DXM overdoses can also be treated with naloxone.

Certain medications can be used to treat heart rhythm problems caused by loperamide overdose. If the heart stops, healthcare providers will perform CPR and other cardiac support therapies.

Can Misuse of These Over-the-Counter Medicines Lead to Addiction?

Yes, misuse of DXM or loperamide can lead to addiction. An addiction develops when continued use of the drug causes issues, such as health problems and failure to meet responsibilities at work, school, or home.

The symptoms of withdrawal from DXM and loperamide have not been well studied.

How Can People Get Treatment for Addiction to These Over-the-Counter Medicines?

There are no medications approved specifically to treat DXM or loperamide addiction. Behavioral therapies, such as cognitive behavioral therapy (CBT) and contingency management, may be helpful. CBT helps modify the patient's drug-use expectations and behaviors, and effectively manage triggers and stress. Contingency management provides vouchers or small cash rewards for positive behaviors such as staying drug-free.

Section 65.2

Kids Are Not Just Small Adults: Tips on Giving Over-the-Counter Medicine to Children

This section includes text excerpted from "Kids Are Not Just Small Adults—Medicines, Children, and the Care Every Child Deserves," U.S. Food and Drug Administration (FDA), December 20, 2017.

Use care when giving any medicine to an infant or a child. Even over-the-counter (OTC) medicines that you buy are serious medicines. The following is advice from the U.S. Food and Drug Administration (FDA) and the makers of OTC medicines for giving OTC medicine to your child:

1. **Always read and follow the Drug Facts label on your OTC medicine.** This is important for choosing and safely using all OTC medicines. Read the label every time, before you give the medicine. Be sure you clearly understand how much medicine to give and when the medicine can be taken again.

2. **Know the "active ingredient" in your child's medicine.** This is what makes the medicine work and is always listed at the top of the Drug Facts label. Sometimes an active ingredient can treat more than one medical condition. For that reason, the same active ingredient can be found in many different medicines that are used to treat different symptoms. For example, a medicine for a cold and a medicine for a headache could each contain the same active ingredient. So, if you are treating a cold and a headache with two medicines and both have the same active ingredient, you could be giving two times the normal dose. If you are confused about your child's medicines, check with a doctor, nurse, or pharmacist.

3. **Give the right medicine, in the right amount, to your child.** Not all medicines are right for an infant or a child. Medicines with the same brand name can be sold in many different strengths, such as infant, children, and adult formulas. The amount and directions are also different for children of different ages or weights. Always use the right medicine and follow the directions exactly. Never use more medicine than directed, even if your child seems sicker than the last time.

4. **Talk to your doctor, pharmacist, or nurse to find out what mixes well and what does not.** Medicines, vitamins, supplements, foods, and beverages do not always mix well with each other. Your healthcare professional can help.

5. **Use the dosing tool that comes with the medicine, such as a dropper or a dosing cup.** A different dosing tool, or a kitchen spoon, could hold the wrong amount of medicine.

6. **Know the difference between a tablespoon (tbsp.) and a teaspoon (tsp.)** Do not confuse them! A tablespoon holds three times as much medicine as a teaspoon. On measuring tools, a teaspoon (tsp.) is equal to "5 cc" or "5 mL."

7. **Know your child's weight.** Directions on some OTC medicines are based on weight. Never guess the amount of

medicine to give to your child or try to figure it out from the adult dose instructions. If a dose is not listed for your child's age or weight, call your doctor or other members of your healthcare team.

8. **Prevent a poison emergency by always using a child-resistant cap.** Relock the cap after each use. Be especially careful with any products that contain iron; they are the leading cause of poisoning deaths in young children.

9. **Store all medicines in a safe place.** Nowadays medicines are tasty, colorful, and many can be chewed. Kids may think that these products are candy. To prevent an overdose or poisoning emergency, store all medicines and vitamins in a safe place out of your child's (and even your pet's) sight and reach. If your child takes too much, call the Poison Center Hotline at 800-222-1222 (open 24 hours every day, 7 days a week) or call 9-1-1.

10. **Check the medicine three times.** First, check the outside packaging for such things as cuts, slices, or tears. Second, once you are at home, check the label on the inside package to be sure you have the right medicine. Make sure the lid and seal are not broken. Third, check the color, shape, size, and smell of the medicine. If you notice anything different or unusual, talk to a pharmacist or another healthcare professional.

Section 65.3

Over-the-Counter Cough and Cold Products for Children

This section includes text excerpted from "OTC Cough and Cold Products: Not for Infants and Children under Two Years of Age," U.S. Food and Drug Administration (FDA), January 17, 2008. Reviewed July 2019.

Frequently Asked Questions

What Is the U.S. Food and Drug Administration Recommending about Use of Over-the-Counter Cough and Cold Products for Infants and Children under Two Years of Age?

The U.S. Food and Drug Administration (FDA) strongly recommends that over-the-counter (OTC) cough and cold products should not be used for infants and children under two years of age because serious and potentially life-threatening side effects could occur.

What Are These Side Effects?

There are a wide variety of serious adverse events reported with cough and cold products. They include death, convulsions, rapid heart rates, and decreased levels of consciousness.

What Ingredients May Cause These Effects, and What Should I Look for on the Label to Tell If These Ingredients Are Present in an Over-the-Counter Product?

Over-the-counter cough and cold products include these ingredients: decongestants (for unclogging a stuffy nose), expectorants (for loosening mucus so that it can be coughed up), antihistamines (for sneezing and runny nose), and antitussives (for quieting coughs). The terms on the label include "nasal decongestants," "cough suppressants," "expectorants," and "antihistamines."

Not Effective? Does "Not Effective" Mean That They Do Not Work?

The FDA does not have any data to support that these products work in children less than two years of age.

My Child Has Allergies. Does This Alert Affect the Medicines for My Child?

This advisory relates only to the use of OTC products for the treatment of cough and cold.

What Should Parents Do If Infants and Children under Two Years of Age Experience Cough and Cold Symptoms?

A cold is a respiratory illness that is usually self-limited and lasts about a week. Cold symptoms typically include sneezing, coughing, a runny or stuffy nose, and a sore throat. Children may also experience a fever. Most of the time, a cold will go away by itself. If you are concerned about making your child feel more comfortable, talk with your doctor about what approaches to take. Your doctor may recommend drinking plenty of fluids to help loosen mucus and to keep children hydrated, and using saline nasal drops and gently suctioning mucus from the nose with a bulb syringe. Your doctor may also recommend fever reducers, such as acetaminophen or ibuprofen. If your child's cold symptoms do not improve or get worse, contact your doctor. A persistent cough may signal a more serious condition, such as bronchitis or asthma.

What Should Parents of Children in Ages 2 through 11 Know about Using Cough and Cold Products?

Giving too much cough and cold medicine can be dangerous. OTC cough and cold products can be harmful if more than the recommended amount is used, if they are given too often, or if more than one product containing the same active ingredient is being used. Parents need to be aware that many OTC cough and cold products contain multiple ingredients (for nasal congestion, cough, and fever). Giving more than one product could result in an overdose. There are many products that have similar names, so it is critical to identify the active ingredient(s) in the product, select the proper medicine, and use the correct dose. Reading the Drug Facts section of the label will help caretakers learn about what active ingredients are in the products. Also, children should not be given medicines that are packaged and made for adults.

The FDA recommends these steps for consumers who use OTC cough and cold products in children two years of age and older:

- Check the "active ingredients" section of the Drug Facts label.

- Be very careful if you are giving more than one OTC cough and cold medicine to a child. If you use two medicines that have the same or similar active ingredients, a child could get too much of an ingredient, which may hurt them.

- Carefully follow the directions in the Drug Facts label.

- Only use the measuring spoons or cups that come with the medicine or those made specially for measuring drugs.

- Choose OTC cough and cold medicines with childproof safety caps, when available, and store the medicines out of reach of children.

- Understand that OTC cough and cold medicines do not cure or shorten the duration of the common cold.

- Do not use these products to sedate your child or to make children sleepy.

- Call a physician, pharmacist, or other healthcare professional if you have any questions about using cough or cold medicines in children two years of age and older.

Chapter 66

Avoiding Drug Interactions

People often combine foods. For example, chocolate and peanut butter might be considered a tasty combination. But, eating chocolate and taking certain drugs might carry risks. In fact, eating chocolate and taking monoamine oxidase (MAO) inhibitors, such as Nardil (phenelzine) or Parnate (tranylcypromine), could be dangerous.

Monoamine oxidase inhibitors treat depression. Someone who eats an excessive amount of chocolate after taking an MAO inhibitor may experience a sharp rise in blood pressure.

Other foods that should be avoided when taking MAO inhibitors include aged cheese, sausage, bologna, pepperoni, and salami. These foods can also cause elevated blood pressure when taken with these medications.

There are three main types of drug interactions:

- Drugs with food and beverages

- Drugs with dietary supplements

- Drugs with other drugs

"Consumers should learn about the warnings for their medications and talk with their healthcare professionals about how to lower the risk of interactions," says Shiew-Mei Huang, Ph.D., deputy director of the Office of Clinical Pharmacology (OCP) in the U.S. Food and Drug

This chapter includes text excerpted from "Avoiding Drug Interactions," U.S. Food and Drug Administration (FDA), November 10, 2008. Reviewed July 2019.

Administration's (FDA) Center for Drug Evaluation and Research (CDER).

Drugs with Food and Beverages

Consequences of drug interactions with food and beverages may include a delayed, decreased, or enhanced absorption of a medication. Food can affect the bioavailability (the degree and rate at which a drug is absorbed into someone's system), metabolism, and excretion of certain medications.

The following are a few examples of drug interactions with food and beverages.

Alcohol: If you are taking any sort of medication, it is recommended that you avoid alcohol, which can increase or decrease the effectiveness of many drugs.

Grapefruit juice: Grapefruit and grapefruit juice are often mentioned as products that can interact negatively with drugs, but the actual number of drugs the juice can interact with is not well-known. Grapefruit juice should not be taken with certain blood pressure-lowering drugs or cyclosporine for the prevention of organ transplant rejection. That is because grapefruit juice can cause higher levels of those medicines in your body, making it more likely that you will have side effects from the medicine. The juice can also interact to cause higher blood levels of the anti-anxiety medicine Buspar (buspirone); the antimalaria drugs Quinerva or Quinite (quinine); and Halcion (triazolam), a medication used to treat insomnia.

Licorice: This would appear to be a fairly harmless snack food. However, for someone taking Lanoxin (digoxin), some forms of licorice may increase the risk for Lanoxin toxicity. Lanoxin is used to treat congestive heart failure and abnormal heart rhythms. Licorice may also reduce the effects of blood pressure drugs or diuretic (urine-producing) drugs, including Hydrodiuril (hydrochlorothiazide) and Aldactone (spironolactone).

Chocolate: MAO inhibitors are just one category of drugs that should not be consumed with excessive amounts of chocolate. The caffeine in chocolate can also interact with stimulant drugs, such as Ritalin (methylphenidate), increasing their effect, or chocolate can decrease the effect of sedative-hypnotics, such as Ambien (zolpidem).

Drugs with Dietary Supplements

Research has shown that 50 percent or more of American adults use dietary supplements on a regular basis, according to a congressional testimony by the Office of Dietary Supplements (ODS) in the National Institutes of Health (NIH).

The law defines "dietary supplements" in part as products taken by mouth that contain a "dietary ingredient." Dietary ingredients include vitamins, minerals, amino acids, and herbs or botanicals, as well as other substances that can be used to supplement the diet.

The following are a few examples of drug interactions with dietary supplements.

St. John's wort (Hypericum perforatum): This herb is considered an inducer of liver enzymes, which means it can reduce the concentration of medications in the blood. St. John's wort can reduce the blood level of medications such as Lanoxin, the cholesterol-lowering drugs Mevacor and Altocor (lovastatin), and the erectile dysfunction drug Viagra (sildenafil).

Vitamin E: Taking vitamin E with a blood-thinning medication, such as Coumadin, can increase anticlotting activity and may cause an increased risk of bleeding.

Ginseng: This herb can interfere with the bleeding effects of Coumadin. In addition, ginseng can enhance the bleeding effects of heparin, aspirin, and nonsteroidal anti-inflammatory drugs, such as ibuprofen, naproxen, and ketoprofen. Combining ginseng with MAO inhibitors such as Nardil or Parnate may cause headache, trouble sleeping, nervousness, and hyperactivity.

Ginkgo biloba: High doses of the herb Ginkgo biloba could decrease the effectiveness of anticonvulsant therapy in patients taking the following medications to control seizures: Tegretol, Equetro or Carbatrol (carbamazepine), and Depakote (valproic acid).

Drugs with Other Drugs

Two out of every three patients who visit a doctor leave with at least one prescription for medication, according to a 2007 report on medication safety issued by the Institute for Safe Medication Practices (ISMP). Close to 40 percent of the U.S. population receive prescriptions for 4 or more medications. And the rate of adverse drug reactions increases dramatically after a patient is on 4 or more medications.

Drug–drug interactions have led to adverse events and withdrawals of drugs from the market, according to an article on drug interactions co-authored by Shiew-Mei Huang, Ph.D., deputy director of the FDA's Office of Clinical Pharmacology. The paper was published in the June 2008 issue of the *Journal of Clinical Pharmacology* (JCP).

However, market withdrawal of a drug is a fairly drastic measure. More often, the FDA will issue an alert, warning the public and health-care providers about risks as the result of drug interactions.

The following are a few examples of drug interactions with other drugs.

Cordarone (amiodarone): The FDA issued an alert in August 2008, warning patients about taking Cordarone to correct abnormal rhythms of the heart and the cholesterol-lowering drug Zocor (Simvastatin). Patients taking Zocor in doses higher than 20 mg while also taking Cordarone run the risk of developing a rare condition of muscle injury called "rhabdomyolysis," which can lead to kidney failure or death. "Cordarone also can inhibit or reduce the effect of the blood thinner Coumadin (warfarin)," said Huang. "So if you are using Cordarone, you may need to reduce the amount of Coumadin you are taking."

Lanoxin (digoxin): "Lanoxin has a narrow therapeutic range. So other drugs, such as Norvir (ritonavir), can elevate the level of Lanoxin," says Huang. "And an increased level of Lanoxin can cause irregular heart rhythms." Norvir is a protease inhibitor used to treat human immunodeficiency virus (HIV), the virus that causes acquired immunodeficiency syndrome (AIDS).

Antihistamines: Over-the-counter (OTC) antihistamines are drugs that temporarily relieve a runny nose or reduce sneezing; itching of the nose or throat; and itchy, watery eyes. If you are taking sedatives, tranquilizers, or a prescription drug for high blood pressure or depression, you should check with a doctor or pharmacist before you start using antihistamines. Some antihistamines can increase the depressant effects (such as sleepiness) of a sedative or tranquilizer. The sedating effect of some antihistamines combined with a sedating antidepressant could strongly affect your concentration level. Operating a car or any other machinery could be particularly dangerous if your ability to focus is impaired. Antihistamines taken in conjunction with blood pressure medication may cause a person's blood pressure to increase and may also speed up the heart rate.

Tips to Avoid Problems

There are lots of things you can do to take prescription or OTC medications in a safe and responsible manner.

- Always read drug labels carefully.

- Learn about the warnings for all the drugs you take.

- Keep medications in their original containers so that you can easily identify them.

- Ask your doctor what you need to avoid when you are prescribed a new medication. Ask about food, beverages, dietary supplements, and other drugs.

- Check with your doctor or pharmacist before taking an OTC drug if you are taking any prescription medications.

- Use one pharmacy for all of your drug needs.

- Keep all of your healthcare professionals informed about everything that you take.

- Keep a record of all prescription drugs, OTC drugs, and dietary supplements (including herbs) that you take. Try to keep this list with you at all times, especially when you go on any medical appointment.

Chapter 67

Complementary and Alternative Medicine for Contagious Diseases

Chapter Contents

Section 67.1—Complementary and Alternative
Medicine for Flu and Colds.................................. 512

Section 67.2—Getting to Know "Friendly
Bacteria"—Probiotics 519

Section 67.3—Herbal Supplements 522

Section 67.4—Dietary Supplements 533

Section 67.5—Hepatitis C and Complementary and
Alternative Medicine... 536

Section 67.1

Complementary and Alternative Medicine for Flu and Colds

This section includes text excerpted from "Flu and Colds: In Depth," National Center for Complementary and Integrative Health (NCCIH), November 2016.

What Do We Know about the Effectiveness of Complementary Approaches for Flu and Colds?

- No complementary health approach has been shown to be helpful for the flu.

- For colds:

  - Complementary approaches that have shown some promise include oral zinc products, rinsing the nose and sinuses (with a neti pot or other device), honey (as a nighttime cough remedy for children), vitamin C (for people under severe physical stress), probiotics, and meditation.

  - Approaches for which the evidence is conflicting, inadequate, or mostly negative include vitamin C (for most people), echinacea, garlic, and American ginseng (Panax quinquefolius).

What Do People Know about the Safety of Complementary Approaches for Colds and Flu?

- People can get severe infections if they use neti pots (a device that comes from the Ayurvedic tradition) or other nasal-rinsing devices improperly. Tap water is not safe for use as a nasal rinse unless it has been filtered, treated, or processed in specific ways.

- Zinc products used in the nose (such as nasal gels and swabs) have been linked to a long-lasting or even permanent loss of the sense of smell.

- Using a dietary supplement to prevent colds often involves taking it for long periods of time. However, little is known about the long-term safety of some dietary supplements studied for the prevention of colds, such as American ginseng and probiotics.

- Complementary approaches that are safe for some people may not be safe for others. Your age, health, special circumstances (such as pregnancy), and medicines or supplements that you take may affect the safety of complementary approaches.

Some Basics about Flu and Colds

Each year, Americans get more than 1 billion colds, and between 5 and 20 percent of Americans get the flu. The 2 diseases have some symptoms in common, and both are caused by viruses. However, they are different conditions, and the flu is more severe. Unlike the flu, colds generally do not cause serious complications, such as pneumonia, or lead to hospitalization.

No vaccine can protect you against the common cold, but vaccines can protect you against the flu. Everyone over the age of six months should be vaccinated against the flu each year. Vaccination is the best protection against getting the flu.

Prescription antiviral drugs may be used to treat the flu in people who are very ill or who are at a high risk of flu complications. They are not a substitute for getting vaccinated. Vaccination is the first line of defense against the flu; antivirals are the second. If you think that you have caught the flu, you may want to check with your healthcare provider to see whether antiviral medicine is appropriate for you. Call promptly. The drugs work best if they are used early in the illness.

What the Science Says about Complementary Health Approaches for the Flu

No complementary approach has been shown to prevent the flu or relieve flu symptoms.

Complementary approaches that have been studied for the flu include the following. In all instances, there is not enough evidence to show whether the approach is helpful.

- American ginseng
- Chinese herbal medicines
- Echinacea
- Elderberry
- Green tea
- Oscillococcinum

- Vitamin C
- Vitamin D

What the Science Says about Complementary Health Approaches for Colds

The following complementary health approaches have been studied for colds:

American Ginseng

- Several studies have evaluated the use of American ginseng to prevent colds. A 2011 evaluation of these studies concluded that the herb has not been shown to reduce the number of colds that people catch, although it may shorten the length of colds. The researchers who conducted the evaluation concluded that there was insufficient evidence to support the use of American ginseng for preventing colds.

- Taking American ginseng in an effort to prevent colds means taking it for prolonged periods of time. However, little is known about the herb's long-term safety. American ginseng may interact with the anticoagulant (blood-thinning) drug warfarin.

Echinacea

- At least 24 studies have tested echinacea to see whether it can prevent colds or relieve cold symptoms. A comprehensive 2014 assessment of this research concluded that echinacea has not been convincingly shown to be beneficial. However, at least some echinacea products might have a weak effect.

- One reason why it is hard to reach definite conclusions about this herb is that echinacea products vary greatly. They may contain different species (types) of the plant and be made from different plant parts (the above-ground parts, the root, or both). They also may be manufactured in different ways, and some products contain other ingredients in addition to echinacea. Research findings on one echinacea product may not apply to other products.

- Few side effects have been reported in studies of echinacea. However, some people are allergic to this herb, and in one study in children, taking echinacea was linked to an increase in rashes.

Garlic

- A 2014 evaluation of the research on garlic concluded that there is not enough evidence to show whether this herb can help prevent colds or relieve their symptoms.

- Garlic can cause bad breath, body odor, and other side effects. Because garlic may interact with anticoagulant drugs (blood thinners), people who take these drugs should consult their healthcare providers before taking garlic.

Honey

- Honey's traditional reputation as a cough remedy has some science to back it up. A small amount of research suggests that honey may help to decrease nighttime coughing in children.

- Honey should never be given to infants younger than one year of age because it may contain spores of the bacterium that causes infant botulism. Honey is considered safe for older children.

Meditation

- Reducing stress and improving general health may protect against colds and other respiratory infections. In a 2012 study funded by the National Center for Complementary and Integrative Health (NCCIH), adults 50 years of age and older were randomly assigned to training in mindfulness meditation, which can reduce stress; an exercise training program, which may improve physical health; or a control group that did not receive any intervention. The study participants kept track of their illnesses during the cold and flu season. People in the meditation group had shorter and less severe acute respiratory infections (most of which were colds) and lost fewer days of work because of these illnesses than those in the control group. Exercise also had some benefit, but not as much as meditation.

- This study is the first to suggest that meditation may reduce the impact of colds. Because it is the only study of its kind, its results should not be regarded as conclusive.

- Meditation is generally considered to be safe for healthy people. However, there have been reports that it might worsen symptoms in people with certain chronic physical or mental-health problems. If you have an ongoing health issue, talk with your healthcare provider before starting meditation.

Probiotics

- A 2015 evaluation of 13 studies found some evidence suggesting that probiotics might reduce the number of colds or other upper respiratory tract infections that people catch and the length of the illnesses, but the quality of the evidence was low or very low.

- In people who are generally healthy, probiotics have a good safety record. Side effects, if they occur at all, usually consist only of mild digestive symptoms, such as gas. However, information on the long-term safety of probiotics is limited, and safety may differ from one type of probiotic to another. Probiotics have been linked to severe side effects, such as dangerous infections, in people with serious underlying medical problems.

Saline Nasal Irrigation

- Saline nasal irrigation means rinsing your nose and sinuses with salt water. People may do this with a neti pot or with other devices, such as bottles, sprays, pumps, or nebulizers. Saline nasal irrigation may be used for sinus congestion, allergies, or colds.

- There is limited evidence that saline nasal irrigation can help relieve cold symptoms. Studies of this technique have been too small to allow researchers to reach definite conclusions.

- Saline nasal irrigation used to be considered safe, with only minor side effects such as nasal discomfort or irritation. However, in 2011, a severe disease caused by an amoeba (a type of microorganism) was linked to nasal irrigation with tap water. The U.S. Food and Drug Administration (FDA) has warned that tap water that is not filtered, treated, or processed in specific ways is not safe for use in nasal rinsing devices and has explained how to use and clean these devices safely.

Vitamin C

- An evaluation of a large amount of research done on vitamin C and colds (29 studies involving more than 11,000 people) concluded that taking vitamin C does not prevent colds in the general population and shortens colds only slightly. Taking vitamin C only after you start to feel cold symptoms does not affect the length or severity of the cold.

- Unlike the situation in the general population, vitamin C does seem to reduce the number of colds in people exposed to short periods of extreme physical stress (such as marathon runners and skiers). In studies of these groups, taking vitamin C cut the number of colds in half.

- Taking too much vitamin C can cause diarrhea, nausea, and stomach cramps. People with the iron storage disease hemochromatosis should avoid high doses of vitamin C. People who are being treated for cancer or taking cholesterol-lowering medications should talk with their healthcare providers before taking vitamin C supplements.

Zinc

- Zinc has been used for colds in forms that are taken orally (by mouth), such as lozenges, tablets, or syrup, or it is used intranasally (in the nose), such as swabs or gels.

Oral Zinc

- A 2012 evaluation of 17 studies of various types of zinc lozenges, tablets, or syrup found that zinc can reduce the duration of colds in adults. 2 evaluations of 3 studies of high-dose zinc acetate lozenges in adults, conducted in 2015 and 2016, found that they shortened colds.

- Some participants in studies that tested zinc for colds reported that the zinc caused a bad taste or nausea.

- Long-term use of high doses of zinc can cause low copper levels, reduced immunity, and low levels of high-density lipoprotein (HDL) cholesterol (the "good" cholesterol). Zinc may interact with drugs, including antibiotics and penicillamine (a drug used to treat rheumatoid arthritis).

Intranasal Zinc

- The use of zinc products inside the nose may cause loss of the sense of smell, which may be long-lasting or permanent. In 2009, the FDA warned consumers to stop using several intranasal zinc products marketed as cold remedies because of this risk.

- Prior to the warnings about effects on the sense of smell, a few studies of intranasal zinc had suggested a possible benefit against cold symptoms. However, the risk of a serious and lasting side effect outweighs any possible benefit in the treatment of a minor illness.

Other Complementary Approaches

In addition to the complementary approaches described above, several other approaches have been studied for colds. In all instances, there is insufficient evidence to show whether these approaches help to prevent colds or relieve cold symptoms.

- Andrographis (Andrographis paniculata)

- Chinese herbal medicines

- Green tea

- Guided imagery

- Hydrotherapy

- Vitamin D

- Vitamin E

Section 67.2

Getting to Know "Friendly Bacteria"—Probiotics

This section includes text excerpted from "Probiotics: In Depth," National Center for Complementary and Integrative Health (NCCIH), October 2016.

Basics of Probiotics

Probiotics are live microorganisms that are intended to have health benefits. Products sold as probiotics include foods (such as yogurt); dietary supplements; and products that are not used orally, such as skin creams.

Although people often think of bacteria and other microorganisms as harmful germs, many microorganisms help our bodies function properly. For example, bacteria that are normally present in our intestines help digest food, destroy disease-causing microorganisms, and produce vitamins. Large numbers of microorganisms live on and in our bodies. Many of the microorganisms in probiotic products are the same as or similar to microorganisms that naturally live in our bodies.

What Do We Know about the Usefulness of Probiotics?

Some probiotics may help to prevent diarrhea that is caused by infections or antibiotics. They may also help with symptoms of irritable bowel syndrome (IBS). However, benefits have not been conclusively demonstrated, and not all probiotics have the same effects.

What Do We Know about the Safety of Probiotics?

In healthy people, probiotics usually have only minor side effects, if any. However, in people with underlying health problems (for example, weakened immune systems), serious complications such as infections have occasionally been reported.

What Kinds of Microorganisms Are in Probiotics?

Probiotics may contain a variety of microorganisms. The most common are bacteria that belong to groups called "*Lactobacillus*" and "*Bifidobacterium*." Each of these two broad groups includes many types

519

of bacteria. Other bacteria may also be used as probiotics and so may yeasts, such as *Saccharomyces boulardii*.

Probiotics, Prebiotics, and Synbiotics

Prebiotics are not the same as probiotics. The term "prebiotics" refers to dietary substances that favor the growth of beneficial bacteria over harmful ones. The term "synbiotics" refers to products that combine probiotics and prebiotics.

What the Science Says about the Effectiveness of Probiotics

Researchers have studied probiotics to find out whether they might help prevent or treat a variety of health problems, including:

- Digestive disorders, such as diarrhea caused by infections, antibiotic-associated diarrhea, IBS, and inflammatory bowel disease

- Allergic disorders, such as atopic dermatitis (eczema) and allergic rhinitis (hay fever)

- Tooth decay, periodontal disease, and other oral health problems

- Colic in infants

- Liver disease

- The common cold

- Prevention of necrotizing enterocolitis in very-low-birth-weight infants

There is preliminary evidence that some probiotics are helpful in preventing diarrhea caused by infections and antibiotics and in improving symptoms of IBS, but more needs to be learned. Still it is not known which probiotics are helpful and which are not. It is also not known how much of the probiotic people would have to take or who would most likely benefit from taking probiotics. Even for the conditions that have been studied the most, researchers are still working toward finding the answers to these questions.

Probiotics are not all alike. For example, if a specific kind of Lactobacillus helps prevent an illness, that does not necessarily mean that another kind of *Lactobacillus* would have the same effect or that any of the *Bifidobacterium* probiotics would do the same thing.

Although some probiotics have shown promise in research studies, strong scientific evidence to support specific uses of probiotics for most health conditions is lacking. The U.S. Food and Drug Administration (FDA) has not approved any probiotics for preventing or treating any health problem. Some experts have cautioned that the rapid growth in marketing and use of probiotics may have outpaced scientific research for many of their proposed uses and benefits.

How Might Probiotics Work?

Probiotics may have a variety of effects in the body, and different probiotics may act in different ways.

Probiotics might:

- Help to maintain a desirable community of microorganisms

- Stabilize the digestive tract's barriers against undesirable microorganisms or produce substances that inhibit their growth

- Help the community of microorganisms in the digestive tract return to normal after being disturbed (for example, by an antibiotic or a disease)

- Outcompete undesirable microorganisms

- Stimulate the immune response

What the Science Says about the Safety and Side Effects of Probiotics

Whether probiotics are likely to be safe for you depends on the state of your health.

- In people who are generally healthy, probiotics have a good safety record. Side effects, if they occur at all, usually consist only of mild digestive symptoms, such as gas.

- On the other hand, there have been reports linking probiotics to severe side effects, such as dangerous infections, in people with serious underlying medical problems. The people who are most at risk of severe side effects include critically ill patients, those who have had surgery, very sick infants, and people with weakened immune systems.

Even for healthy people, there are uncertainties about the safety of probiotics. Because many research studies on probiotics have not looked closely at safety, there is not enough information right now to answer some safety questions. Most of our knowledge about safety comes from studies of *Lactobacillus* and *Bifidobacterium*; less is known about other probiotics. Information on the long-term safety of probiotics is limited, and safety may differ from one type of probiotic to another. For example, even though a National Center for Complementary and Integrative Health (NCCIH)-funded study showed that a particular kind of *Lactobacillus* appears safe in healthy adults 65 years of age and older, this does not mean that all probiotics would necessarily be safe for people in this age group.

Section 67.3

Herbal Supplements

This section includes text excerpted from "Herbs at a Glance," National Center for Complementary and Integrative Health (NCCIH), June 20, 2019.

This section provides basic information about specific herbs or botanicals, including common names, what the science says, and potential side effects and cautions.

Echinacea
Background

- There are nine known species of echinacea, all of which are native to North America. They were used by Native Americans of the Great Plains region as traditional medicines.

- Echinacea is used as a dietary supplement for the common cold and other infections, based on the idea that it might stimulate the immune system to more effectively fight infection. Echinacea preparations have been used topically (applied to the skin) for wounds and skin problems.

- The roots and above-ground parts of the echinacea plant are used fresh or dried to make teas, squeezed (expressed) juice, extracts, capsules and tablets, and preparations for external use. Several species of echinacea, most commonly *Echinacea purpurea* or *Echinacea angustifolia*, may be included in dietary supplements.

How Much Do We Know?

- Many studies have been done on echinacea and the common cold. Much less research has been done on the use of echinacea for other health purposes.

What Have We Learned?

- Taking echinacea after you catch a cold has not been shown to shorten the time that you will be sick.

- Taking echinacea while you are well may slightly reduce your chances of catching a cold. However, the evidence on this point is not completely certain. The National Center for Complementary and Integrative Health (NCCIH) is funding research to identify the active constituents in echinacea and to study the effects on the human immune system of substances in bacteria that live within echinacea plants.

What Do We Know about Safety?

- There are many different echinacea products. They may contain different species of plants or different parts of the plant, be manufactured in different ways, and have other ingredients in addition to echinacea. Most of these products have not been tested in people.

- For most people, short-term oral (by mouth) use of echinacea is probably safe; the safety of long-term use is uncertain.

- The most common side effects of echinacea are digestive tract symptoms, such as nausea or stomach pain.

- Some people have allergic reactions to echinacea, which may be severe. Some children participating in a clinical trial of echinacea developed rashes, which may have been caused by an allergic reaction. People with atopy (a genetic tendency toward allergic reactions) may be more likely to have an allergic reaction when taking echinacea.

- Evidence indicates that the risk of interactions between echinacea supplements and most medications is low.

Goldenseal
Background

- Goldenseal is a plant native to North America. Overharvesting and a loss of habitat have decreased the availability of wild goldenseal, but the plant is now grown commercially in the United States, especially in the Blue Ridge Mountains.

- Historically, Native Americans used goldenseal for skin disorders, ulcers, fevers, and other conditions. European settlers adopted it as a medicinal plant, using it for a variety of conditions.

- Goldenseal is used as a dietary supplement for colds and other respiratory tract infections; allergic rhinitis (hay fever); ulcers; and digestive upsets, such as diarrhea and constipation. It is also used as a mouthwash for sore gums and as an eyewash for eye inflammation, and it is applied to the skin for rashes and other skin problems.

- The roots of goldenseal are dried and used to make teas, extracts, tablets, or capsules. Goldenseal is often combined with echinacea in commercial products.

How Much Do We Know?

Very little research has been done on the health effects of goldenseal.

What Have We Learned?

- The scientific evidence does not support the use of goldenseal for any health-related purpose.

- Berberine, a substance found in goldenseal, has been studied for heart failure, diarrhea, infections, and other health conditions. However, when people take goldenseal orally, very little berberine may be absorbed by the body or enter the bloodstream, so study results on berberine may not apply to goldenseal.

- The NCCIH is funding research to study how goldenseal may act against bacteria and to develop research-grade goldenseal for use in human studies.

What Do We Know about Safety?

- There is not much reliable information on the safety of goldenseal.

- Women who are pregnant or breastfeeding should not use goldenseal, and it should not be given to infants. Berberine can cause or worsen jaundice in newborn infants and could lead to a life-threatening problem called "kernicterus."

- Goldenseal contains substances that may change the way your body processes many medications. If you are taking medication, consult your healthcare provider before using goldenseal.

Licorice Root
Background

- Most licorice root grows in Greece, Turkey, and Asia. Anise oil is often used instead of licorice root to flavor licorice candy.

- Centuries ago, licorice root was used in Greece, China, and Egypt for stomach inflammation and upper respiratory problems. Licorice root also has been used as a sweetener.

- People use licorice root as a dietary supplement for digestive problems, menopausal symptoms, cough, and bacterial and viral infections. People also use it as a shampoo.

- Licorice is harvested from the plants' roots and underground stems. Licorice supplements are available as capsules, tablets, and liquid extracts.

How Much Do We Know?

A number of studies of licorice root in people have been published, but not enough support the use for any specific health condition.

What Have We Learned?

- Glycyrrhizin—a compound found in licorice root—has been tested in a few clinical trials in hepatitis C patients, but there is not enough evidence to determine if it is helpful. Laboratory studies were done in Japan (where an injectable glycyrrhizin compound is used in people with chronic hepatitis C who do not respond to conventional treatment) suggest that glycyrrhizin may have some effect against hepatitis C.

- There is some evidence that topical licorice extract may improve skin rash symptoms, such as redness, swelling, and itching.

- A Finnish study of mothers and their young children suggested that eating a lot of actual licorice root during pregnancy may harm a fetus's developing brain, leading to reasoning and behavioral issues, such as attention problems, rule-breaking, and aggression.

- Studies of licorice root extracts in people for cavities, mouth ulcers, and oral yeast infections have returned mixed results.

What Do We Know about Safety?

- In large amounts and with long-term use, licorice root can cause high blood pressure and low potassium levels, which could lead to heart and muscle problems. Some side effects are thought to be due to a chemical called "glycyrrhizic acid." Licorice that has had this chemical removed (called "DGL" for deglycyrrhizinated licorice) may not have the same degree of side effects.

- Taking licorice root containing glycyrrhizinic acid with medications that reduce potassium levels, such as diuretics, might be bad for your heart.

- Pregnant women should avoid using licorice root as a supplement or consuming large amounts of it as food.

Milk Thistle
Background

- Milk thistle is native to southern Europe, southern Russia, Asia Minor, and northern Africa. It also grows in North America, South America, and South Australia.

- Silymarin is considered to be the main component of milk thistle seeds, but the terms "milk thistle" and "silymarin" often are used interchangeably.

- Historically, people have used milk thistle for liver disorders, such as hepatitis and cirrhosis, and gallbladder problems.

- Silymarin is the most commonly used herbal supplement in the United States for liver problems.

- Milk thistle products are available as capsules, powders, and extracts.

How Much Do We Know?

- We know little about whether milk thistle is effective in people, as only a few well-designed clinical studies have been conducted.

What Have We Learned?

- Results from clinical trials of milk thistle for liver diseases have been mixed, and two rigorously designed studies found no benefit.

- The 2008 Hepatitis C Antiviral Long-Term Treatment Against Cirrhosis (HALT-C) study, sponsored by the National Institutes of Health (NIH), found that hepatitis C patients who used silymarin had fewer and milder symptoms of liver disease and somewhat better quality of life, but there was no change in virus activity or liver inflammation.

- A 2012 clinical trial, cofounded by the NCCIH and the National Institute of Diabetes and Digestive and Kidney Diseases (NIDDK), showed that two higher-than-usual doses of silymarin were no better than placebo for chronic hepatitis C in people who had not responded to standard antiviral treatment.

- Results from a 2013 clinical study suggest that milk thistle may enhance standard treatment in young people with a particular form of anemia (Cooley's anemia).

What Do We Know about Safety?

- In clinical trials, milk thistle appears to be well tolerated in recommended doses. Occasionally, people report various gastrointestinal side effects.

- Milk thistle may produce allergic reactions, which tend to be more common among people who are allergic to plants in the same family (for example, ragweed, chrysanthemum, marigold, and daisy).

- Compounds in milk thistle may lower blood sugar levels in people with type 2 diabetes. People with diabetes should use caution.

Turmeric
What Is Turmeric?

- Turmeric, a plant related to ginger, is grown throughout India, other parts of Asia, and Central America.

- Historically, turmeric has been used in Ayurvedic medicine, primarily in South Asia, for many conditions, including breathing problems, rheumatism, serious pain, and fatigue.

- Turmeric is used as a dietary supplement for inflammation; arthritis; stomach, skin, liver, and gallbladder problems; cancer; and other conditions.

- Turmeric is a common spice and a major ingredient in curry powder. Its primary active ingredients, curcuminoids, are yellow and used to color foods and cosmetics.

- Turmeric's underground stems (rhizomes) are dried and made into capsules, tablets, teas, or extracts. Turmeric powder is also made into a paste for skin conditions.

What Are The Health Effects of Turmeric?

- Claims that curcuminoids found in turmeric help to reduce inflammation are not supported by strong studies.

- Preliminary studies found that curcuminoids may:
  - Reduce the number of heart attacks bypass patients had after surgery
  - Control knee pain from osteoarthritis, as well as ibuprofen, did
  - Reduce the skin irritation that often occurs after radiation treatments for breast cancer

- Other preliminary studies in people have looked at curcumin, a type of curcuminoid, for different cancers, colitis, diabetes, surgical pain, and as an ingredient in mouthwash for reducing plaque.

- The NCCIH has studied curcumin for Alzheimer's disease, rheumatoid arthritis, and prostate and colon cancer.

Is Turmeric Safe?

- Turmeric in amounts tested for health purposes is generally considered safe when taken by mouth or applied to the skin.

- High doses or long-term use of turmeric may cause gastrointestinal problems.

Aloe Vera
Background

- Aloe vera's use can be traced back 6,000 years to early Egypt, where the plant was depicted on stone carvings. Known as the "plant of immortality," aloe was presented as a funeral gift to pharaohs.

- Historically, Aloe vera has been used for a variety of purposes, including treatment of wounds, hair loss, and hemorrhoids; it has also been used as a laxative.

- Two substances from Aloe vera, the clear gel and the yellow latex, are used in health products. Aloe gel is primarily used topically (applied to the skin) as a remedy for skin conditions, such as burns, frostbite, psoriasis, and cold sores, but it may also be taken orally (by mouth) for conditions including osteoarthritis, bowel diseases, and fever. Aloe latex is taken orally, usually for constipation.

How Much Do We Know?

- There is not enough evidence to show whether Aloe vera is helpful for most of the purposes for which people use it.

What Have We Learned?

- Aloe latex contains strong laxative compounds. Products made with aloe were at one time regulated by the U.S. Food and Drug Administration (FDA) as over-the-counter (OTC) laxatives. In 2002, the FDA required that all OTC aloe laxative products be removed from the U.S. market or reformulated because the companies that manufactured them did not provide the safety data necessary for continued approval.

- There is some evidence that the topical use of aloe products might be helpful for symptoms of certain conditions such as psoriasis and certain rashes.

- There is not enough high-quality scientific evidence to show whether topical use of aloe helps to heal wounds.

- There is not enough scientific evidence to support Aloe vera for any of its other uses.

What Do We Know about Safety?

- Use of topical Aloe vera is likely to be safe.

- A two year National Toxicology Program study on oral consumption of nondecolorized whole leaf extract of Aloe vera found clear evidence of carcinogenic activity in male and female rats, based on tumors of the large intestine. Another study in rats showed that decolorized whole leaf Aloe vera did not cause harmful effects. This suggests that a component called "aloin," most of which is removed by the decolorization process, may be responsible for the tumors seen in rats fed nondecolorized whole leaf Aloe vera. More information, including what products are actually in the marketplace and how individuals use different types of Aloe vera products, is needed to determine the potential risks to humans.

- Abdominal cramps and diarrhea have been reported with oral use of aloe latex. Also, because aloe latex is a laxative, it may reduce the absorption and, therefore, the effectiveness of some drugs that are taken orally.

- People with diabetes who use glucose-lowering medication should be cautious if also taking aloe orally because aloe may lower blood glucose levels.

- There have been a few reported cases of acute hepatitis in people who took Aloe vera orally. However, the evidence is not definitive.

Pomegranate
Background

- The pomegranate fruit has a leathery rind (or husk) with many little pockets of edible seeds and juice inside.

- Since ancient times, the pomegranate has been a symbol of fertility.

- Researchers have studied all parts of the pomegranate for their potential health benefits. Those parts include the fruit, seed, seed oil, tannin-rich peel, root, leaf, and flower.

- The pomegranate has been used as a dietary supplement for many conditions, including wounds, heart conditions, intestinal problems, and as a gargle for a sore throat.

- Pomegranate is made into capsules, extracts, teas, powders, and juice products.

How Much Do We Know?

- We do not have a lot of strong scientific evidence on the effects of pomegranate for people's health.

What Have We Learned?

- A 2012 clinical trial of about 100 dialysis patients suggested that pomegranate juice may help ward off infections. In the study, the patients who were given pomegranate juice three times a week for a year had fewer hospitalizations for infections and fewer signs of inflammation when compared with patients who got the placebo.

- Pomegranate extract in mouthwash may help control dental plaque, according to a small 2011 clinical trial with 30 healthy participants.

- Pomegranate may help improve some signs of heart disease, but the research is not definitive.

What Do We Know about Safety?

Some people, particularly those with plant allergies, may be allergic to pomegranate.

- It is unclear whether pomegranate interacts with the anticoagulant (blood-thinning) medicine warfarin or drugs that work similarly in the body to warfarin.

- Federal agencies have taken action against companies selling pomegranate juice and supplements for deceptive advertising and making drug-like claims about the products.

Ginger
Background

- Ginger is a tropical plant that has green-purple flowers and a fragrant underground stem (called a "rhizome"). It is widely used as a flavoring or fragrance in foods, beverages, soaps, and cosmetics.

- Ancient Sanskrit, Chinese, Greek, Roman, and Arabic texts discussed the use of ginger for health-related purposes. In Asian medicine, dried ginger has been used for thousands of years to treat stomach ache, diarrhea, and nausea.

- Ginger is used as a dietary supplement for postsurgery nausea; nausea caused by motion, chemotherapy, or pregnancy; rheumatoid arthritis; and osteoarthritis.

- Common forms of ginger include the fresh or dried root, tablets, capsules, liquid extracts, and teas.

How Much Do We Know?

- There is some information from studies in people on the use of ginger for nausea and vomiting.

- Much less is known about other uses of ginger for other health conditions.

What Have We Learned?

- Some evidence indicates that ginger may help relieve pregnancy-related nausea and vomiting.

- Ginger may help to control nausea related to cancer chemotherapy when used in addition to conventional anti-nausea medication.

- It is unclear whether ginger is helpful for postsurgery nausea, motion sickness, rheumatoid arthritis, or osteoarthritis.

What Do We Know about Safety?

- Ginger, when used as a spice, is believed to be generally safe.

- In some people, ginger can have mild side effects, such as abdominal discomfort, heartburn, diarrhea, and gas.

- Some experts recommend that people with gallstone disease use caution with ginger because it may increase the flow of bile.

- Research has not definitely shown whether ginger interacts with medications, but concerns have been raised that it might interact with anticoagulants.

- Although several studies have found no evidence of harm from taking ginger during pregnancy, it is uncertain whether ginger is always safe for pregnant women. If you are considering using ginger while you are pregnant, consult your healthcare provider.

Section 67.4

Dietary Supplements

This section contains text excerpted from the following sources:
Text under the heading "What Is a Dietary Supplement?" is
excerpted from "Dietary Supplements," National Institute on Aging
(NIA), National Institutes of Health (NIH), November 30, 2017;
Text beginning with the heading "Federal Regulation of Dietary
Supplements" is excerpted from "Using Dietary Supplements
Wisely," National Center for Complementary and
Integrative Health (NCCIH), January 2019.

What Is a Dietary Supplement?

Dietary supplements are substances you might use to add nutrients to your diet or to lower your risk of health problems, such as osteoporosis or arthritis. Dietary supplements come in the form of pills, capsules, powders, gel tabs, extracts, or liquids. They might contain vitamins, minerals, fiber, amino acids, herbs or other plants, or enzymes. Sometimes, the ingredients in dietary supplements are added to foods, including drinks. A doctor's prescription is not needed to buy dietary supplements.

Federal Regulation of Dietary Supplements

- Federal regulations state that companies are responsible for having evidence that their dietary supplements are safe and for ensuring that product labels are truthful and not misleading. Manufacturers are required to produce dietary supplements in a quality manner, ensure that they do not contain contaminants or impurities, and label them accurately.

- However, rules for manufacturing and distributing dietary supplements are less strict than those for prescription or over-the-counter (OTC) drugs.

- The U.S. Food and Drug Administration (FDA), which regulates dietary supplements, requires that companies submit safety data about any new ingredient not sold in the United States in a dietary supplement before 1994. In all other cases, the FDA is not authorized to review dietary supplements for safety and effectiveness before they are marketed.

- The FDA can take action against adulterated or misbranded dietary supplements only after the product is on the market. In contrast, companies must show the FDA evidence that their prescription and OTC drugs are safe and effective before the drugs are marketed.

- Once a dietary supplement is on the market, the FDA tracks side effects reported by consumers, supplement companies, and others. You can report any safety concerns you may have about a dietary supplement through the U.S. Health and Human Services (HHS) Safety Reporting Portal.

- If the FDA finds a product to be unsafe, it can take legal action against the manufacturer or distributor, and the FDA may issue a warning or require that the product be removed from the marketplace. However, the FDA says it cannot test all products marketed as dietary supplements that may have potentially harmful hidden ingredients.

What the Science Says about the Safety and Side Effects of Dietary Supplements

- What is on the label may not be what is in the product. For example, the FDA has found prescription drugs, including anticoagulants (e.g., warfarin), anticonvulsants (e.g., phenytoin), and others, in products being sold as dietary supplements. You can see a list of some of those products on the FDA's Tainted Supplements webpage.

- A 2012 government study of 127 dietary supplements marketed for weight loss or to support the immune system found that 20 percent made illegal claims.

- Some dietary supplements may harm you if you have a particular medical condition or risk factor, or if you are taking certain prescription or OTC medications. For example, the herbal supplement St. John's wort makes many medications less effective.

- Dietary supplements result in an estimated 23,000 emergency room visits every year in the United States, according to a 2015 study. Many of the patients are young adults having heart problems from weight-loss or energy products and older adults having swallowing problems from taking large vitamin pills.

- Although it is still rare, more cases are being reported of acute (sudden) liver damage in people taking dietary supplements in the United States and elsewhere. The liver injury can be severe, can require an emergency liver transplant, and is sometimes fatal.

- Many dietary supplements (and some prescription drugs) come from natural sources, but "natural" does not always mean "safe." For example, the kava plant is a member of the pepper family, but taking kava supplements can cause liver disease.

- A manufacturer's use of the term "standardized" (or "verified" or "certified") does not necessarily guarantee product quality or consistency.

Safety Considerations

- If you are going to have surgery, be aware that certain dietary supplements may increase the risk of bleeding or affect your response to anesthesia. Talk to your healthcare providers as far in advance of the operation as possible, and tell them about all dietary supplements that you are taking.

- If you are pregnant, nursing a baby, trying to get pregnant, or considering giving a child a dietary supplement, consider that many dietary supplements have not been tested in pregnant women, nursing mothers, or children.

- If you are taking a dietary supplement, follow the instructions on the label. If you have side effects, stop taking the supplement and contact your healthcare provider. You may also want to contact the supplement manufacturer.

Section 67.5

Hepatitis C and Complementary and Alternative Medicine

This section includes text excerpted from "Hepatitis C: A Focus on Dietary Supplements," National Center for Complementary and Integrative Health (NCCIH), November 2014. Reviewed July 2019.

What Is Hepatitis C?

Hepatitis C is a contagious liver disease. It is caused by the hepatitis C virus. People can get hepatitis C through contact with blood from a person who is already infected or, less commonly, through having sex with an infected person. The infection usually becomes chronic. Chronic hepatitis C often is treated with drugs that can eliminate the virus. This may slow or stop liver damage, but the drugs may cause side effects, and for some people, treatment is ineffective. An estimated 3.2 million Americans have chronic hepatitis C.

Use of Herbal Supplements and Other Complementary Approaches for Hepatitis C

Several herbal supplements have been studied for hepatitis C, and a substantial number of people with hepatitis C has tried herbal supplements. For example, a survey of 1,145 participants in the Hepatitis C Long-Term Treatment Against Cirrhosis (HALT-C) trial, a study supported by the National Institutes of Health (NIH), found that 23 percent of the participants were using herbal products. Although participants reported using many different herbal products, silymarin (milk thistle) was by far the most common. Another study, which surveyed 120 adults with hepatitis C, found that many used a variety of complementary health approaches, including multivitamins, herbal remedies, massage, deep breathing exercises, meditation, progressive relaxation, and yoga*.

* *A mind and body practice with origins in ancient Indian philosophy. The various styles of yoga typically combine physical postures, breathing techniques, and meditation or relaxation.*

What the Science Says

No dietary supplement has been shown to be effective for hepatitis C. This section summarizes what is known about the safety and effectiveness of milk thistle and some of the other dietary supplements studied for hepatitis C.

- Milk thistle (scientific name: *Silybum marianum*) is a plant from the aster family. Silymarin is an active component of milk thistle that is believed to be responsible for the herb's health-related properties. Milk thistle has been used in Europe for treating liver disease and jaundice since the sixteenth century. In the United States, silymarin is the most popular dietary supplement taken by people with liver disease. However, two rigorously designed studies of silymarin in people with hepatitis C did not show any benefit.

- A 2012 controlled clinical trial, cofounded by the National Center for Complementary and Integrative Health (NCCIH) and the National Institute of Diabetes and Digestive and Kidney Diseases (NIDDK), showed that 2 higher-than-usual doses of silymarin were no better than placebo in reducing the high blood levels of an enzyme that indicates liver damage. In the study, 154 people who had not responded to standard antiviral treatment for chronic hepatitis C were randomly assigned to receive 420 mg of silymarin, 700 mg of silymarin, or placebo 3 times per day for 24 weeks. At the end of the treatment period, blood levels of the enzyme were similar in all 3 groups.

- Results of the HALT-C study mentioned above suggested that silymarin used by hepatitis C patients was associated with fewer and milder symptoms of liver disease and a somewhat better quality of life, but there was no change in virus activity or liver inflammation. The researchers emphasized that this was a retrospective study (one that examined the medical and lifestyle histories of the participants). It is finding of improved quality of life in patients taking silymarin was not confirmed in the more rigorous 2012 study described above.

What Do We Know about Safety?

- **Safety.** Available evidence from clinical trials in people with liver disease suggests that milk thistle is generally well-tolerated. Side effects can include a laxative effect, nausea, diarrhea, abdominal bloating and pain, and occasional allergic reactions. In NIH-funded studies of silymarin in people with hepatitis C that were completed in 2010 and 2012, the frequency of side effects was similar in people taking silymarin and those taking placebos. However, these studies were not large enough to show with certainty that silymarin is safe for people with chronic hepatitis C.

Other supplements have been studied for hepatitis C, but overall, no benefits have been clearly demonstrated. These supplements include the following:

- Probiotics are live microorganisms that are intended to have a health benefit when consumed. Research has not produced any clear evidence that probiotics are helpful in people with hepatitis C. Most people can use probiotics without experiencing any side effects—or with only mild gastrointestinal side effects, such as intestinal gas—but there have been some case reports of serious adverse effects in people with underlying serious health conditions.

- Preliminary studies, most of which were conducted outside the United States, have examined the use of zinc for hepatitis C. Zinc supplements might help to correct zinc deficiencies associated with hepatitis C or reduce some symptoms, but the evidence for these possible benefits is limited. Zinc is generally considered to be safe when used appropriately, but it can be toxic if taken in excessive amounts.

- A few preliminary studies have looked at the effects of combining supplements such as lactoferrin, S-Adenosyl-L-methionine (SAMe) or zinc with conventional drug therapy for hepatitis C. The evidence is not sufficient to draw clear conclusions about benefit or safety.

- Glycyrrhizin—a compound found in licorice root—has been tested in a few clinical trials in hepatitis C patients, but there is not enough evidence to determine if it is helpful. In large amounts, glycyrrhizin or licorice can be dangerous in people with a history of hypertension (high blood pressure), kidney failure, or cardiovascular diseases.

- Preliminary studies have examined the potential of the following products for treating chronic hepatitis C: TJ-108 (a mixture of herbs used in Japanese Kampo medicine), Schisandra, oxymatrine (an extract from the sophora root), and thymus extract. The limited research on these products has not produced convincing evidence that they are helpful for hepatitis C.

- Colloidal silver has been suggested as a treatment for hepatitis C, but there is no research to support its use for this purpose. Colloidal silver is known to cause serious side effects, including permanent bluish discoloration of the skin, called "argyria."

Part Six

Medical Diagnosis and Treatment of Contagious Diseases

Chapter 68

Diagnostic Tests for Contagious Diseases

Chapter Contents

Section 68.1—Medical Tests That Diagnose Infection.............. 544

Section 68.2—Testing for Influenza.. 546

Section 68.3—Strep Throat Testing and Treatment................. 552

Section 68.4—Rapid and Home Tests for Human
           Immunodeficiency Virus 556

Section 68.1

Medical Tests That Diagnose Infection

"Medical Tests That Diagnose Infection,"
© 2019 Omnigraphics. Reviewed July 2019.

The medical tests that are required to diagnose an infection begin with a physical examination. The doctor conducts a physical examination in order to evaluate your health or to identify the cause of infection. However, sometimes, the doctor may suggest more tests to study the infection. Below are some common tests and what they involve:

Blood Tests

Blood tests usually can be performed in a doctor's office or in a lab with a trained technician. Blood tests are conducted on blood samples that are taken through a vein in your body. The common blood tests that are used to detect an infection in your body are as follows:

Complete Blood Count

A complete blood count (CBC) is a type of blood test that is performed to evaluate your overall health and to detect disorders such as anemia, leukemia, and infection.

The CBC test measures various components and features of your blood including:

- White blood cells (WBCs)—cells that fight and prevent infection

- Red blood cells (RBCs)—cells that carry oxygen and remove carbon dioxide from organs

- Hemoglobin—protein that carry oxygen in RBCs

- Platelets—cells that are involved in blood clotting

If the result of the CBC test shows an abnormal increase or decrease in cell counts, it may indicate that you have an underlying medical condition that requires further evaluation.

Blood Culture Test

The blood culture test helps the doctor to figure out the presence of an infection in your bloodstream and whether it affects your body.

This test checks for foreign invaders, such as bacteria, yeast, or any other micro-organism, in your body. This test will help the doctor to determine the type of germ causing the infection in your body and how to combat it.

Throat Culture Test

The throat culture test may be suggested by the doctor in order to find and identify the germs that cause strep throat, which are called group A Streptococcus, or strep. The doctor may take a sample from the back of your throat to conduct a throat culture test. This test is not painful, but it may make you uncomfortable for a few minutes.

Urine Culture Test

The doctor performs a urine culture test to find the presence of germs, such as bacteria, in the urine that causes infection. This test is also suggested to identify any problems with the kidney, such as an infection. The collected urine sample is added to a substance that promotes the growth of the germ. If no germ growth is found, the test is negative. If the test is positive, the type of germ is examined under a microscope.

Stool Culture Test

The stool culture test helps the doctor to determine the presence of any bacterial infections in the intestine or any part of the gastro-intestinal system. A technician places the collected stool samples with nutrients to encourage the growth of the bacteria. If present, the samples are examined under a microscope to identify the type of germ.

Biopsy Test

Sometimes, the doctor may suggest a biopsy test to find any infections or abnormalities, such as anemia, leukemia, etc., in your body. There are many types of biopsies; however, the doctor will choose the type based upon the condition of the illness. A biopsy involves collecting tissue samples from bone marrow, lymph nodes, or the kidney. The doctor analyzes the tissue under a microscope to find the presence of germs.

References

1. "Complete Blood Count (CBC)," Mayo Clinic, December 19, 2018.

2. "What Is a Blood Culture Test?" WebMD, December 19, 2018.

3. "What Is a Throat Culture? When Do I Need One?" WebMD, September 18, 2018.

4. "Urine Culture," Michigan Medicine, July 30, 2018.

Section 68.2

Testing for Influenza

This section includes text excerpted from "Overview of Influenza Testing Methods," Centers for Disease Control and Prevention (CDC), March 4, 2019.

Influenza virus testing is not required to make a clinical diagnosis of influenza in outpatients with suspected influenza, particularly during increased influenza activity when seasonal influenza A and B viruses are circulating in the local community. However, influenza virus testing can inform clinical management when the results may influence clinical decisions, such as whether to initiate antiviral treatment, perform other diagnostic testing, or to implement infection prevention and control measures for influenza. Influenza virus testing is recommended for all patients with suspected influenza who are being admitted to the hospital. Most importantly, clinicians should understand the limitations of influenza virus tests and how to properly interpret the results, especially negative results. During a respiratory illness outbreak in a closed setting (such as hospitals, long-term care facilities, cruise ships, boarding schools, and summer camps), testing for influenza virus infection can be very helpful in determining if influenza is the cause of the outbreak.

Influenza Virus Tests

Diagnostic tests available for the detection of influenza viruses in respiratory specimens include molecular assays (including rapid molecular assays, reverse transcription polymerase chain reaction (RT-PCR), and other nucleic acid amplification tests (NAAT)) and antigen detection tests (including rapid influenza diagnostic tests (RIDTs) and immunofluorescence assays (IFAs)). Viral culture is important for public health purposes but does not provide timely results to inform clinical management. Sensitivity and specificity of any test for influenza viruses in respiratory specimens might vary by the type of testing method and specific test used, the time from illness onset to specimen collection, the quality of the specimen collected, the respiratory source of the specimen, the handling and processing of the specimen, and the time from specimen collection to testing. The posttest probability or predictive values (positive and negative predictive values) of an influenza virus test depend upon the prevalence of circulating seasonal influenza viruses in the patient population and the specific test characteristics (sensitivity and specificity) when compared to a "gold standard" comparison test (molecular assay or viral culture). As with any diagnostic test, results should be evaluated in the context of other clinical and epidemiologic information available to healthcare providers. Serological testing does not provide timely results to inform clinical management decisions.

The Infectious Diseases Society of America (IDSA) recommends the use of rapid influenza molecular assays over rapid influenza diagnostic tests for the detection of influenza viruses in respiratory specimens of outpatients. The IDSA recommends the use of RT-PCR or other molecular assays for the detection of influenza viruses in respiratory specimens of hospitalized patients.

Rapid Molecular Assays

Rapid molecular assays are a kind of molecular influenza diagnostic test to detect influenza virus nucleic acids in upper respiratory tract specimens with high sensitivity (90 to 95%) and specificity. U.S. Food and Drug Administration (FDA)-cleared rapid molecular assays are available that produce results in approximately 15 to 30 minutes. Some of these rapid molecular assays are Clinical Laboratory Improvement Amendments (CLIA)-waived for point-of-care (POC) use.

Table 68.1. Influenza Virus Testing Methods

Method[1]	Types Detected	Acceptable Specimens[2]	Test Time	CLIA Waived[3]
Rapid Influenza Diagnostic Tests[4] (antigen detection)	A and B	NP[5] swab, aspirate or wash, nasal swab, aspirate or wash, throat swab	<15 min.	Yes/No
Rapid Molecular Assay (influenza viral RNA or nucleic acid detection)	A and B	NP[5] swab, nasal swab	15 to 30 minutes[6]	Yes/No[6]
Immunofluorescence, Direct (DFA) or Indirect (IFA) Fluorescent Antibody Staining (antigen detection)	A and B	NP[4] swab or wash, bronchial wash, nasal or endotracheal aspirate	1 to 4 hours	No
RT-PCR[7] (singleplex and multiplex; real-time and other RNA-based) and other molecular assays (influenza viral RNA or nucleic acid detection)	A and B	NP[5] swab, throat swab, NP[5] or bronchial wash, nasal or endotracheal aspirate, sputum	Varies (1 to 8 hours, varies by the assay)	No
Rapid cell culture (shell vials; cell mixtures; yields live virus)	A and B	NP[5] swab, throat swab, NP[5] or bronchial wash, nasal or endotracheal aspirate, sputum; (specimens placed in VTM[8])	1 to 3 days	No

Table 68.1. Continued

Method[1]	Types Detected	Acceptable Specimens[2]	Test Time	CLIA Waived[3]
Viral tissue cell culture (conventional; yields live virus)	A and B	NP[5] swab, throat swab, NP[5] or bronchial wash, nasal or endotracheal aspirate, sputum (specimens placed in VTM[8])	3 to 10 days	No

1. Serologic (antibody detection) testing is not recommended for routine patient diagnosis, and it cannot inform clinical management. A single acute serum specimen for seasonal influenza serology is uninterpretable and should not be collected. Serological testing for the detection of antibodies to seasonal influenza viruses is useful for research studies and requires the collection of appropriately timed acute and convalescent serum specimens and testing of paired sera at specialized research or public health laboratories.

2. Approved clinical specimens vary by influenza test. Consult the manufacturer's package insert for the approved clinical specimens for each test. Approved respiratory specimens vary among the U.S. Food and Drug Administration (FDA)-cleared influenza assays.

3. Clinical Laboratory Improvement Amendments (CLIA) of 1988. Information on CLIA can be found on the Centers for Medicare & Medicaid Services (CMS) website under Regulations and Guidance.

4. Chromatographic- and/or fluorescence-based lateral flow and membrane-based immunoassays. Some approved rapid influenza diagnostic assays utilize an analyzer reader device.

5. NP = nasopharyngeal

6. Rapid molecular assays can provide results in approximately 15 to 30 minutes.

7. Reverse transcription polymerase chain reaction, including FDA-approved test systems, reference laboratory testing using analyte specific reagent (ASR) or lab-developed reagents. Some approved molecular assays can produce results in approximately 60 to 80 minutes.

8. VTM = Viral transport media

Other Molecular Assays

Reverse transcription-polymerase chain reaction (RT-PCR) and other molecular assays can identify the presence of influenza viral ribonucleic acid (RNA) or nucleic acids in respiratory specimens with very high sensitivity and specificity. Some molecular assays are able to detect and discriminate between infections with influenza A and B viruses; other tests can identify specific seasonal influenza A virus subtypes [A(H1N1)pdm09, or A(H3N2)]. These assays can yield results in approximately 45 minutes to several hours, depending upon the assay. Notably, the detection of influenza viral RNA or nucleic acids by these assays does not necessarily indicate the detection of viable infectious virus or ongoing influenza viral replication. It is important to note that not all assays have been cleared by the FDA for diagnostic use. Some multiplex molecular assays are available that can detect influenza viral nucleic acids and distinguish influenza virus infection from other respiratory pathogens, and they may also be useful for the management of severely immunosuppressed patients or for use in identifying the cause of an institutional outbreak of respiratory illness.

Rapid Influenza Diagnostic Tests

Rapid influenza diagnostic tests are antigen detection assays that can detect influenza viral antigens in 10 to 15 minutes with high specificity. Some tests are CLIA-waived and approved for use in any outpatient setting, whereas others must be used in a moderately complex clinical laboratory. Some RIDTs utilize an analyzer reader device to standardize results to improve sensitivity (75 to 80%). The detection of an influenza virus antigen does not necessarily indicate the detection of viable infectious virus or ongoing influenza viral replication.

None of the rapid influenza diagnostic tests provide any information about influenza A virus subtypes. The types of specimens acceptable for use (i.e., nasopharyngeal, or nasal aspirates, swabs, or washes) also vary by test. The specificity and, in particular, the sensitivity of rapid influenza diagnostic tests are lower than for viral culture and RT-PCR, and they vary by test. Most of the rapid influenza diagnostic tests that can be done in a physician's office are approximately 50 to 70 percent sensitive for detecting influenza virus antigens and greater than 90 percent specific. The FDA has reclassified the RIDTs and published requirements for improved accuracy, including higher sensitivity. Tests with low-to-moderate sensitivity and high specificity can produce false negative results more commonly than false positive results, especially during peak influenza activity in the community. Because of the lower sensitivity of the rapid influenza diagnostic tests, clinicians should consider confirming negative test results with molecular assays, especially during periods of peak community influenza activity and/or during suspected institutional influenza outbreaks because of the possibility of false-negative RIDT results. In contrast, false-positive RIDT results are less likely but can occur, and they are more common during periods of low influenza activity. Therefore, when interpreting the results of a rapid influenza diagnostic test, clinicians should consider the test in the context of the level of influenza activity in their community. Package inserts and the laboratory performing the test should be consulted for more details regarding the use of rapid influenza diagnostic tests.

Immunofluorescence

Immunofluorescence assays (IFAs) are antigen detection assays that generally require the use of a fluorescent microscope to produce results in approximately 2 to 4 hours with moderate sensitivity and high specificity. Both direct fluorescent antibody (DFA) and indirect fluorescent antibody (IFA) staining assays are available to detect influenza A and B viral antigens in respiratory tract specimens. Subtyping or further identification of influenza A virus is not possible by immunofluorescence assays. One rapid immunofluorescence assay is an RIDT and utilizes an analyzer device to produce results in approximately 15 minutes.

Viral Culture

Viral culture results do not yield timely results to inform clinical management. Shell-vial tissue culture results may take 1 to 3 days, while traditional tissue-cell viral culture results may take 3 to 10 days. However, viral culture allows for extensive antigenic and genetic characterization of influenza viruses. The collection of some respiratory samples for viral culture is essential for surveillance and antigenic characterization of new seasonal influenza A and B virus strains that may need to be included in the next year's influenza vaccine.

Serologic Testing

Routine serological testing for influenza requires paired acute and convalescent sera, does not provide timely results to help with clinical decision-making, is only available at a limited number of public health or research laboratories, and is not generally recommended, except for research and public health investigations. Serological testing results for antibodies to human influenza viruses on a single serum specimen is not interpretable and not recommended.

Novel Influenza A Virus Infections

If human infection with a novel influenza A virus of animal origin (e.g., avian influenza A virus or swine influenza A virus) is suspected, the local and state health department should be contacted to perform RT-PCR for seasonal influenza viruses and novel influenza A viruses. Commercially available influenza diagnostic tests do not specifically detect novel influenza A viruses, and a positive result for influenza A virus cannot distinguish seasonal influenza A virus from avian or swine influenza A virus infections.

Section 68.3

Strep Throat Testing and Treatment

This section includes text excerpted from "Group A Streptococcal (GAS) Disease—Pharyngitis (Strep Throat)," Centers for Disease Control and Prevention (CDC), November 1, 2018.

Diagnosis and Testing

The differential diagnosis of acute pharyngitis includes multiple viral and bacterial pathogens. Viruses are the most common cause of pharyngitis in all age groups. Experts estimate that group A strep, the most common bacterial cause, causes 20 to 30 percent of pharyngitis episodes in children. In comparison, experts estimate it causes approximately 5 to 15 percent of pharyngitis infections in adults.

History and clinical examination can be used to diagnose viral pharyngitis when clear viral symptoms are present. Viral symptoms include:

- Cough
- Rhinorrhea

- Hoarseness
- Oral ulcers
- Conjunctivitis

Patients with clear viral symptoms do not need testing for group A strep. However, clinicians cannot use clinical examination to differentiate viral and group A strep pharyngitis in the absence of viral symptoms.

Clinicians need to use either a rapid antigen detection test (RADT) or throat culture to confirm group A strep pharyngitis. RADTs have high specificity for group A strep but varying sensitivities when compared to throat culture. The throat culture is the gold standard diagnostic test.

Special Considerations

Clinicians should confirm group A strep pharyngitis in children older than three years of age to appropriately guide treatment decisions. Giving antibiotics to children with confirmed group A strep pharyngitis can reduce their risk of developing sequela (acute rheumatic fever). Testing for group A strep pharyngitis is not routinely indicated for:

- Children younger than three years of age
- Adults

Acute rheumatic fever is very rare in those age groups.

Clinicians can use a positive RADT as confirmation of group A strep pharyngitis in children. However, clinicians should follow up a negative RADT in a child with symptoms of pharyngitis with a throat culture. Clinicians should have a mechanism to contact the family and initiate antibiotics if the back-up throat culture is positive.

Treatment

The use of a recommended antibiotic regimen to treat group A strep pharyngitis:

- Shortens the duration of symptoms
- Reduces the likelihood of transmission to family members, classmates, and other close contacts

- Prevents the development of complications, including acute rheumatic fever

When left untreated, the symptoms of group A strep pharyngitis are usually self-limited. However, acute rheumatic fever and suppurative complications (e.g., peritonsillar abscess, mastoiditis) are more likely to occur after an untreated infection. Patients, regardless of age, who have a positive RADT or throat culture need antibiotics. Clinicians should not treat viral pharyngitis with antibiotics.

Penicillin or amoxicillin is the antibiotic of choice to treat group A strep pharyngitis. There has never been a report of a clinical isolate of group A strep that is resistant to penicillin. However, resistance

Table 68.2. Antibiotic Regimens Recommended for Group A Streptococcal Pharyngitis

Drug, Route	Dose or Dosage	Duration or Quantity
For individuals without penicillin allergy		
Penicillin V, oral	Children: 250 mg twice daily or 3 times daily; adolescents and adults: 250 mg 4 times daily or 500 mg twice daily	10 days
Amoxicillin, oral	50 mg/kg once daily (max = 1000 mg); alternate: 25 mg/kg (max = 500 mg) twice daily	10 days
Benzathine penicillin G, intramuscular	<27 kg: 600 000 U; ≥27 kg: 1 200 000 U	1 dose
For individuals with penicillin allergy		
Cephalexin,[a] oral	20 mg/kg/dose twice daily (max = 500 mg/dose)	10 days
Cefadroxil,[a] oral	30 mg/kg once daily (max = 1 g)	10 days
Clindamycin, oral	7 mg/kg/dose 3 times daily (max = 300 mg/dose)	10 days
Azithromycin,[b] oral	12 mg/kg once (max = 500 mg), then 6 mg/kg (max=250 mg) once daily for the next 4 days	5 days
Clarithromycin,[b] oral	7.5 mg/kg/dose twice daily (max = 250 mg/dose)	10 days

Abbreviation: Max, maximum.
[a] Avoid in individuals with immediate-type hypersensitivity to penicillin.
[b] Resistance of group A strep to these agents is well-known and varies geographically and temporally.

to azithromycin and clarithromycin is common in some communities. For patients with a penicillin allergy, recommended regimens include narrow-spectrum cephalosporins (cephalexin, cefadroxil), clindamycin, azithromycin, and clarithromycin.

Carriage

Asymptomatic group A strep carriers usually do not require treatment. Carriers have positive throat cultures or are RADT positive, but they do not have clinical symptoms or immunologic response to group A strep antigens on laboratory testing. Compared to people with symptomatic pharyngitis, carriers are much less likely to transmit group A strep to others. Carriers are also very unlikely to develop suppurative or nonsuppurative complications.

Some people with recurrent episodes of acute pharyngitis with evidence of group A strep by RADT or throat culture actually have recurrent episodes of viral pharyngitis with concurrent streptococcal carriage. Repeated use of antibiotics among this subset of patients is unnecessary. However, identifying carriers clinically or by laboratory methods can be very difficult. The Infectious Diseases Society of America guidelines and Red Book address determining if someone is a carrier and their management.

Prognosis and Complications

Rarely, suppurative and nonsuppurative complications can occur after group A strep pharyngitis. Suppurative complications result from the spread of group A strep from the pharynx to adjacent structures. They can include:

- Peritonsillar abscess

- Retropharyngeal abscess

- Cervical lymphadenitis

- Mastoiditis

Other focal infections or sepsis are even less common.

Acute rheumatic fever is a nonsuppurative sequelae of group A strep pharyngitis. Poststreptococcal glomerulonephritis is a nonsuppurative sequelae of group A strep pharyngitis or skin infections. These complications occur after the original infection resolves and involve sites distant to the initial group A strep infection site. They are thought to be the result of the immune response and not of direct group A strep infection.

Prevention

Good hand hygiene and respiratory etiquette can reduce the spread of all types of group A strep infection. Hand hygiene is especially important after coughing and sneezing and before preparing foods or eating. Good respiratory etiquette involves covering your cough or sneeze. Treating an infected person with an antibiotic for 24 hours or longer generally eliminates their ability to transmit the bacteria. Thus, people with group A strep pharyngitis should stay home from work, school, or day care until:

- They are afebrile

- At least 24 hours after starting appropriate antibiotic therapy

Section 68.4

Rapid and Home Tests for Human Immunodeficiency Virus

This section includes text excerpted from "Information Regarding the OraQuick In-Home HIV Test," U.S. Food and Drug Administration (FDA), February 2, 2018.

How the OraQuick In-Home Human Immunodeficiency Virus Test Works
What Is the OraQuick In-Home Human Immunodeficiency Virus Test and How Does It Work?

The OraQuick In-Home Human Immunodeficiency Virus (HIV) Test is a rapid, self-administered, over-the-counter (OTC) test. The OraQuick In-Home HIV Test kit consists of a test stick (device) to collect the specimen, a test tube (vial) to insert the test stick (device) and complete the test, testing directions, two information booklets ("HIV,

Testing and Me" and "What your results mean to you"), a disposal bag, and phone numbers for consumer support.

This approved test uses oral fluid to check for antibodies to HIV type 1 and HIV type 2, the viruses that cause acquired immunodeficiency syndrome (AIDS). The kit is designed to allow you to take the HIV test anonymously and in private with the collection of an oral fluid sample by swabbing your upper and lower gums with the test device. After collecting the sample, you insert the device into the kit's vial, which contains a developer solution, wait 20 to 40 minutes, and read the test result. A positive result with this test does not mean that an individual is definitely infected with HIV but rather that additional testing should be done in a medical setting to confirm the test result. Additionally, a negative test result does not mean that an individual is definitely not infected with HIV, particularly when exposure may have been within the previous three months. Again, an individual should obtain a confirmatory test in a medical setting.

When Should I Take a Test for Human Immunodeficiency Virus?

If you actively engage in behavior that puts you at risk for HIV infection, or your partner engages in such behavior, then you should consider testing on a regular basis. It can take some time for the immune system to produce enough antibodies for the test to detect, and this time period can vary from person to person. This timeframe is commonly referred to as the "window period," when a person is infected with HIV but antibodies to the virus cannot be detected; however, the person may be able to infect others. According to the Centers for Disease Control and Prevention (CDC), although it can take up to six months to develop antibodies for HIV, most people (97%) will develop detectable antibodies in the first three months following the time of their infection.

How Reliable Is the OraQuick In-Home Human Immunodeficiency Virus Test?

As noted in the package insert, clinical studies have shown that the OraQuick In-Home HIV Test has an expected performance of approximately 92 percent for test sensitivity (i.e., the percentage of results that will be positive when HIV is present). This means that 1 false-negative result would be expected out of every 12 test results in HIV-infected individuals. The clinical studies also showed that the

OraQuick In-Home HIV Test has an expected performance of 99.98 percent for test specificity (i.e., the percentage of results that will be negative when HIV is not present). This means that 1 false-positive result would be expected out of every 5,000 test results in uninfected individuals.

It is extremely important for those who self-test using the OraQuick In-Home HIV Test to carefully read and follow all labeled directions. Even when used according to the labeled directions, there will be some false-negative results and a small number of false-positive results. The OraQuick test package contains step-by-step instructions, and there is also an OraQuick Consumer Support Center to assist users in the testing process.

Results

If the Test Says I Am Human Immunodeficiency Virus-Positive, What Should I Do?

A positive test result does not necessarily mean that you are infected with HIV. If you test positive for HIV using the OraQuick In-Home Test, you should see your healthcare provider or call the OraQuick Consumer Support Center, which has support center representatives available 24 hours a day/7 days a week to answer your questions and provide referrals to local healthcare providers for follow-up care. You will be advised to obtain confirmatory testing to confirm a positive result or to inform you that the initial result was a false-positive result. The test kit also contains an information booklet, "What your results mean to You," which is designed to instruct individuals on what to do once they have obtained their test results.

Do I Need a Confirmatory Test?

A positive test result on the OraQuick In-Home HIV Test indicates that you may be infected with HIV. Additional testing in a medical setting will either confirm a positive test result or inform you that the initial result was a false-positive result.

What Is a False-Positive Result?

A false-positive result occurs when an individual not infected with the HIV virus receives a test result that indicates that she or he is infected with HIV.

If the Test Says I Am Human Immunodeficiency Virus-Negative, What Should I Do?

A negative result on this test does not necessarily mean that you are not infected with HIV. The OraQuick test kit contains an information booklet, "What your results mean to You," which is designed to instruct individuals on what to do once they have obtained their test results. The test is relatively reliable if there has been sufficient time for the HIV antibodies to develop in the infected person. For the Ora-Quick In-Home HIV Test, the window period is about three months. If you have recently been engaging in behavior that puts you at high risk for HIV infection, you should take the test again at a later time. Alternatively, you should see your healthcare provider who can discuss other options for HIV testing.

What Is a False-Negative Result?

A false-negative result occurs when an HIV-infected individual receives a test result that incorrectly indicates that she or he is not infected with HIV.

How Quickly Will I Get the Results of the OraQuick Test?

You can read the results of the OraQuick In-Home HIV Test within 20 to 40 minutes.

Chapter 69

Prescription Medicines That Treat Contagious Diseases (Antibiotics, Antivirals, and Other Prescription Medicines)

Although evidence suggests that the use of medicines to treat infections, also known as "antimicrobial chemotherapy," may date back to ancient times, the modern use of this treatment begins in the early twentieth century when researchers in the lab of Paul Ehrlich, a German physician and scientist, synthesized an arsenical compound called "arsphenamine." This drug, manufactured under the trade name Salvarsan, went on to become the first chemotherapeutic agent proven effective against human parasitic disease and was widely used in the treatment of syphilis.

This was followed by the discovery of penicillin in 1928 by Alexander Fleming, a Scottish scientist, who noticed that the accidental growth of *Penicillium* mold in a petri dish inhibited the growth of *Staphylococcus aureus* bacteria. By the forties, this wonder drug was

"Antibiotics, Antivirals, and Other Prescription Medicines," © 2017 Omnigraphics. Reviewed July 2019.

being used to treat a number of infections—some life-threatening—of skin, blood, bone, and vital organs caused by *Staphylococcus*. During the Second World War, penicillin saved millions of lives and prevented the debilitating effects of wounds from dangerous infections. These early discoveries set the stage for the development of numerous anti-infective agents capable of preventing and treating a wide range of microbial infections.

Infections are generally caused when infective agents, such as bacteria, virus, or fungi, invade the tissues of an organism, sometimes called the "host." These organisms multiply inside the host and produce toxins, provoking a reaction in the host tissues that could either result in an acute infection (short term) or a chronic infection (long term). There are a number of anti-infective agents that are used to treat infections. These agents work either by killing the infectious agent or pathogen, or by inhibiting its growth. While antimicrobial chemotherapy refers to the treatment of infections caused by infective agents, antimicrobial prophylaxis is used to prevent the spread of infection caused by pathogens. Anti-infective agents are classified on the basis of the infective agents they fight. For example, antibacterials are pharmacologic agents generally used to treat infections caused by bacteria. Antifungals are primarily effective against fungi and include fungistats (which inhibit fungal growth and proliferation) and fungicides (which kill fungal cells and spores). Antivirals and antiprotozoals act against viruses and protozoa, respectively.

Antibiotics

The discovery of antimicrobial agents, particularly the antibiotics, is often regarded as one of the greatest achievements of modern medicine, since it led to a significant decline in mortality rates from infectious diseases. The term "antibiotic" was first suggested by Selman Waksman, a Russian-born American biochemist and microbiologist credited with the discovery of several antibiotics, including streptomycin and neomycin, which have found extensive use in the treatment of many infectious diseases. The term is used to define the activity or application of a chemical compound and it includes any molecule that kills or inhibits the growth of bacteria.

Classes of Antibiotics

Antibiotics may be derived from certain classes of microorganisms or living systems and are used to fight against one or more types of disease-causing microorganisms. They may also be derived from nonorganic sources, as in the case of sulphonamides and quinolones. Some antibiotics are effective against a number of bacteria, both gram-positive and gram-negative; these are termed as broad-spectrum antibiotics. Other antibiotics, called "narrow-spectrum," are used to treat infections caused by specific families of bacteria.

Mode of Action

Most antibiotics work by disrupting the bacteria's metabolic processes. Although the exact mechanism of how this is brought about is still under study, it is believed that most antibacterial action either targets enzymes that regulate biosynthesis of the cell wall or cell proteins; others target enzymes that regulate nucleic acid metabolism of the bacterial cell. Some, like ionophores, work by interfering with cell membrane integrity. Antibiotics like penicillin and cephalosporins act on the bacterial cell wall, while quinolones and sulphonamides target the bacterial enzymes. Lincosamides and tetracyclines are examples of antibiotics that interfere with protein synthesis in bacterial cells.

Although the discovery of antibiotics was thought to herald the end of infectious diseases, their rampant misuse and overuse in humans, as well as in food-producing animals, in the last few decades have led to the emergence of antibiotic-resistant strains of bacteria. Antibiotics that were used successfully in the treatment of many infections in the past have now become inefficient against the same infection, and the dire need for new antibiotics—along with a slowdown in antibiotic discovery programs in the pharmaceutical industry—poses a serious challenge to public health worldwide.

Antivirals

Drugs used to treat infections caused by viruses are called "antiviral drugs." Unlike bacteria, viruses are difficult to treat because they are obligate parasites, meaning they can grow and multiply only within living hosts. This makes it impossible to use prophylactic measures to contain viral infections. Contrary to popular belief, antibiotics do not treat viral infections, such as influenza, bronchitis, ear infection, or chest cold in otherwise healthy people. Most of the antiviral remedies currently in use include vaccines, which have successfully controlled—and in some cases eradicated—such serious viral infections as smallpox and poliomyelitis. The last few decades have seen growing interest in developing antiviral drugs to prevent the multiplication of the virus and cause the illness to run its course rapidly. Unfortunately, these drugs are only partially effective and work only on a very few specific viruses. The most difficult aspect of developing antiviral agents is the astounding diversity in the structural characteristic of viruses, of which there can be more than 50 different types for any given virus. In addition, the viral antigen, a protein coded by the viral genome that provokes an immune response in the host cell, periodically mutates, making it particularly difficult to contain the infection with specific therapy.

Mentioned below are few classes of antiviral drugs.

Anti-Hepatitis

Viral hepatitis can be treated with several antiviral medications, most of which work by preventing viral replication in infected cells. Ribavirin is commonly used to treat hepatitis C, while lamivudine and adefovir are used to treat chronic hepatitis B infections. In addition to treating viral hepatitis, these drugs are used to treat HIV infections. Interferons are another important class of drugs used in the treatment regimen for hepatitis, and they are commonly used in combination with other antiviral agents, such as ribavirin.

Anti-Herpes

Anti-herpes medications like acyclovir, penciclovir, and their respective prodrugs (an inactive form of medication that is metabolized into a pharmacologically active drug inside the body) interfere with viral DNA replication and help control their spread to new cells. While anti-herpes drugs cannot eradicate the virus, they can help control symptoms and reduce the course of infections.

Anti-Influenza

Anti-influenza medications are not substitutes for vaccination but are used in conjunction with vaccines. Some strains of the influenza virus have become resistant to older antiviral drugs, such as amantadine and rimantadine, and are no longer used, although their potential use against new strains of virus that may be susceptible to these drugs cannot be ruled out. Some of the FDA-approved anti-influenza drugs include oseltamivir (Tamiflu®), zanamivir (Relenza®), and peramivir (Rapivab®). These drugs can ease the severity of symptoms and reduce the course of infection. The government maintains a stockpile of anti-influenza medications in preparation for a pandemic emergency.

Antiretroviral

Antiretroviral drugs work by suppressing a virus and retarding the progression of the disease. Although the antiretroviral drugs do not kill the virus or cure the disease, they slow down viral replication and substantially reduce the amount of virus in the body. This helps the immune system stay healthy and also reduces the risk of transmission to other people. More often than not, a cocktail of drugs from three or more classes of antiretroviral drugs is used for maximum effect. Referred to as "Highly Active AntiRetroviral Therapy (HAART)," this treatment regimen has substantially reduced HIV-related morbidity and mortality around the world.

Antiprotozoals

These are drugs that are used to treat infections caused by single-celled protozoans, such as *Entamoeba histolytica*, which causes amoebiasis, and *plasmodium*, the pathogen that causes malaria. Like many other infective agents, antiprotozoals work on specific targets and inhibit their growth and reproduction. Antimalarial drugs, which include a diverse class of quinoline derivatives, act by targeting the erythrocytic (red blood cell) stage of the infection, which can be life-threatening, since blood circulates through all tissues and organs. In addition to antimalarials, there are several other classes of antiprotozoals, some of which may also be used to treat certain bacterial infections. Two of the most commonly used drugs in this group are metronidazole and tinidazole, which are used to treat a variety of parasitic and amoebic infections.

Antifungal Drugs

This class of medication controls a diverse range of infections caused by fungi, from simple infections like athlete's foot to extremely dangerous infections, such as cryptococcal meningitis, which affects the brain and spinal cord. Antifungal medications are based on mechanisms that inhibit vital cell processes in the organism. They work by either disrupting the integrity of the fungal cell membrane or cell wall, or by interfering with cell division by preventing DNA replication.

Antifungal agents are broadly classified as topical and systemic drugs. While topical antifungal agents may be directly applied to skin, nails, or hair to treat superficial fungal infections, systemic antifungal agents are used to treat invasive fungal infections that affect body tissues or internal organs. Antifungal drugs come as lotions, sprays, creams, tablets, injections, and pessaries (for vaginal use).

As in the case of antibiotics, drug resistance has become a major concern with a number of antifungal drugs as a result of their indiscriminate use in healthcare settings. For example, low dosage or short-term treatments may be a common cause of antifungal resistance in candidemia—one of the most common bloodstream infections in hospital settings—which incurs substantial healthcare costs. Although drug resistance in several species of *Candida* is a serious problem, studies show that drug resistance in other fungal species, such as *Aspergillus*, is also becoming a cause for concern. Some studies also show that the overuse of antibiotics could lead to resistance by inhibiting gut bacteria and favoring the growth of fungal species like *Candida*.

References

1. "Antiviral Drug," Encyclopaedia Britannica, n.d.

2. Davies, Julian, and Dorothy Davies. "Origins and Evolution of Antibiotic Resistance," Microbiology and Molecular Biology Reviews, September 2010.

3. "Mechanisms of Action," Sigma-Aldrich, n.d.

4. Coates, R.M., Gerry Halls and Yanmin Hu. "Novel Classes of Antibiotics or More of the Same?" British Journal of Pharmacology, May 2011.

Chapter 70

Antiviral Drugs for Seasonal Flu

The information in this chapter should be considered current for the 2018–2019 influenza season for clinical practice regarding the use of influenza antiviral medications.

Neuraminidase Inhibitors

Neuraminidase inhibitors are chemically-related antiviral medications that block the viral neuraminidase enzyme and have activity against both influenza A and B viruses. The neuraminidase inhibitors include:

- **Oseltamivir** (available as a generic or under the trade name "Tamiflu®" for oral administration) is U.S. Food and Drug Administration (FDA)-approved for early treatment of uncomplicated influenza in people 2 weeks of age and older, and for chemoprophylaxis to prevent influenza in people 1 year of age and older. Although not part of FDA-approved indications, use of oral oseltamivir for treatment of influenza in infants younger than 14 days of age, and for chemoprophylaxis in infants 3 months to 1 year of age, is recommended by the

---

This chapter includes text excerpted from "Antiviral Drugs for Seasonal Influenza: Additional Links and Resources," Centers for Disease Control and Prevention (CDC), November 29, 2018.

Centers for Disease Control and Prevention (CDC) and the American Academy of Pediatrics. If a child is younger than 3 months of age, the use of oseltamivir for chemoprophylaxis is not recommended unless the situation is judged critical, due to the limited data in this age group.

- **Zanamivir** (trade name Relenza®) for oral inhalation is FDA-approved for early treatment of uncomplicated influenza in people 7 years of age and older and to prevent influenza in people 5 years of age and older. It is not recommended for use in people with underlying respiratory disease, including people with asthma.

- **Peramivir** (trade name Rapivab®) for intravenous administration is FDA-approved for early treatment of uncomplicated influenza in people 2 years of age and older.

Cap-Dependent Endonuclease Inhibitor

An endonuclease inhibitor has a different mechanism of action than a neuraminidase inhibitor. Endonuclease inhibitors interfere with viral ribonucleic acid (RNA) transcription, and they block virus replication in both influenza A and B viruses. There is only one approved cap-dependent endonuclease inhibitor:

- **Baloxavir marboxil** (trade name Xofluza®) for oral administration is FDA-approved for early treatment of uncomplicated influenza in people 12 years of age and older. Baloxavir is not recommended for pregnant women, breastfeeding mothers, outpatients with complicated or progressive illness, or hospitalized patients.

Adamantanes

The adamantanes target the M2 ion channel protein of influenza A viruses. (Therefore, these medications are active against influenza A viruses but not influenza B viruses.) The adamantanes are not currently recommended for use in the United States because of widespread antiviral resistance in circulating influenza A viruses. The adamantanes include:

- **Amantadine** (generic) for oral administration is FDA-approved to treat and prevent only influenza A viruses in people older than 1 year of age.

- **Rimantadine** (generic or under the trade name "Flumadine") for oral administration is FDA-approved to prevent only influenza A virus infection among people older than 1 year of age. It is approved to treat only influenza A virus infections in people 17 years of age and older.

Chapter 71

Drug Resistance

Chapter Contents

Section 71.1—Antibiotic Safety and Drug Resistance.............. 572

Section 71.2—Antimicrobial (Drug) Resistance........................ 575

Section 71.3—Surveillance of Antimicrobial
Resistance Patterns and Rates........................... 580

Section 71.4—Influenza Antiviral Drug Resistance 583

Section 71.1

Antibiotic Safety and Drug Resistance

This section contains text excerpted from the following sources:
Text beginning with the heading "What Is the Right Way to Take
Antibiotics?" is excerpted from "Antibiotics Aren't Always the
Answer," Centers for Disease Control and Prevention (CDC),
November 12, 2017; Text under the heading "What the U.S. Food and
Drug Administration Is Doing" is excerpted from
"Combating Antibiotic Resistance," U.S. Food and Drug
Administration (FDA), November 15, 2011.
Reviewed July 2019.

What Is the Right Way to Take Antibiotics?

If you need antibiotics, take them exactly as prescribed.

Improving the way healthcare professionals prescribe antibiotics, and the way we take antibiotics, helps keep us healthy now, helps fight antibiotic resistance, and ensures that these life-saving drugs will be available for future generations.

Talk with your doctor if you have any questions about your antibiotics, or if you develop any side effects, especially diarrhea, since that could be *Clostridium difficile* infection (also called "*C. difficile*" or "*C. diff*"), which needs to be treated. *C.diff* can lead to severe colon damage and death.

What Are the Side Effects?

Common side effects range from minor to very severe health problems and can include:

- Rash
- Dizziness
- Nausea
- Diarrhea
- Yeast infections

More serious side effects can include:

- *Clostridium difficile* infection
- Severe and life-threatening allergic reactions

Why Does Taking Antibiotics Lead to Antibiotic Resistance?

Any time antibiotics are used, they can cause side effects and lead to antibiotic resistance. Antibiotic resistance is one of the most urgent threats to public health. Always remember:

* Antibiotic resistance does not mean the body is becoming resistant to antibiotics; it is that bacteria have become resistant to the antibiotics designed to kill them.

* When bacteria become resistant, antibiotics cannot fight them, and the bacteria multiply.

* Some resistant bacteria can be harder to treat and can spread to other people.

Each year in the United States, at least 2 million people get infected with antibiotic-resistant bacteria. At least 23,000 people die as a result.

How Can I Stay Healthy?

You can stay healthy and keep others healthy by:

* Cleaning your hands

* Covering your coughs

* Staying home when you are sick

* Getting recommended vaccines for the flu, for example

Talk to your doctor or nurse about the steps you can take to prevent infections.

What Do Antibiotics Treat?

Antibiotics are only needed for treating certain infections caused by bacteria. Antibiotics are critical tools for treating common infections, such as pneumonia, and for life-threatening conditions including sepsis, the body's extreme response to an infection.

What Do Not Antibiotics Treat?

Antibiotics do not work on viruses, such as colds and flu, or runny noses, even if the mucus is thick, yellow or green. Antibiotics also would not help some common bacterial infections, including most cases of bronchitis, many sinus infections, and some ear infections.

Why Is It Important to Be Antibiotics Aware?

Antibiotics save lives. When a patient needs antibiotics, the benefits outweigh the risks of side effects or antibiotic resistance.

When antibiotics are not needed, they would not help you and the side effects could still hurt you. Reactions from antibiotics cause one out of five medication-related visits to the emergency department.

In children, reactions from antibiotics are the most common cause of medication-related emergency department visits.

What the U.S. Food and Drug Administration Is Doing

The FDA is combating antibiotic resistance through activities that include:

- **Labeling regulations addressing proper use of antibiotics.** Antibiotic labeling contains required statements in several places, advising healthcare professionals that these drugs should be used only to treat infections that are believed to be caused by bacteria. Labeling also encourages healthcare professionals to counsel patients about proper use.

- **Partnering to promote public awareness.** The FDA is partnering with the Centers for Disease Control and Prevention (CDC) on "Get Smart: Know When Antibiotics Work," a campaign that offers web pages, brochures, fact sheets, and other information sources aimed at helping the public learn about preventing antibiotic-resistant infections.

- **Encouraging the development of new antibiotics.** The FDA is actively engaged in developing guidance for industries on the types of clinical studies that could be performed to evaluate how an antibacterial drug works for the treatment of different types of infections.

Section 71.2

Antimicrobial (Drug) Resistance

This section includes text excerpted from "Understanding
Antimicrobial (Drug) Resistance," National Institute of Allergy and
Infectious Diseases (NIAID), April 3, 2012. Reviewed July 2019.

Antimicrobial Resistance Quick Facts

- Many infectious diseases are increasingly difficult to treat
  because of antimicrobial-resistant organisms, including human
  immunodeficiency virus (HIV) infection, staphylococcal infection,
  tuberculosis, influenza, gonorrhea, *Candida* infection, and
  malaria.

- Between 5 and 10 percent of all hospital patients develop
  an infection. About 90,000 of these patients die each year as
  a result of their infection, up from 13,300 patient deaths in
  1992.

- According to the Centers for Disease Control and Prevention
  (CDC), antibiotic resistance in the United States costs an
  estimated $20 billion a year in excess healthcare costs, $35
  billion in other societal costs, and more than 8 million additional
  days that people spend in the hospital.

- People infected with antimicrobial-resistant organisms are
  more likely to have longer hospital stays and may require more
  complicated treatment.

- The Antibiotic Resistance Threats in the United States, a report
  from the CDC, gives a first-ever snapshot of the burden and
  threats posed by the antibiotic-resistant germs having the most
  impact on human health.

Definition of Terms, Antimicrobial Resistance
Microbes

Microbes are living organisms that multiply frequently and spread
rapidly. They include bacteria (e.g., *Staphylococcus aureus*, which
causes some staph infections), viruses (e.g., influenza, which causes the
flu), fungi (e.g., *Candida albicans*, which causes some yeast infections),
and parasites (e.g., *Plasmodium falciparum*, which causes malaria).

575

Some microbes cause disease, and others exist in the body without causing harm and may actually be beneficial.

Antimicrobial Resistance

Microbes are constantly evolving, enabling them to efficiently adapt to new environments. Antimicrobial resistance is the ability of microbes to grow in the presence of a chemical (drug) that would normally kill them or limit their growth.

Antimicrobial resistance makes it harder to eliminate infections from the body, as existing drugs become less effective. As a result, some infectious diseases are now more difficult to treat than they were just a few decades ago. As more microbes become resistant to antimicrobials, the protective value of these medicines is reduced. Overuse and misuse of antimicrobial medicines are among the factors that have contributed to the development of drug-resistant microbes.

Examples of Antimicrobial Resistance

- Drug-resistant Mycobacterium tuberculosis (TB)
- Methicillin-resistant *Staphylococcus aureus* (MRSA)
- Vancomycin-resistant enterococci (VRE)
- Gram-negative bacteria

Examples of Antimicrobials

- Tetracycline, an antibiotic that treats urinary tract infections
- Oseltamivir, also known as "Tamiflu," an antiviral that treats the flu
- Terbinafine, also known as "Lamisil," an antifungal that treats athlete's foot

Causes of Antimicrobial Resistance

Microbes, such as bacteria, viruses, fungi, and parasites, are living organisms that evolve over time. Their primary function is to reproduce, thrive, and spread quickly and efficiently. Therefore, microbes adapt to their environments and change in ways that ensure their survival. If something stops their ability to grow, such as antimicrobial, genetic changes can occur that enable the microbe to survive. There are several ways this happens.

Natural Causes
Selective Pressure

In the presence of an antimicrobial, microbes are either killed or, if they carry resistance genes, survive. These survivors will replicate, and their progeny will quickly become the dominant type throughout the microbial population.

Gene Transfer

Microbes also may get genes from each other, including genes that make the microbe drug-resistant. Bacteria multiply by the billions. Bacteria that have drug-resistant deoxyribonucleic acid (DNA) may transfer a copy of these genes to other bacteria. Nonresistant bacteria receive new DNA and become resistant to drugs. In the presence of drugs, only drug-resistant bacteria survive. The drug-resistant bacteria multiply and thrive.

Societal Pressures

The use of antimicrobials, even when used appropriately, creates selective pressure for resistant organisms. However, there are additional societal pressures that act to accelerate the increase of antimicrobial resistance.

Inappropriate Use

The selection of resistant microorganisms is exacerbated by inappropriate use of antimicrobials. Sometimes, healthcare providers will prescribe antimicrobials inappropriately, wishing to placate an insistent patient who has a viral infection or an as-yet-undiagnosed condition.

Inadequate Diagnostics

More often, healthcare providers must use incomplete or imperfect information to diagnose an infection and, thus, prescribe an antimicrobial just-in-case or prescribe a broad-spectrum antimicrobial when a specific antibiotic might be better. These situations contribute to selective pressure and accelerate antimicrobial resistance.

Hospital Use

Critically ill patients are more susceptible to infections and, thus, often require the aid of antimicrobials. However, the heavier use of antimicrobials in these patients can worsen the problem by selecting for antimicrobial-resistant microorganisms. The extensive use of antimicrobials and close contact among sick patients creates a fertile environment for the spread of antimicrobial-resistant germs.

Agricultural Use

Scientists also believe that the practice of adding antibiotics to agricultural feed promotes drug resistance. More than half of the antibiotics produced in the United States are used for agricultural purposes. However, there is still much debate about whether drug-resistant microbes in animals pose a significant public-health burden.

Diagnosis of Antimicrobial Resistance

Diagnostic tests are designed to determine which microbe is causing infection and to which antimicrobials the microbe might be resistant. This information would be used by a healthcare provider to choose an appropriate antimicrobial treatment. However, current diagnostic tests often take a few days or weeks to give results. This is because many of today's tests require the microbe to grow over a period of time before it can be identified.

Oftentimes, healthcare providers need to make treatment decisions before the results are known. While waiting for test results, healthcare providers may prescribe a broad-spectrum antimicrobial when a more specific treatment might be better. The common practice of treating unknown infections with broad-spectrum antimicrobials can accelerate the emergence of antimicrobial resistance.

Treatment of Antimicrobial Resistance

If you think you have an infection of any type—bacterial, viral, or fungal—talk with your healthcare provider. Some infections will go away without medical intervention. Others will not and can become extremely serious. Ear infections are a good example: Some middle-ear infections are caused by a virus and will get better without treatment. However, other middle-ear infections caused by bacteria can cause perforated eardrums or worse, if left untreated.

The decision to use antimicrobials should be left to your healthcare provider. In some cases, antimicrobials will not shorten the course of the disease, but they might reduce your chance of transmitting it to others, as is the case with pertussis (whooping cough).

Antibiotics are designed to kill or slow the growth of bacteria and some fungi. Antibiotics are commonly used to fight bacterial infections but cannot fight against infections caused by viruses.

Antibiotics are appropriate to use when:

- There is a known bacterial infection.

- The cause of the infection is unknown, and bacteria are suspected. In that case, the consequences of not treating a condition could be devastating (e.g., in early meningitis).

Of note, the color of your sputum (saliva) does not indicate whether you need antibiotics. For example, most cases of bronchitis are caused by viruses. Therefore, a change in sputum color does not indicate a bacterial infection.

Prevention of Antimicrobial Resistance

To prevent antimicrobial resistance, you and your healthcare provider should discuss the appropriate medicine for your illness. Strictly follow prescription medicine directions, and never share or take medicine that was prescribed for someone else. Talk with your healthcare provider so that she or he has a clear understanding of your symptoms and can decide whether an antimicrobial drug, such as an antibiotic, is appropriate.

Do not save your antibiotic for the next time you get sick. Take the medicine exactly as directed by your healthcare provider. If your healthcare provider has prescribed more than the required dose, appropriately discard leftover medicines once you have completed the prescribed course of treatment.

Healthy lifestyle habits—including proper diet; exercise; and sleeping patterns; as well as good hygiene, such as frequent handwashing—can help prevent illness, therefore, also preventing overuse or misuse of medications.

Section 71.3

Surveillance of Antimicrobial Resistance Patterns and Rates

This section includes text excerpted from "Surveillance for Antimicrobial Drug Resistance in Under-Resourced Countries," Centers for Disease Control and Prevention (CDC), February 19, 2014. Reviewed July 2019.

Antimicrobial drug resistance has become such a global concern that it was the focus of the 2011 World Health Day sponsored by the World Health Organization (WHO). Although antimicrobial drug resistance is well-mapped and tightly monitored in some well-resourced countries, such processes do not exist in under-resourced countries. An increasing body of evidence reveals accelerating rates of antimicrobial drug resistance in these countries. Resistance may arise in the absence of any surveillance and threatens the achievement of the Millenium Goals for Development in terms of reduction of maternal and infant deaths. The problem is even more pressing because, in a globalized world, microorganisms and their resistance genes travel faster and farther than ever before, and the pipeline of new drugs is faltering.

Mapping antimicrobial drug resistance in under-resourced countries is urgently needed so that measures can be set up to curb it. Such mapping must rely on efficient surveillance networks, endowed with adequate laboratory capacity, and take into account up-to-date diagnostic techniques. The way forward is to assess the effects of resistance, its clinical effects, and any increase in deaths, with the ultimate objective of providing achievable guidelines for surveillance and control.

What Are the Main Threats?
Tuberculosis

Resistance of *Mycobacterium tuberculosis* to antimycobacterial drugs is a global concern. In 2010, an estimated 650,000 cases of multidrug-resistant tuberculosis (MDR-TB) (i.e., infections with strains resistant to, at minimum, rifampin, and isoniazid) occurred worldwide. An estimated 10 percent of cases were extensively drug-resistant (XDR) (i.e., MDR strains that are also resistant to second-line drugs). Almost no surveillance system is in place, and no data exist on TB resistance in sub-Saharan Africa (apart from South Africa) and Asia.

Malaria

Plasmodium falciparum strains resistant to chloroquine, fansidar, and mefloquine are widespread. Interventions using artemisinin and insecticide-treated bed nets have led to a drop of 40 percent of malaria cases since 2004, according to the WHO. An estimated 750,000 lives were saved in Africa alone. Those efforts are potentially hindered by the emergence of resistance to artemisinin, which was first reported in 2008 at the Thailand–Cambodia border and subsequently reported in neighboring countries, although not in Africa so far. Resistance mechanisms to artemisinin are poorly understood, although mutations in some parasite genes have been partially correlated with resistance.

Severe Acute Respiratory Infections

Severe acute respiratory infections (SARIs) kill an estimated 1.4 million children younger than 5 years of age every year. The emergence of resistance to neuraminidase inhibitors would potentially have dramatic consequences because they are the first-line response to pandemics caused by a highly virulent influenza virus. Resistance of *Streptococcus pneumoniae* to antimicrobial drugs is also a concern. The extent of outpatient penicillin usage correlates with level of resistance. A prospective surveillance study of 2,184 patients hospitalized with pneumococcal pneumonia in 11 Asian countries in 2008–2009 found that high-level penicillin resistance was rare, that resistance to erythromycin was highly prevalent (72.7%), and that MDR was observed for 59.3 percent of *S. pneumoniae* isolates. Of 20,100 cases of invasive pneumococcal diseases identified in South Africa during 2003–2008, a total of 3,708 (18%) were caused by isolates resistant to at least 3 antimicrobial drugs.

Gram-Negative Bacteria Infections

Gram-negative bacteria resistant to β-lactams are spreading worldwide. CTX-M-15, a heterogeneous and mobile resistance gene first described in 2001 in India, has since been reported all over the world and is transmissible between different species of *Enterobacteriaceae*. New Delhi metallo-β-lactamase-1 (NDM-1) is a gene that confers resistance to all β-lactams, including carbapenems, which are the only alternative for treating severe infections, such as neonatal sepsis caused by MDR strains. First identified in 2008, it is now widespread in *Escherichia coli* (*E.coli*) and *Klebsiella pneumoniae* isolates from the Indian subcontinent and is found in many countries. Spread of gram-negative resistant bacteria from the hospital to the environment by direct person-to-person contact or through unsanitized water is a concern in under-resourced countries. The worldwide increase of the number of travelers, some of whom have diarrhea, is a major cause of the spread of resistance. A study conducted in Barcelona, Spain showed that nalidixic acid resistance in enterotoxigenic or enteroaggregative E. coli strains isolated from patients returning from India increased from 6 percent during 1994–1997 to 64 percent during 2001–2004. Sixty-five percent of strains isolated from patients who had traveled to India were resistant to quinolones.

Methicillin-Resistant **Staphylococcus aureus Infections**

Methicillin-resistant *Staphylococcus aureus* (MRSA) infections have become widespread even in under-resourced countries. Pakistan and India have reported MRSA percentages of 42 to 54.9, with an increasing trend.

The above sections describing antimicrobial drug resistance in various diseases is not exhaustive. Careful attention must be given to the potential spread of antimicrobial drug resistance in the drugs used to treat highly prevalent infectious diseases, such as typhoid, meningitis, HIV, and hepatitis, in under-resourced countries.

Who Are the Most Vulnerable Populations?

Antimicrobial drug resistance accounts for excess deaths in infants and childbearing women because of poor intrapartum and postnatal infection-control practices. In 2005, infections in hospital-born babies were estimated to account for 4 to 56 percent of all deaths in the neonatal period in some under-resourced countries. *K. pneumoniae, E. coli, Pseudomonas* spp., *Acinetobacter* spp., and *S. aureus* were the most frequent causative pathogens of neonatal sepsis; 70 percent of these isolates would not be eliminated by an empiric regimen of ampicillin and gentamicin. Many infections might be untreatable in resource-constrained environments. Fifty-one percent of *Klebsiella* spp. were extended-spectrum β-lactamase (ESBL) producers, 38 percent of *S. aureus* strains were methicillin-resistant, and 64 percent were resistant to co-trimoxazole. Preliminary data from Kilifi District Hospital (Kenya) also show alarming rates of ESBL positivity: 180 (39%) of 459 *Enterobacteriaceae* clinical isolates from child and adult patients (including 115 isolates of *K. pneumoniae*) collected from August 2010 to August 2012 were ESBL positive.

The Division of Women and Child Health at the Aga Khan University Medical College in Karachi, Pakistan has proposed a model for monitoring the development of neonatal infections and outcomes in southern Asia, on the basis of a cohort of 69,450 births. Resistance rates are constantly increasing. Antimicrobial drug resistance is estimated to result in an additional 96,000 (about 26%, range 16% to 37%) deaths each year from neonatal sepsis in southern Asia, highlighting the toll that children pay for drug resistance.

Section 71.4

Influenza Antiviral Drug Resistance

This section includes text excerpted from "Influenza Antiviral Drug Resistance," Centers for Disease Control and Prevention (CDC), February 20, 2019.

What Are Reduced Susceptibility and Antiviral Resistance?

When an antiviral drug is fully effective against a virus, that virus is said to be susceptible to that antiviral drug. Influenza viruses are constantly changing and can sometimes change in ways that might make antiviral drugs work less well or not work at all against these viruses. When an influenza virus changes in the active site where an antiviral drug works, that virus shows reduced susceptibility to that antiviral drug. Reduced susceptibility can be a sign of potential antiviral drug resistance. Antiviral drugs may not work as well in viruses with reduced susceptibility. Influenza viruses can show reduced susceptibility to one or more influenza antiviral drugs.

In the United States, there are four U.S. Food and Drug Administration (FDA)-approved antiviral drugs recommended by the Centers for Disease Control and Prevention (CDC). Three are neuraminidase inhibitor antiviral drugs: oseltamivir (available as a generic version or under the trade name "Tamiflu®") for oral administration, zanamivir (trade name "Relenza®") for oral inhalation using an inhaler device, and peramivir (trade name "Rapivab®") for intravenous administration. The fourth is a cap-dependent endonuclease (CEN) inhibitor, baloxavir marboxil (trade name "Xofluza®") for oral administration, approved for use in the United States during the 2018–2019 season by FDA in October 2018.

There is another class of influenza antiviral drugs (amantadine and rimantadine) called the "adamantanes" (which have activity against only influenza A viruses) that are not recommended for use in the United States at this time because of widespread antiviral resistance in circulating influenza A viruses.

How Widespread Are Reduced Susceptibility and Antiviral Resistance in the United States?

In the United States, the majority of the circulating influenza viruses have been fully susceptible to the neuraminidase inhibitor antiviral medications and to baloxavir. On the other hand, many flu A viruses are resistant to the adamantane drugs, which is why they are not recommended for use at this time.

How Does Reduced Susceptibility and Antiviral Resistance Happen?

Influenza viruses are constantly changing; they can change from one season to the next and can even change within the course of one flu season. As a flu virus replicates (i.e., make copies of itself), the genetic makeup may change in a way that results in the virus becoming less susceptible to one or more of the antiviral drugs used to treat or prevent influenza. Influenza viruses can become less susceptible to antiviral drugs spontaneously or emerge during the course of antiviral treatment. Viruses that are less susceptible or resistant vary in their ability to transmit to other people.

How Are Reduced Susceptibility and Antiviral Resistance Detected?

The CDC routinely tests flu viruses collected through domestic and global surveillance to see if they have indications of reduced susceptibility to any of the FDA-approved flu antiviral drugs, as this can suggest the potential for antiviral resistance. This data informs public-health policy recommendations about the use of flu antiviral medications.

Detection of reduced susceptibility and antiviral resistance involves several laboratory tests, including specific functional assays and molecular techniques (sequencing and pyrosequencing) to look for genetic changes that are associated with reduced antiviral susceptibility.

How Has the Centers for Disease Control and Prevention Prepared to Test for Reduced Susceptibility and Antiviral Resistance to the New Flu Antiviral Baloxavir?

The CDC's Influenza Division has taken specific laboratory actions to incorporate the new antiviral drug baloxavir into routine virologic surveillance. This includes the creation and validation of new assays to determine baloxavir susceptibility, and training of laboratorians to conduct baloxavir susceptibility testing.

Seasonal influenza A and B viruses in humans, as well as several influenza A viruses that circulate in animals, were tested to establish baseline susceptibility to baloxavir. In addition, the susceptibility of other distantly related influenza viruses to baloxavir was tested. The CDC also is collaborating with the Association of Public Health Laboratories (APHL) and the Wadsworth Center New York State Department of Health (NYSDOH), a National Influenza Reference Center (NIRC), to establish laboratory-testing capacity for baloxavir susceptibility. The CDC has trained staff within these partner organizations to use its new method for assessing baloxavir susceptibility.

What Is Oseltamivir Resistance, and What Does Cause It?

Flu viruses are constantly changing. Changes that occur in circulating flu viruses typically involve the structures of the viruses' two primary surface proteins: neuraminidase (NA) and hemagglutinin (HA).

Oseltamivir is the most commonly prescribed of the recommended antiviral drugs in the United States that is used to treat flu illness. Oseltamivir is known as a "NA inhibitor" because this antiviral drug binds to NA proteins of a flu virus and inhibits the enzymatic activity of these proteins. By inhibiting NA activity, oseltamivir prevents flu viruses from spreading from infected cells to other healthy cells.

If the NA proteins of the flu virus change, oseltamivir can lose its ability to bind to and inhibit the function of the virus's NA proteins.

This results in oseltamivir resistance (nonsusceptibility). A particular genetic change known as the "H275Y" mutation is the only known mutation to confer oseltamivir resistance in 2009 H1N1 flu viruses. The H275Y mutation makes oseltamivir ineffective in treating illnesses with that flu virus by preventing oseltamivir from inhibiting NA activity, which then allows the virus to spread to healthy cells. The H275Y mutation also reduces the effectiveness of peramivir to treat influenza virus infections with this mutation.

How Does the Centers for Disease Control and Prevention Improve Monitoring of Influenza Viruses for Reduced Susceptibility and Antiviral Resistance?

The CDC continually improves the ability to rapidly detect influenza viruses with antiviral reduced susceptibility and antiviral resistance through improvements in laboratory methods, increasing the number of surveillance sites domestically and globally, and increasing the number of laboratories that can test for reduced susceptibility and antiviral resistance. Enhanced surveillance efforts have provided the CDC with the capability to detect resistant viruses more quickly and enabled it to monitor for changing trends over time.

How Did Influenza Antiviral Susceptibility Patterns Change during the Previous (2017–2018) Influenza Season?

Antiviral susceptibility patterns changed very little in 2017–2018 when compared with the previous season (2016–2017). During the 2016–2017 season, no oseltamivir resistance was found. During the 2017–2018 influenza season, only a small number of viruses were resistant to oseltamivir. Most of the influenza viruses tested during 2017–2018 continued to be susceptible to the antiviral drugs recommended for influenza by the CDC and the Advisory Committee on Immunization Practices (ACIP) (oseltamivir, zanamivir, and peramivir). Resistance to the adamantane class of antiviral drugs among A/H3N2 and A/H1N1 viruses remained widespread (influenza B viruses are not susceptible to adamantane drugs).

Specifically, for the 2017–2018 season:

- The CDC tested 1,147 influenza A(H1N1)pdm09, 2,354 influenza A(H3N2), and 1,118 influenza B viruses for reduced susceptibility and resistance to antiviral medications (i.e., oseltamivir, zanamivir, or peramivir).

- While the majority of the tested viruses showed susceptibility to the antiviral drugs, 11 (1.0%) A(H1N1)pdm09 viruses were resistant to both oseltamivir and peramivir but were sensitive to zanamivir.

- As indicated by these results, oseltamivir, zanamivir, and peramivir remained recommended antiviral treatment options for flu illness during the 2017–2018 flu season.

- High levels of resistance to the adamantanes (amantadine and rimantadine) persisted among circulating influenza A viruses. And, as adamantanes are not effective against influenza B viruses, adamantane drugs were not recommended for use against influenza at this time.

The CDC conducts ongoing surveillance and testing of influenza viruses for antiviral reduced susceptibility and resistance among seasonal and novel influenza viruses, and guidance is updated as needed.

Because there were no dramatic changes in antiviral susceptibility patterns during the 2017–2018 flu season, the guidance for the 2018–2019 flu season on the use of influenza antiviral drugs remains unchanged.

What Can People Do to Protect Themselves against Flu Viruses with Reduced Susceptibility and Antiviral Resistance?

Getting a yearly seasonal flu vaccination is the best way to reduce the risk of flu and its potentially serious complications. Flu vaccines protect against an influenza A(H1N1) virus, an influenza A(H3N2) virus, and one or two influenza B viruses (depending on the vaccine). The CDC recommends that everyone six months of age and older gets vaccinated each year. If you are in a group at a high risk of serious flu-related complications and become ill with flu symptoms, call your doctor right away; you may benefit from early treatment with an influenza antiviral drug. If you are not at high risk, if possible, stay home from work, school, and errands when you are sick. This will help prevent you from spreading your illness to others.

What Implications Do Reduced Susceptibility and Antiviral Resistance Have for the U.S. Antiviral Stockpile That Was Created as Part of the United States Pandemic Plan?

Antiviral drugs are one component of a multifaceted approach to pandemic preparedness planning and response. The U.S. Strategic National Stockpile (SNS) contains supplies of three neuraminidase inhibitor (NAI) antiviral medications, including oseltamivir (for oral administration), zanamivir (for oral inhalation), and peramivir (for intravenous administration). These medications are to be used in the event that a novel influenza A virus, such as avian influenza A(H7N9) virus, gains the ability to spread easily among people in a sustained manner, and is susceptible to NAI antiviral drugs. During the 2009 H1N1 pandemic, antiviral drugs were released from the SNS and used to treat infection with the pandemic virus, now referred to as "influenza A(H1N1)pdm09 virus." Information about how antiviral drugs from the SNS were used during the 2009 H1N1 pandemic is available in "The 2009 H1N1 Pandemic: Summary Highlights, April 2009 to April 2010" (www.cdc.gov/h1n1flu/cdcresponse.htm). Antivirals in the SNS are for use during public health emergencies in the United States, such as an influenza pandemic, but not for seasonal influenza epidemics. Since antiviral drug resistance can emerge in influenza viruses, including to the NAI antivirals, new antivirals with mechanisms of action that are different than the NAIs are needed for the SNS.

Part Seven

Preventing
Contagious Diseases

Chapter 72

Handwashing Prevents the Spread of Germs

Handwashing can help prevent illness. It involves five simple and effective steps (wet, lather, scrub, rinse, and dry) you can use to reduce the spread of diarrheal and respiratory illness so you can stay healthy. Regular handwashing, particularly before and after certain activities, is one of the best ways to remove germs, avoid getting sick, and prevent the spread of germs to others. It is quick, simple, and it can keep us all from getting sick. Handwashing is a win for everyone, except the germs.

When and How to Wash Your Hands

Keeping our hands clean through improved hand hygiene is one of the most important steps we can take to avoid getting sick and spreading germs to others. Many diseases and conditions are spread by not washing your hands with soap and clean, running water. If clean, running water is not accessible, as is common in many parts of the world, use soap and available water. If soap and water are unavailable,

This chapter contains text excerpted from the following sources: Text in this chapter begins with excerpts from "Handwashing: Clean Hands Save Lives," Centers for Disease Control and Prevention (CDC), June 13, 2019; Text beginning with the heading "How Germs Get onto Hands and Make People Sick" is excerpted from "Show Me the Science—Why Wash Your Hands?" Centers for Disease Control and Prevention (CDC), September 17, 2018.

use an alcohol-based hand sanitizer that contains at least 60 percent alcohol to clean your hands.

When Should You Wash Your Hands?

- Before, during, and after preparing food
- Before eating food
- Before and after caring for someone who is sick
- Before and after treating a cut or wound
- After using the toilet
- After changing diapers or cleaning up a child who has used the toilet
- After blowing your nose, coughing, or sneezing
- After touching an animal, animal feed, or animal waste
- After handling pet food or pet treats
- After touching garbage

How Should You Wash Your Hands?

- Wet your hands with clean, running water (warm or cold), turn off the tap, and apply soap.
- Lather your hands by rubbing them together with the soap. Be sure to lather the backs of your hands, between your fingers, and under your nails.
- Scrub your hands for at least 20 seconds. Need a timer? Hum the "Happy Birthday" song from beginning to end twice.
- Rinse your hands well under clean, running water.
- Dry your hands using a clean towel, or air dry them.

What Should You Do If You Do Not Have Soap and Clean, Running Water?

Washing your hands with soap and water is the best way to reduce the number of germs on them in most situations. If soap and water are not available, use an alcohol-based hand sanitizer that contains at least 60 percent alcohol. Alcohol-based hand sanitizers can quickly reduce the number of germs on your hands in some situations, but sanitizers do not eliminate all types of germs and might not remove harmful chemicals.

Hand sanitizers are not as effective when hands are visibly dirty or greasy.

How Do You Use Hand Sanitizers?

- Apply the product to the palm of one hand (read the label to learn the correct amount).

- Rub your hands together.

- Rub the product over all surfaces of your hands and fingers until your hands are dry.

How Germs Get onto Hands and Make People Sick

Feces from people or animals is an important source of germs—such as Salmonella, *E. coli* O157, and norovirus that cause diarrhea—and it can spread some respiratory infections, such as adenovirus and hand-foot-mouth disease (HFMD). These kinds of germs can get onto the hands after people use the toilet or change a diaper but also in less obvious ways, such as after handling raw meats that have invisible amounts of animal poop on them. A single gram of human feces—which is about the weight of a paper clip—can contain one trillion germs. Germs can also get onto hands if people touch any object that has germs on it because someone coughed or sneezed on it or it was touched by some other contaminated object. When these germs get onto our hands and are not washed off, they can be passed from person to person and make people sick.

Washing Hands Prevents Illnesses and the Spread of Infections to Others

Handwashing with soap removes germs from hands. This helps prevent infections because:

- People frequently touch their eyes, nose, and mouth without even realizing it. Germs can get into the body through the eyes, nose, and mouth and make us sick.

- Germs from unwashed hands can get into foods and drinks while people prepare or consume them. Germs can multiply in some types of foods or drinks, under certain conditions, and make people sick.

- Germs from unwashed hands can be transferred to other objects, such as handrails, table tops, or toys, and then transferred to another person's hands.

- Removing germs through handwashing, therefore, helps prevent diarrhea and respiratory infections, and it may even help prevent skin and eye infections.

Teaching people about handwashing helps them and their communities stay healthy. Handwashing education in the community:

- Reduces the number of people who get sick with diarrhea by 23 to 40 percent

- Reduces diarrheal illness in people with weakened immune systems by 58 percent

- Reduces respiratory illnesses, such as colds, in the general population by 16 to 21 percent

- Reduces absenteeism due to gastrointestinal illness in schoolchildren by 29 to 57 percent

Not Washing Hands Harms Children around the World

About 1.8 million children under the age of 5 die each year from diarrheal diseases and pneumonia, the top 2 killers of young children around the world.

- Handwashing with soap could protect about one out of every three young children who get sick with diarrhea and almost 1 out of 5 young children with respiratory infections, such as pneumonia.

- Although people around the world clean their hands with water, very few use soap to wash their hands. Washing your hands with soap removes germs much more effectively.

- Handwashing education and access to soap in schools can help improve attendance.

- Good handwashing early in life may help improve child development in some settings.

- Estimated global rates of handwashing after using the toilet are only 19 percent.

Handwashing Helps Battle the Rise in Antibiotic Resistance

Preventing sickness reduces the amount of antibiotics people use and the likelihood that antibiotic resistance will develop. Handwashing can prevent about 30 percent of diarrhea-related sicknesses and about 20 percent of respiratory infections (e.g., colds). Antibiotics are often prescribed unnecessarily for these health issues. Reducing the number of these infections by washing our hands frequently helps prevent the overuse of antibiotics—the single most important factor leading to antibiotic resistance around the world. Handwashing can also prevent people from getting sick with germs that are already resistant to antibiotics, which can be difficult to treat.

Chapter 73

Vaccines: What They Are and How They Work

Chapter Contents

Section 73.1—Understanding How Vaccines Work 598

Section 73.2—Making the Vaccine Decision 601

Section 73.1

Understanding How Vaccines Work

This section includes text excerpted from "Understanding How Vaccines Work," Centers for Disease Control and Prevention (CDC), August 17, 2018.

The Immune System—The Body's Defense against Infection

To understand how vaccines work, it helps to first look at how the body fights illness. When germs, such as bacteria or viruses, invade the body, they attack and multiply. This invasion, called an "infection," is what causes illness. The immune system uses several tools to fight infection. Blood contains red blood cells, for carrying oxygen to tissues and organs, and white or immune cells, for fighting infection. These white cells consist primarily of macrophages, B-lymphocytes, and T-lymphocytes:

- **Macrophages** are white blood cells that swallow up and digest germs, in addition to dead or dying cells. The macrophages leave behind parts of the invading germs called "antigens." The body identifies antigens as dangerous and stimulates antibodies to attack them.

- **B-lymphocytes** are defensive white blood cells. They produce antibodies that attack the antigens left behind by the macrophages.

- **T-lymphocytes** are another type of defensive white blood cell. They attack cells in the body that have already been infected.

The first time the body encounters a germ, it can take several days to make and use all the germ-fighting tools needed to get over the infection. After the infection, the immune system remembers what it learned about how to protect the body against that disease.

The body keeps a few T-lymphocytes, called "memory cells," that go into action quickly if the body encounters the same germ again. When the familiar antigens are detected, B-lymphocytes produce antibodies to attack them.

How Vaccines Work

Vaccines help develop immunity by imitating an infection. This type of infection, however, almost never causes illness, but it does cause the immune system to produce T-lymphocytes and antibodies. Sometimes, after getting a vaccine, the imitation infection can cause minor symptoms, such as fever. Such minor symptoms are normal and should be expected as the body builds immunity.

Once the imitation infection goes away, the body is left with a supply of "memory" T-lymphocytes, as well as B-lymphocytes, that will remember how to fight that disease in the future. However, it typically takes a few weeks for the body to produce T-lymphocytes and B-lymphocytes after vaccination. Therefore, it is possible that a person infected with a disease just before or just after vaccination could develop symptoms and get a disease because the vaccine has not had enough time to provide protection.

Vaccines Require More than One Dose

There are four reasons that babies—and even teens or adults— who receive a vaccine for the first time may need more than one dose:

- For some vaccines (primarily inactivated vaccines), the first dose does not provide as much immunity as possible. So, more than one dose is needed to build more complete immunity. The vaccine that protects against the bacteria Hib, which causes meningitis, is a good example.

- For some vaccines, after a while, immunity begins to wear off. At that point, a booster dose is needed to bring immunity levels back up. This booster dose usually occurs several years after the initial series of vaccine doses is given. For example, in the case of the DTaP vaccine, which protects against diphtheria, tetanus, and pertussis, the initial series of 4 shots that children receive as part of their infant immunizations helps build immunity. But, a booster dose is needed between the ages of 4 and 6. Another booster against these diseases is needed between 11 and 12 years of age. This booster for older children—and teens and adults, too—is called "Tdap."

- For some vaccines (primarily live vaccines), studies have shown that more than one dose is needed for everyone to develop the best immune response. For example, after one dose of the measles, mumps, and rubella (MMR) vaccine, some people may not develop enough antibodies to fight off infection. The second dose helps make sure that almost everyone is protected.

- Finally, in the case of flu vaccines, adults and children (six months and older) need to get a dose every year. Children between six months and eight years of age who have never gotten a flu vaccine in the past, or have only gotten one dose in past years, need two doses the first year they are vaccinated. Then, an annual flu vaccine is needed because the flu viruses causing disease may be different from season to season. Every year, flu vaccines are made to protect against the viruses that research suggests will be most common. Also, the immunity a child gets from a flu vaccination wears off over time. Getting a flu vaccine every year helps keep a child protected, even if the vaccine viruses do not change from one season to the next.

The Bottom Line

Some people believe that naturally acquired immunity—immunity from having the disease itself—is better than the immunity provided by vaccines. However, natural infections can cause severe complications, and they can be deadly. This is true even for diseases that many people consider mild, such as chickenpox. It is impossible to predict who will get serious infections that may lead to hospitalization.

Vaccines, as with any medication, can cause side effects. The most common side effects are mild. However, many vaccine-preventable disease symptoms can be serious or even deadly. Although many of these diseases are rare in this country, they do circulate around the world and can be brought into the United States, putting unvaccinated children at risk. Even with advances in healthcare, the diseases that vaccines prevent can still be very serious— and vaccination is the best way to prevent them.

Section 73.2

Making the Vaccine Decision

This section includes text excerpted from "Making the
Vaccine Decision," Centers for Disease Control and
Prevention (CDC), March 18, 2019.

How Vaccines Prevent Diseases

The diseases vaccines prevent can be dangerous or even deadly. Vaccines reduce your child's risk of infection by working with their body's natural defenses to help them safely develop immunity to disease.

When germs, such as bacteria or viruses, invade the body, they attack and multiply. This invasion is called an "infection," and the infection is what causes illness. The immune system then has to fight the infection. Once it fights off the infection, the body has a supply of cells that help recognize and fight that disease in the future. These supplies of cells are called "antibodies."

Vaccines help develop immunity by imitating an infection, but this imitation infection does not cause illness. Instead, it causes the immune system to develop the same response as it does to a real infection, so the body can recognize and fight the vaccine-preventable disease in the future. Sometimes, after getting a vaccine, imitation infection can cause minor symptoms, such as fever. Such minor symptoms are normal and should be expected as the body builds immunity.

As children get older, they require additional doses of some vaccines for best protection. Older kids also need protection against additional diseases they may encounter.

Vaccines and Your Child's Immune System

As a parent, you may get upset or concerned when you watch your child get 3 or 4 shots during a doctor's visit. But, all of those shots add up to protection against 14 infectious diseases. Young babies can get very ill from vaccine-preventable diseases.

The Advisory Committee on Immunization Practices (ACIP), a group of medical and public health experts that develops recommendations on how to use vaccines to control diseases in the United States, designs the vaccination schedule. The ACIP designs the vaccination schedule to protect young children before they are likely to be exposed to potentially serious diseases and when they are most vulnerable to serious infections. This is the schedule that the Centers for Disease Control and Prevention (CDC) recommends.

Although children continue to get several vaccines up to their second birthday, these vaccines do not overload the immune system. Every day, your child's healthy immune system successfully fights off thousands of antigens—the parts of germs that cause their immune system to respond. The antigens in vaccines come from weakened or killed germs so they cannot cause serious illness. Even if your child receives several vaccines in one day, vaccines contain only a tiny amount of antigens, compared to the antigens your baby encounters every day.

This is the case even if your child receives combination vaccines. Combination vaccines take two or more vaccines that could be given individually and put them into one shot. Children get the same protection as they do from individual vaccines given separately but with fewer shots.

Vaccine Side Effects/Risks

As with any medication, vaccines can cause side effects. The most common side effects are mild. On the other hand, many vaccine-preventable disease symptoms can be serious or even deadly. Even though many of these diseases are rare in this country, they still occur around the world. Unvaccinated U.S. citizens who travel abroad can bring these diseases to the United States, putting unvaccinated children at risk.

The side effects of vaccines are almost always minor (such as redness and swelling where the shot was given) and go away within a few days. If your child experiences a reaction at the injection site, use a cool, wet cloth to reduce redness, soreness, and swelling.

Serious side effects after vaccination, such as a severe allergic reaction, are very rare, and doctors and clinic staff are trained to deal with them. Pay extra attention to your child for a few days after vaccination. If you see something that concerns you, call your child's doctor.

Vaccine Ingredients

Vaccines contain antigens, which cause the body to develop immunity. Vaccines also contain very small amounts of other ingredients. All ingredients either help make the vaccine or ensure the vaccine is safe and effective. These types of ingredients are listed below.

Table 73.1. Types of Ingredients in Vaccines

Type of Ingredient	Examples	Purpose
Preservatives	Thimerosal (only in multi-dose vials of flu vaccine)*	To prevent contamination
Adjuvants	Aluminum salts	To help stimulate the body's response to the antigens
Stabilizers	Sugars, gelatin	To keep the vaccine potent during transportation and storage
Residual cell culture materials	Egg protein	To grow enough of the virus or bacteria to make the vaccine
Residual inactivating ingredients	Formaldehyde	To kill viruses or inactivate toxins during the manufacturing process
Residual antibiotics	Neomycin	To prevent contamination by bacteria during the vaccine manufacturing process

The only childhood vaccines used routinely in the United States that contain thimerosal (mercury) are flu vaccines in multidose vials. These vials have very tiny amounts of thimerosal as a preservative. This is necessary because each time an individual dose is drawn from a multidose vial with a new needle and syringe, there is the potential to contaminate the vial with harmful microbes (toxins).

There is no evidence that the small amounts of thimerosal in flu vaccines cause any harm, except for minor reactions, such as redness and swelling at the injection site. Although no evidence suggests that there are safety concerns with thimerosal, vaccine manufacturers have stopped using it as a precautionary measure. Flu vaccines that do not contain thimerosal are available (in single-dose vials).

Ensuring Vaccine Safety

The United States' long-standing vaccine safety system ensures vaccines are as safe as possible. In fact, the United States has the safest vaccine supply in its history.

Safety monitoring begins with the U.S. Food and Drug Administration (FDA), which ensures the safety, effectiveness, and availability of vaccines for the United States. Before the FDA approves a vaccine for use by the public, highly trained FDA scientists and doctors evaluate the results of studies on the safety and effectiveness of the vaccine. The FDA also inspects the sites where vaccines are made to make sure they follow strict manufacturing guidelines.

Although scientists identify the most common side effects of a vaccine in studies before the vaccine is licensed, they may not detect rare adverse events in these studies. Therefore, the U.S. vaccine safety system continuously monitors for possible side effects after the FDA licenses a vaccine. When millions of people receive a vaccine, less common side effects that studies did not identify earlier may occur.

If the CDC and the FDA find a link between a possible side effect and a vaccine, public health officials take appropriate action. They will weigh the benefits of the vaccine against its risks to determine if recommendations for using the vaccine should change.

The Vaccine Adverse Event Reporting System (VAERS) is a national system used by scientists at the FDA and the CDC to collect reports of adverse events (possible side effects) that happen after vaccination.

Chapter 74

Vaccine Types and Ingredients

Vaccine Types

Scientists take many approaches to design vaccines against a microbe. These choices are typically based on fundamental information about the microbe, such as how it infects cells and how the immune system responds to it, as well as practical considerations, such as regions of the world where the vaccine would be used. The following are some of the options that researchers might pursue:

- Live, attenuated vaccines

- Inactivated vaccines

- Subunit vaccines

- Toxoid vaccines

- Conjugate vaccines

- Deoxyribonucleic acid (DNA) vaccines

- Recombinant vector vaccines

This chapter includes text excerpted from "Vaccine Types," National Institute of Allergy and Infectious Virus (NIAID), July 1, 2019.

Live, Attenuated Vaccines

Live, attenuated vaccines contain a version of the living microbe that has been weakened in the lab, so it cannot cause disease. Because a live, attenuated vaccine is the closest thing to a natural infection, these vaccines are good "teachers" of the immune system; they elicit strong cellular and antibody responses and often confer lifelong immunity with only one or two doses.

Despite the advantages of live, attenuated vaccines, there are some downsides. It is the nature of living things to change or mutate, and the organisms used in live, attenuated vaccines are no different. The remote possibility exists that an attenuated microbe in the vaccine could revert to a virulent form and cause disease. Also, not everyone can safely receive live, attenuated vaccines. For their own protection, people who have damaged or weakened immune systems—because they have undergone chemotherapy or have human immunodeficiency virus (HIV), for example—cannot be given live vaccines.

Another limitation is that live, attenuated vaccines usually need to be refrigerated to stay potent. If the vaccine needs to be shipped overseas and stored by healthcare workers in developing countries that lack widespread refrigeration, a live vaccine may not be the best choice.

Live, attenuated vaccines are relatively easy to create for certain viruses. Vaccines against measles, mumps, and chickenpox, for example, are made by this method. Viruses are simple microbes containing a small number of genes, and scientists can, therefore, more readily control their characteristics. Viruses often are attenuated through a method of growing generations of them in cells in which they do not reproduce very well. This hostile environment takes the fight out of viruses; as they evolve to adapt to the new environment, they become weaker with respect to their natural host, human beings.

Live, attenuated vaccines are more difficult to create for bacteria. Bacteria have thousands of genes and thus are much harder to control. Scientists working on a live vaccine for a bacterium, however, might be able to use recombinant DNA technology to remove several key genes. This approach has been used to create a vaccine against the bacterium that causes cholera, *Vibrio cholerae*, although the live cholera vaccine has not been licensed in the United States.

Inactivated Vaccines

Scientists produce inactivated vaccines by killing the disease-causing microbe with chemicals, heat, or radiation. Such vaccines are more stable and safer than live vaccines; the dead microbes cannot mutate back to their disease-causing state. Inactivated vaccines usually do not require refrigeration, and they can be easily stored and transported in a freeze-dried form, which makes them accessible to people in developing countries.

Most inactivated vaccines, however, stimulate a weaker immune system response than live vaccines. So it would likely take several additional doses, or booster shots, to maintain a person's immunity. This could be a drawback in areas where people do not have regular access to healthcare and cannot get booster shots on time.

Subunit Vaccines

Instead of the entire microbe, subunit vaccines include only the antigens that best stimulate the immune system. In some cases, these vaccines use epitopes—the very specific parts of the antigen that antibodies or T cells recognize and bind to. Because subunit vaccines contain only the essential antigens and not all the other molecules that make up the microbe, the chances of adverse reactions to the vaccine are lower.

Subunit vaccines can contain anywhere from 1 to 20 or more antigens. Of course, identifying which antigens best stimulate the immune system is a tricky, time-consuming process. Once scientists do that, however, they can make subunit vaccines in 1 of 2 ways:

- They can grow the microbe in the laboratory and then use chemicals to break it apart and gather the important antigens.

- They can manufacture the antigen molecules from the microbe using recombinant DNA technology. Vaccines produced this way are called "recombinant subunit vaccines."

A recombinant subunit vaccine has been made for the hepatitis B virus. Scientists inserted hepatitis B genes that code for important antigens into common baker's yeast. The yeast then produced the antigens, which the scientists collected and purified for use in the vaccine. Research is continuing on a recombinant subunit vaccine against hepatitis C virus.

Toxoid Vaccines

For bacteria that secrete toxins, or harmful chemicals, a toxoid vaccine might be the answer. These vaccines are used when a bacterial toxin is the main cause of illness. Scientists have found that they can inactivate toxins by treating them with formalin, a solution of formaldehyde and sterilized water. Such "detoxified" toxins, called "toxoids," are safe for use in vaccines.

When the immune system receives a vaccine containing a harmless toxoid, it learns how to fight off the natural toxin. The immune system produces antibodies that lock onto and block the toxin. Vaccines against diphtheria and tetanus are examples of toxoid vaccines.

Conjugate Vaccines

If a bacterium possesses an outer coating of sugar molecules called "polysaccharides," as many harmful bacteria do, researchers may try making a conjugate vaccine for it. Polysaccharide coatings disguise a bacterium's antigens so that the immature immune systems of infants and younger children cannot recognize or respond to them. Conjugate vaccines, a special type of subunit vaccine, get around this problem.

When making a conjugate vaccine, scientists link antigens or toxoids from a microbe that an infant's immune system can recognize to the polysaccharides. The linkage helps the immature immune system react to polysaccharide coatings and defend against the disease-causing bacterium.

The vaccine that protects against *Haemophilus influenzae type b* (Hib) is a conjugate vaccine.

Deoxyribonucleic Acid Vaccines

Once the genes from a microbe have been analyzed, scientists could attempt to create a DNA vaccine against it.

Still, in the experimental stages, these vaccines show great promise, and several types are being tested in humans. DNA vaccines take immunization to a new technological level. These vaccines dispense with both the whole organism and its parts and get right down to the essentials: the microbe's genetic material. In particular, DNA vaccines use the genes that code for those all-important antigens.

Researchers have found that when the genes for a microbe's antigens are introduced into the body, some cells will take up that DNA. The DNA then instructs those cells to make the antigen molecules. The cells secrete the antigens and display them on their surfaces. In other words, the body's own cells become vaccine-making factories, creating the antigens necessary to stimulate the immune system.

A DNA vaccine against a microbe would evoke a strong antibody response to the free-floating antigen secreted by cells, and the vaccine also would stimulate a strong cellular response against the microbial antigens displayed on cell surfaces. The DNA vaccine could not cause the disease because it would not contain the microbe, just copies of a few of its genes. In addition, DNA vaccines are relatively easy and inexpensive to design and produce.

So-called "naked DNA vaccines" consist of DNA that is administered directly into the body. These vaccines can be administered with a needle and syringe or with a needleless device that uses high-pressure gas to shoot microscopic gold particles coated with DNA directly into cells. Sometimes, the DNA is mixed with molecules that facilitate its uptake by the body's cells. Naked DNA vaccines being tested in humans include those against the viruses that cause influenza and herpes.

Recombinant Vector Vaccines

Recombinant vector vaccines are experimental vaccines similar to DNA vaccines, but they use an attenuated virus or bacterium to introduce microbial DNA to cells of the body. "Vector" refers to the virus or bacterium used as the carrier.

In nature, viruses latch on to cells and inject their genetic material into them. In the lab, scientists have taken advantage of this process. They have figured out how to take the roomy genomes of certain harmless or attenuated viruses and insert portions of the genetic material from other microbes into them. The carrier viruses then ferry that microbial DNA to cells. Recombinant vector vaccines closely mimic a natural infection and, therefore, do a good job of stimulating the immune system.

Attenuated bacteria also can be used as vectors. In this case, the inserted genetic material causes the bacteria to display the antigens of other microbes on its surface. In effect, the harmless bacteria mimic a harmful microbe, provoking an immune response.

Researchers are working on both bacterial- and viral-based recombinant vector vaccines for HIV, rabies, and measles.

Vaccine Ingredients
Suspending Fluid

Active vaccine components typically are suspended in sterile water, saline, or protein-containing liquids. Some vaccines are stored as freeze-dried powders and must be mixed with a liquid called a diluent before they can be administered. Diluents are specifically designed for each vaccine to ensure proper safety and potency.

Stabilizers

Stabilizers are additives that protect vaccines from adverse conditions like high temperatures. Commonly used stabilizers include the sugars sucrose and lactose, the amino acid glycine, and monosodium glutamate, an amino acid salt. Proteins such as human or bovine serum albumin and gelatin also are used as stabilizers.

Preservatives

Preservatives such as phenol, phenoxyethanol, and thimerosal may be included in vaccines to prevent bacterial or fungal contamination. Phenol is a disinfectant and antiseptic. Phenoxyethanol is chemically related to phenol and also is used as a preservative in many cosmetics. Thimerosal is a mercury-containing compound that has been used as a preservative in some vaccines since the 1930s.

One product of the metabolism, or degradation within the body, of thimerosal is ethyl mercury, an organic derivative of mercury. A related compound found in many fish and shellfish, called methyl mercury, can be toxic to people at high levels. Due to concerns about mercury exposure, thimerosal was removed from most childhood vaccines by 2001 as a precautionary measure. Subsequent studies have shown that, unlike methyl mercury, ethyl mercury is quickly eliminated from the body and does not build up to toxic levels.

Trace Components

Some vaccines may contain residual quantities of components used during the manufacturing process, including inactivating agents, antibiotics, and cellular residuals. These agents are removed at the end of the manufacturing process, but trace amounts may be present in some vaccines.

Inactivating agents are used to eliminate the harmful effects of bacterial toxins or to render viruses incapable of causing disease. Examples of inactivating agents include formaldehyde and β-propiolactone. Formaldehyde is a naturally occurring chemical found in plants, animals, and the human body, where it plays a role in the synthesis of DNA and amino acids (the building blocks of proteins). Although prolonged exposure to high levels of formaldehyde can be harmful, the amount of the chemical present in certain vaccines is much lower than the amount naturally present in the body. Exposure to β-propiolactone also has been linked to health concerns. However, the chemical breaks down quickly in water-based solutions, and the very small amount of residual β-propiolactone in some vaccines is completely broken down and harmless.

Antibiotics sometimes are added to vaccines to ensure that bacterial contamination does not occur during the manufacturing process. Antibiotics used for this purpose include neomycin, streptomycin, polymyxin B, chlortetracycline, and amphotericin B. The antibiotics that are most likely to cause allergic reactions—penicillins, cephalosporins, and sulfonamides—are not used in vaccine manufacture.

Vaccine viruses can be produced in cells or cell culture, and trace amounts of cellular materials may be present in the final vaccine. The viruses incorporated into influenza and yellow fever vaccines, for example, are grown in chicken eggs, and the vaccines may contain traces of egg proteins. In general, people with egg allergy can receive these vaccines safely. In January 2013, the Food and Drug Administration approved the first egg-free flu vaccine, called Flublok. The antigens included in Flublok are produced in laboratory-grown insect cells.

Measles and mumps vaccine viruses are grown in chicken embryo tissue cultures. Studies have shown that the measles, mumps, and rubella (MMR) and measles, mumps, rubella, and varicella (MMRV) vaccines can be given safely to egg-allergic children, including those with severe allergy.

Other vaccine antigens, such as those used in hepatitis B vaccines and the human papillomavirus (HPV) vaccine Gardasil, are manufactured in yeast cells. These vaccines may contain small amounts of yeast proteins, which have not been shown to cause allergic reactions in people.

Chapter 75

Childhood Immunizations: Ten Vaccines for Fourteen Diseases

Immunization is one of the best ways parents can protect their children from 14 serious childhood diseases before the age of 2. Vaccinate your child according to the Centers for Disease Control and Prevention's (CDC) recommended immunization schedule for safe, proven disease protection.

Diseases that vaccines prevent can be very serious—even deadly—especially for infants and young children. Vaccines work with your child's natural defenses to help them safely build immunity to these diseases.

Most parents have never seen first-hand the devastating consequences that vaccine-preventable diseases have on a family or community. Some diseases that are prevented by vaccines, such as pertussis (whooping cough) and chickenpox, remain common in the United States.

This chapter contains text excerpted from the following sources: Text in this chapter begins with excerpts from "Vaccinate Your Baby for Best Protection," Centers for Disease Control and Prevention (CDC), April 29, 2019; Text under the heading "14 Diseases You Almost Forgot About" is excerpted from "14 Diseases You Almost Forgot about (Thanks to Vaccines)," Centers for Disease Control and Prevention (CDC), May 30, 2018.

Protect Your Child from Serious Diseases

Measles is an example of how serious vaccine-preventable diseases can be. Cases and outbreaks still occur when the disease is brought into the United States by unvaccinated travelers (Americans or foreign visitors) who get infected when they are in other countries. Measles is still a common disease in many parts of the world. The viral disease is highly contagious and can spread easily when it reaches a community in the U.S. where groups of people are unvaccinated. Measles can be serious, and it can cause pneumonia, encephalitis (swelling of the brain), and even death. Young children are at the highest risk for serious complications from measles.

Another example is whooping cough. The United States has experienced an increase in whooping cough cases and outbreaks reported over the last few decades. Whooping cough can be deadly, especially for young babies who are too young to get their own vaccines. Since 2010, there have been tens of thousands of whooping cough cases reported each year nationwide, with a peak of more than 48,000 cases reported in 2012.

14 Diseases You Almost Forgot About
1. Diphtheria

Most of us only know diphtheria as an obscure disease from long ago, thanks to the diphtheria vaccine babies get. This vaccine, called "diphtheria, tetanus, and pertussis" (DTaP), provides protection against diphtheria, tetanus, and pertussis. While preventable, diphtheria does still exist. It can cause a thick covering in the back of the nose or throat that makes it hard to breathe or swallow. Diphtheria can also lead to heart failure, paralysis, and even death. Make sure to vaccinate to help keep this dangerous infection away from your kids.

Doctors recommend that your child get 5 doses of DTaP vaccine for best protection. Your child will need 1 dose at each of the following ages: 2 months, 4 months, 6 months, 15 through 18 months, and 4 through 6 years.

2. Chickenpox

Chickenpox is a disease that causes an itchy rash of blisters and a fever. A person with chickenpox may have a lot of blisters — as many as 500 all over their body. Chickenpox can be serious and even life-threatening, especially in babies, adults, and people with weakened immune systems. Even healthy children can get really sick. Vaccinating kids at an early age is especially important to keep your children healthy.

Doctors recommend that your child get 2 doses of the chickenpox shot for best protection. Your child will need 1 dose at each of the following ages: 12 through 15 months and 4 through 6 years.

3. Mumps

Mumps is best known for causing puffy cheeks and a swollen jaw. This is due to swelling of the salivary glands. Other symptoms include fever, head and muscle aches, and tiredness. Mumps is a contagious disease and there is no treatment. Mumps is still a threat—every year, people in the United States get mumps. Mumps outbreaks have occurred in settings where there was close, extended contact with infected people, such as being in the same classroom or playing on the same sports team. The measles, mumps, and rubella (MMR) vaccine protects you and your family against mumps, measles, and rubella.

Doctors recommend that your child get 2 doses of the MMR shot for best protection. Your child will need one dose at each of the following ages: 12 through 15 months and 4 through 6 years.

4. Rotavirus

Rotavirus is contagious and can cause severe watery diarrhea, often with vomiting, fever, and abdominal pain, mostly in infants and young children. Children can become severely dehydrated from the disease and need to be hospitalized. If a dehydrated child does not get needed care, they could die. Rotavirus is one of the first vaccines an infant can get; it is the best way to protect your child from rotavirus disease.

Doctors recommend that your child get two or three doses of the vaccine (depending on the brand) for best protection. For both brands, babies should get their first dose at two months of age and a second dose at four months. If they are getting the RotaTeq vaccine, they will need a third dose at six months.

5. Pneumococcal Disease

This disease is caused by bacteria called "*Streptococcus pneumoniae*." It causes ear infections, sinus infections, pneumonia, and even meningitis, making it very dangerous for children. The germs can invade parts of the body—such as the brain or spinal cord—that are normally free from germs. Make sure you keep kids safe from this dangerous disease by vaccinating.

Doctors recommend that your child get 4 doses of the pneumococcal conjugate vaccine (also called "PCV13") for best protection. Your child will need 1 dose at each of the following ages: 2 months, 4 months, 6 months, and at 12 through 15 months.

6. Whooping Cough

Whooping cough, or pertussis, is a highly contagious disease that can be deadly for babies. Whooping cough can cause uncontrollable, violent coughing, which often makes it hard to breathe. Its "whooping" name comes from the sharp breath intake sound right after a coughing fit. In babies, this disease also can cause life-threatening pauses in breathing with no cough at all. Whooping cough is especially dangerous to babies who are too young to be vaccinated themselves. Mothers should get the whooping cough vaccine during each pregnancy to pass some protection to their babies before birth. It is very important for your baby to get the whooping cough vaccine on time so she or he can start building her or his own protection against the disease. Since 2010, between 15,000 and 50,000 cases of whooping cough were reported each year in the United States, with cases reported in every state.

The DTaP vaccine provides protection against whooping cough, diphtheria, and tetanus. Doctors recommend that your child get 5 doses of the DTaP shot for best protection. Your child will need 1 dose at each of the following ages: 2 months, 4 months, 6 months, 15 through 18 months, and 4 through 6 years.

7. Measles

Did you know that your child can get measles by being in a room where a person with measles has been, even up to two hours after that person has left? Measles is very contagious, and it can be serious, especially for young children. Because measles is common in other parts of the world, unvaccinated people can get measles while traveling and bring it into the United States. Anyone who is not protected is at risk, so make sure to stay up to date on your child's vaccines to minimize the risk of coming into contact with an imported case.

Doctors recommend that your child get two doses of the MMR shot for best protection. Your child will need 1 dose at each of the following ages: 12 through 15 months and 4 through 6 years.

Infants 6 to 11 months old should have 1 dose of the MMR shot before traveling abroad. Infants vaccinated before 12 months of age should be revaccinated on or after their first birthday with 2 doses, each dose separated by at least 28 days.

8. Haemophilus influenzae Type B

Hib (or its official name, "*Haemophilus influenzae type b*") is not as well-known as some of the other diseases. Hib can do some serious damage to our kids' immune systems and cause brain damage, hearing loss, or even death. Hib mostly affects kids under 5 years of age. Before the vaccine, over 20,000 kids were infected each year. That is about 400 yellow school buses worth of kids. Of these kids, 1 in 5 suffered brain damage or became deaf. Even with treatment, as many as 1 out of 20 kids with Hib meningitis dies. Get your child vaccinated to help them beat the odds.

Doctors recommend that your child get 4 doses of the Hib vaccine for best protection. Your child will need 1 dose at each of the following ages: 2 months, 4 months, 6 months (for some brands), and 12 through 15 months.

9. Rubella

Rubella is spread by coughing and sneezing. It is especially dangerous for a pregnant woman and the fetus. If an unvaccinated pregnant woman gets infected with rubella, she can have a miscarriage, or her baby could die just after birth. Also, she can pass the disease to the fetus, who can develop serious birth defects. Make sure you and your child are protected from rubella by getting vaccinated on schedule.

Doctors recommend that your child get 2 doses of the MMR vaccine for best protection. Your child will need 1 dose at each of the following ages: 12 through 15 months and 4 through 6 years.

10. Hepatitis A

The hepatitis A vaccine was developed in 1995 and since then has cut the number of cases dramatically in the United States. Hepatitis A is a contagious liver disease and is transmitted through person-to-person contact or through contaminated food and water. Vaccinating against hepatitis A is a good way to help your baby stay hepatitis A-free and healthy.

617

Doctors recommend that your child get 2 doses of the hepatitis A shot for best protection. Your child should get the first dose at 12 through 23 months and the second dose 6 months after the last dose.

11. Hepatitis B

Did you know that worldwide more than 780,000 people per year die from complications to hepatitis B? Hepatitis B is spread through blood or other bodily fluids. It is especially dangerous for babies, since the hepatitis B virus can spread from an infected mother to child during birth. About 9 out of every 10 infants who contract it from their mothers become chronically infected, which is why babies should get the first dose of the hepatitis B vaccine shortly after birth. All pregnant women should be tested, and all babies should be vaccinated.

Doctors recommend that your child get three doses of the Hepatitis B shot for best protection. Typically, your child will need one dose at each of the following ages: shortly after birth, one through two months, and six months.

12. The Flu

Flu is a respiratory illness caused by the influenza virus that infects the nose, throat, and lungs. Flu can affect people differently based on their immune system, age, and health. Did you know that flu can be dangerous for children of any age? Flu symptoms in children can include coughing, fever, aches, fatigue, vomiting, and diarrhea. Not to mention, every year in the United States, otherwise healthy children are hospitalized or die from flu complications. In fact, the CDC estimates that since 2010, flu-related hospitalizations among children younger than 5 years of age have ranged from 6,000 to 26,000 in the United States. It is important to know that children younger than 6 months of age are more likely to end up in the hospital from flu, but they are too young to get a flu vaccine. The best way to protect babies against flu is for the mother to get a flu vaccine during pregnancy and for all caregivers and close contacts of the infant to be vaccinated. Everyone 6 months of age and older should get a flu vaccine every year.

Doctors recommend that your child get the flu vaccine every year starting when they are 6 months of age. Children younger than 9 years of age who are getting vaccinated for the first time need 2 doses of flu vaccine, spaced at least 28 days apart.

13. Tetanus

Tetanus causes painful muscle stiffness and lockjaw, and it can be fatal. Parents used to warn kids about tetanus every time we scratched, scraped, poked, or sliced ourselves on something metal. Lately, the tetanus vaccine is part of a disease-fighting vaccine DTaP, which provides protection against tetanus, diphtheria, and pertussis.

Doctors recommend that your child get 5 doses of the DTaP shot for best protection. Your child will need 1 dose at each of the following ages: 2 months, 4 months, 6 months, 15 through 18 months, and 4 through 6 years.

14. Polio

Polio is a crippling and potentially deadly infectious disease that is caused by the poliovirus. The virus spreads from person to person and can invade an infected person's brain and spinal cord, causing paralysis. Polio was eliminated in the United States with vaccination, and continued use of polio vaccine has kept this country polio-free. But, polio is still a threat in some other countries. Making sure that infants and children are vaccinated is the best way to prevent polio from returning. Make sure your baby is protected with the polio vaccine.

Doctors recommend that your child get 4 doses of the polio vaccine (also called "inactivated polio vaccine" (IPV)) for best protection. Your child will need 1 dose at each of the following ages: 2 months, 4 months, 6 through 18 months, and 4 through 6 years.

Chapter 76

Questions and Answers about Immunizations

Are Vaccines Safe?

Yes. Vaccines are very safe. The United States' long-standing vaccine safety system ensures that vaccines are as safe as possible. The United States has the safest vaccine supply in its history. Millions of children safely receive vaccines each year. The most common side effects are typically very mild, such as pain or swelling at the injection site.

What Are the Side Effects of Vaccines? How Do I Treat Them?

Vaccines, as with any medication, may cause some side effects. Most of these side effects are very minor, such as soreness where the shot was given, fussiness, or a low-grade fever. These side effects typically only last a couple of days and are treatable. For example, you can apply a cool, wet washcloth on the sore area to ease discomfort. Serious reactions are very rare. However, if your child experiences any reactions that concern you, call the doctor's office.

This chapter includes text excerpted from "Vaccination FAQs," Centers for Disease Control and Prevention (CDC), May 14, 2019.

What Are the Risks and Benefits of Vaccines?

Vaccines can prevent infectious diseases that once killed or harmed many infants, children, and adults. Without vaccines, your child is at risk of getting seriously ill and pain, disability, and even death from diseases such as measles and whooping cough. The main risks associated with getting vaccines are side effects, which are almost always mild (redness and swelling at the injection site) and go away within a few days. Serious side effects after vaccination, such as a severe allergic reaction, are very rare, and doctors and clinic staff are trained to deal with them. The disease-prevention benefits of getting vaccines are much greater than the possible side effects for almost all children. The only exceptions to this are cases in which a child has a serious chronic medical condition, such as cancer; has a disease that weakens the immune system; or has had a severe allergic reaction to a previous vaccine dose.

Is There a Link between Vaccines and Autism?

No. Scientific studies and reviews continue to show no relationship between vaccines and autism. Some people have suggested that thimerosal (a compound that contains mercury) in vaccines given to infants and young children might be a cause of autism. Others have suggested that the measles-mumps-rubella (MMR) vaccine may be linked to autism. However, numerous scientists and researchers have studied and continue to study the MMR vaccine and thimerosal, and they reach the same conclusion: there is no link between MMR vaccine or thimerosal and autism.

Can Vaccines Overload My Child's Immune System?

Vaccines do not overload the immune system. Every day, a child's healthy immune system successfully fights off thousands of germs. Antigens are parts of germs that cause the body's immune system to go to work to build antibodies, which fight off diseases.

The antigens in vaccines come from the germs themselves, but the germs are weakened or killed so they cannot cause serious illness. Even if babies receive several vaccinations in one day, vaccines contain only a tiny fraction of the antigens they encounter every day in their environment. Vaccines give your child the antibodies they need to fight off serious vaccine-preventable diseases.

Why Are so Many Doses Needed for Each Vaccine?

Getting every recommended dose of each vaccine provides your child with the best protection possible. Depending on the vaccine, your child will need more than one dose to build high enough immunity to prevent disease or to boost immunity that fades over time. Your child may also receive more than one dose to make sure they are protected if they did not get immunity from the first dose, or to protect them against germs that change over time, such as the flu. Every dose is important because each protects against infectious diseases that can be especially serious for infants and very young children.

Why Do Vaccines Start so Early?

The recommended schedule protects infants and children by providing immunity early in life before they come into contact with life-threatening diseases. Children receive immunization early because they are susceptible to diseases at a young age. The consequences of these diseases can be very serious, even life-threatening, for infants and young children.

What Do You Think of Delaying Some Vaccines or Following a Nonstandard Schedule?

Children do not receive any known benefits from following schedules that delay vaccines. Infants and young children who follow immunization schedules that spread out or leave out shots are at risk of developing diseases during the time you delay their shots. Some vaccine-preventable diseases remain common in the United States, and children may be exposed to these diseases during the time they are not protected by vaccines, placing them at risk for a serious case of the disease that might cause hospitalization or death.

Haven't We Gotten Rid of Most of These Diseases in This Country?

Some vaccine-preventable diseases, such as pertussis (whooping cough) and chickenpox, remain common in the United States. On the other hand, other diseases vaccines prevent are no longer common in this country because of vaccines. However, if we stopped vaccinating, the few cases we have in the United States could very quickly become tens or hundreds of thousands of cases. Even though many serious vaccine-preventable diseases are uncommon in the United States, some are common in other parts of the world. Even if your family does not travel internationally, you could come into contact with international travelers anywhere in your community. Children who do not receive all vaccinations and are exposed to a disease can become seriously sick and spread it through a community.

What Are Combination Vaccines? Why Are They Used?

Combination vaccines protect your child against more than one disease with a single shot. They reduce the number of shots and office visits your child would need, which not only saves you time and money but is also easier on your child. Some common combination vaccines are Pediarix®, which combines DTaP, Hep B, and IPV (polio), and ProQuad®, which combines MMR and varicella (chickenpox).

Can't I Just Wait until My Child Goes to School to Catch Up on Immunizations?

Before entering school, young children can be exposed to vaccine-preventable diseases from parents and other adults, brothers, and sisters, on a plane, at child care, or even at the grocery store. Children under the age of five are especially susceptible to diseases because their immune systems have not built up the necessary defenses to fight infection. Do not wait to protect your baby and risk getting these diseases when she or he needs protection.

Why Does My Child Need a Chickenpox Shot? Isn't It a Mild Disease?

Your child needs a chickenpox vaccine because chickenpox can actually be a serious disease. In many cases, children may experience a mild case of chickenpox, but other children may have blisters that become infected. Some others may develop pneumonia. There is no way of telling in advance how severe your child's symptoms may be. Before a vaccine was made available, about 50 children died every year from chickenpox, and about 1 in 500 children who got chickenpox was hospitalized.

My Child Is Sick Right Now. Is It Okay for Her or Him to Still Get Shots?

Talk with your child's doctor, but children can usually get vaccinated even if they have a mild illness, such as cold, earache, mild fever, or diarrhea. If the doctor says it is okay, your child can still get vaccinated.

What Are the Ingredients in Vaccines and What Do They Do?

Vaccines contain ingredients that cause the body to develop immunity. They also contain very small amounts of other ingredients. All the ingredients play the necessary roles either in making the vaccine or in ensuring that the final product is safe and effective.

Don't Infants Have Natural Immunity? Isn't Natural Immunity Better Than the Kind from Vaccines?

Infants may get some temporary immunity from their mother during the last few weeks of pregnancy but only for diseases to which the mother is immune. Added to this, breastfeeding may also protect your child temporarily from minor infections, such as colds. However, antibodies do not last long, leaving your child vulnerable to disease.

Natural immunity occurs when your child gets exposed to a disease and becomes infected. It is true that natural immunity usually results in better immunity than vaccination, but the risks are much greater. A natural chickenpox infection may result in pneumonia, whereas the vaccine might only cause a sore arm for a couple of days.

Can't I Just Wait to Vaccinate My Child, since She or He Isn't in Child care, Where She or He Could Be Exposed to Diseases?

No, even young children who are cared for at home can be exposed to vaccine-preventable diseases, so it is important for them to get all their vaccines at the recommended ages. Children can catch these illnesses from any number of people or places, including from parents, brothers, or sisters, visitors to their home, on playgrounds, or even at the grocery store. Regardless of whether or not your baby is cared for outside the home, she or he comes in contact with people throughout the day, some of whom may be sick but not know it yet.

If someone has a vaccine-preventable disease, they may not have symptoms or the symptoms may be mild, and they can end up spreading the disease to babies or young children. Remember, many of these diseases can be especially dangerous to young children, so it is safest to vaccinate your child at the recommended ages to protect her or him, whether or not she or he is in child care.

Do I Have to Vaccinate My Child on Schedule If I Am Breastfeeding Her or Him?

Yes, even breastfed babies need to be protected with vaccines at the recommended ages. The immune system is not fully developed at birth, which puts newborns at a greater risk for infections.

Breast milk provides important protection from some infections as your baby's immune system is developing. For example, babies who are breastfed have a lower risk of ear infections, respiratory tract infections, and diarrhea. However, breast milk does not protect children against all diseases. Even in breastfed infants, vaccines are the most effective way to prevent many diseases. Your baby needs the long-term protection that can only come from making sure she or he receives all her or his vaccines according to the recommended schedule of the Centers for Disease Control and Prevention (CDC).

What Is Wrong with Delaying Some of My Child's Vaccines If I Am Planning to Get Them All Eventually?

Young children have the highest risk of having a serious case of disease that could cause hospitalization or death. Delaying or spreading out vaccine doses leaves your child unprotected during the time when they need vaccine protection the most. For example, diseases such as *Haemophilus influenzae type b* (Hib) or pneumococcus almost always occur in the first two years of a baby's life. And some diseases, such as hepatitis B and whooping cough, are more serious when babies get them at a younger age. Vaccinating your child according to the recommended immunization schedule of the CDC means that you can help protect her or him at a young age.

I Got Whooping Cough and Flu Vaccines during My Pregnancy. Why Does My Child Need These Vaccines Too?

The protection (antibodies) you passed to your baby before birth will give her or him some early protection against whooping cough and flu. However, these antibodies will only give her or him short-term protection. It is very important for your baby to get vaccines on time so that she or he can start building her or his own protection against these serious diseases.

Chapter 77

Facts about Adolescent Immunization

What Vaccines Do Adolescents Need?

Starting at the age of 11 or 12, the Centers for Disease Control and Prevention (CDC) recommends 4 vaccines for almost all children.

Meningococcal: Children should get their first dose of this vaccine at the age of 11 or 12, and they should get a second dose at 16 years of age. The shots protect them from bacteria and viruses that cause meningitis, a serious condition that happens when the tissues around the brain and spinal cord get infected and swell. Meningococcal diseases are rare, but they can spread through casual contacts, such as sharing food and drinks or kissing. They can also spread in places where people are living in close quarters, such as college dorms, and as a result, teens and young adults are at a particularly high risk when compared with other age groups.

Human papillomavirus (HPV): The HPV vaccine is licensed, safe, and effective for both females and males between the ages of 9 and 26, and the Advisory Committee on Immunization Practices (ACIP) recommends that all adolescents begin receiving the vaccine

This chapter includes text excerpted from "What Vaccines Do Adolescents Need?" U.S. Department of Health and Human Services (HHS), April 16, 2018.

at the age of 11 or 12. Older adolescents who did not begin the series at the age of 11 or 12 are encouraged to start as soon as possible to "catch up." These catch-up vaccines are recommended up until the age of 26 for females and until the age of 21 for males (or 26 years of age for males who have sex with other males). The ACIP recommends 3 doses for those who start the vaccination series at the ages of 15 to 26. Despite evidence that the vaccine has cut HPV infections in teen girls by two-thirds, researchers say that too few girls and boys are getting vaccinated.

For full protection, those that are 11 or 12 years of age need 2 doses of the vaccine, which they should receive within a 6- to 12-month window. Teens and young adults who start the series between the ages of 15 and 26, younger adolescents (between the ages of 9 and 14) who received 2 doses of the vaccine less than 6 months apart, and young people with weakened immune systems need 3 doses. There are 2 reasons as to why the HPV vaccine series is recommended to start at the age of 11 or 12. First, ideally, adolescents should complete all doses before any sexual activity with another person. Second, the human body produces more antibodies against HPV when the vaccine is given early in adolescence, as opposed to later in the teen years or in early adulthood.

HPV is a virus that is very common. It infects about 14 million people every year. Some strains of the virus can cause cervical cancer in women, penile cancer in men, and anal or oropharyngeal (throat) cancers in both sexes. Some HPV strains can also cause genital warts through skin-to-skin contact.

Tdap: All adolescents who are 11 or 12 years of age should get this single shot to protect against 3 diseases: tetanus, diphtheria, and pertussis. Children get protection for these as babies with a shot called "DTaP," but this follow-up booster shot gives them more protection since the first one wears off over time.

Tetanus is a bacterial disease that kids can get through cuts or wounds (such as stepping on a rusty nail). The infection can cause painful muscle spasms, breathing problems, paralysis, and even death. The Tdap vaccine also prevents diphtheria and pertussis, which both spread through the air by coughs and sneezes. Both can cause dangerous breathing problems. Pertussis, also known as "whooping cough," can be especially deadly for babies. If an adolescent has younger siblings or spends time around small children, Tdap can keep them from passing whooping cough on to them.

Influenza: All children age 6 months of age and older should get a flu shot every year because the flu virus changes every year. Scientists tailor the vaccine to fight the strains they think will be the most common that season. It is especially important for those with diabetes and asthma since the flu is more dangerous for them.

The Importance of Following Through

For some vaccines, it takes only one shot to protect adolescents. Others require two or three doses to fully guard against diseases or infections. Each shot is important. Not following through means that adolescents are at risk for serious diseases.

When One Dose Is Not Enough

Sometimes, the first dose of a vaccine is a primer, preparing the body to build its full response with the second or third dose. A single dose might give protection for a while, but it will not last nearly as long as the series will. Some childhood vaccines wear off over time. To stay protected from tetanus, diphtheria, and pertussis, adolescents need the booster shot, Tdap, at the age of 11 or 12. The influenza virus changes from year to year, meaning that scientists have to make a new vaccine for each flu season. Adolescents who do not get a flu shot each year will not be protected from that season's strains.

Vaccines for Some Preteens

If adolescents have chronic health problems, are getting certain kinds of medical treatment, or will be traveling abroad in the near future, they may need different vaccines than other kids their age. Their doctor can advise whether these immunizations are needed:

Adolescents with chronic health problems may need different vaccines than other kids their age.

Pneumococcal: Children between the ages of 6 and 18 who are at a high risk for pneumonia may need a pneumococcal conjugate vaccine (PCV13) or a pneumococcal polysaccharide vaccine (PPSV23), or both.

Hepatitis A: Doctors recommend this vaccine for people of all ages who are at a high risk of hepatitis A virus or those who live in communities that have had outbreaks of it. Healthy people can also receive this shot. A doctor can advise whether an adolescent is at risk of hepatitis A.

Other vaccines: People planning to travel abroad may need extra shots, depending on where they are going. For example, an adolescent may need shots for hepatitis A, yellow fever, or typhoid if they are spending time in countries where these illnesses are common.

Catch-Up Vaccinations

If an adolescent is more than a month behind on their vaccines, they can catch up. Even if kids have missed the second or third dose in a series, like the ones for the HPV vaccine, they can usually finish the series without starting over.

Vaccines for Traveling Abroad

Adolescents should visit their doctor before they travel to discuss any vaccines, medicines, and other recommendations. It is best to do this at least four to six weeks before traveling to ensure the completion of recommended vaccine series and/or to get any medications they might need.

Pediatricians often carry most of the vaccines that adolescents will need for travel, including the standard adolescent vaccines. There are certain vaccines that may need to be called into a pharmacy, such as the oral typhoid vaccine. Travel clinics and health departments can also provide vaccines if adolescents or their families are not able to get them at a doctor's office. The travel website of the CDC has listings of travel clinics (wwwnc.cdc.gov/travel).

Chapter 78

Adult Immunization Recommendations

Adult Immunization Schedule

Vaccine	19-21 years	22-26 years	27-49 years	50-64 years	≥65 years
Influenza inactivated (IIV) or Influenza recombinant (RIV)	1 dose annually				
Influenza live attenuated (LAIV)	1 dose annually				
Tetanus, diphtheria, pertussis (Tdap or Td)	1 dose Tdap, then Td booster every 10 yrs				
Measles, mumps, rubella (MMR)	1 or 2 doses depending on indication (if born in 1957 or later)				
Varicella (VAR)	2 doses (if born in 1980 or later)				
Zoster recombinant (RZV) (preferred)					2 doses
Zoster live (ZVL)					1 dose
Human papillomavirus (HPV) Female	2 or 3 doses depending on age at initial vaccination				
Human papillomavirus (HPV) Male	2 or 3 doses depending on age at initial vaccination				
Pneumococcal conjugate (PCV13)					1 dose
Pneumococcal polysaccharide (PPSV23)	1 or 2 doses depending on indication				1 dose
Hepatitis A (HepA)	2 or 3 doses depending on vaccine				
Hepatitis B (HepB)	2 or 3 doses depending on vaccine				
Meningococcal A, C, W, Y (MenACWY)	1 or 2 doses depending on indication, then booster every 5 yrs if risk remains				
Meningococcal B (MenB)	2 or 3 doses depending on vaccine and indication				
Haemophilus influenzae type b (Hib)	1 or 3 doses depending on indication				

Figure 78.1. *Recommended Immunization Schedule for Adults Aged 19 Years or Older, by Vaccine and Age Group*

This chapter includes text excerpted from "Immunization Schedules," Centers for Disease Control and Prevention (CDC), February 5, 2019.

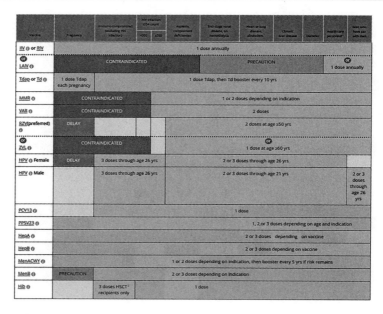

Figure 78.2. *Vaccines That Might Be Indicated for Adults Aged 19 Years or Older Based on Medical and Other Indications*

Haemophilus Influenzae *Type B Vaccination*
Special Situations

- **Anatomical or functional asplenia (including sickle cell disease):** 1 dose Hib if previously did not receive Hib; if elective splenectomy, 1 dose Hib, preferably at least 14 days before splenectomy

- **Hematopoietic stem cell transplant (HSCT):** Three-dose series Hib 4 weeks apart starting 6 to 12 months after a successful transplant, regardless of Hib vaccination history

Hepatitis A Vaccination
Routine Vaccination

Not at risk but want protection from hepatitis A (identification of risk factor not required): 2-dose series HepA (Havrix 6 to 12 months apart or Vaqta 6 to 18 months apart [minimum interval: 6 months]) or 3-dose series HepA-HepB (Twinrix at 0, 1, 6 months [minimum intervals: 4 weeks between doses 1 and 2, 5 months between doses 2 and 3])

Special Situations

- **At risk for hepatitis A virus infection:** two-dose series HepA as above:

  - Chronic liver disease

  - Clotting factor disorders

  - Men who have sex with men

  - Injection or noninjection drug use

  - Homelessness

  - Work with hepatitis A virus in a research laboratory or nonhuman primates with hepatitis A virus infection

  - Travel in countries with high or intermediate endemic hepatitis A

Close personal contact with an international adoptee (e.g., household, regular babysitting) in the first 60 days after arrival from a country with high or intermediate endemic hepatitis A (administer dose 1 as soon as adoption is planned, at least 2 weeks before adoptee's arrival)

Hepatitis B Vaccination
Routine Vaccination

Not at risk but want protection from hepatitis B (identification of risk factor not required): 2- or 3-dose series HepB (2-dose series Heplisav-B at least 4 weeks apart [2-dose series HepB only applies when 2 doses of Heplisav-B are used at least 4 weeks apart] or 3-dose series Engerix-B or Recombivax HB at 0, 1, 6 months [minimum intervals: 4 weeks between doses 1 and 2, 8 weeks between doses 2 and 3, 16 weeks between doses 1 and 3]) or 3-dose series HepA-HepB (Twinrix at 0, 1, 6 months [minimum intervals: 4 weeks between doses 1 and 2, 5 months between doses 2 and 3])

Special Situations

- **At risk for hepatitis B virus infection:** two-dose (Heplisav-B) or three-dose (Engerix-B, Recombivax HB) series HepB, or three-dose series HepA-HepB as above:

  - Hepatitis C virus infection

- Chronic liver disease (e.g., cirrhosis, fatty liver disease, alcoholic liver disease, autoimmune hepatitis, alanine aminotransferase [ALT] or aspartate aminotransferase [AST] level greater than twice the upper limit of normal)

- Human immunodeficiency virus (HIV) infection

- Sexual exposure risk (e.g., sex partners of hepatitis B surface antigen (HBsAg)-positive persons; sexually active persons not in mutually monogamous relationships, persons seeking evaluation or treatment for a sexually transmitted infection, men who have sex with men)

- Current or recent injection drug use

- Percutaneous or mucosal risk for exposure to blood (e.g., household contacts of HBsAg-positive persons; residents and staff of facilities for developmentally disabled persons; healthcare and public safety personnel with reasonably anticipated risk for exposure to blood or blood-contaminated body fluids; hemodialysis, peritoneal dialysis, home dialysis, and predialysis patients; persons with diabetes mellitus age younger than 60 years of age and, at the discretion of the treating clinician, those 60 years of age or older)

- Incarcerated persons

- Travel in countries with high or intermediate endemic hepatitis B

Human Papillomavirus Vaccination
Routine Vaccination

- **Females up to 26 years of age and males up to 21 years of age:** 2- or 3-dose series human papillomavirus vaccination (HPV) vaccine depending on age at initial vaccination; males between 22 and 26 years of age may be vaccinated based on an individual clinical decision (HPV vaccination routinely recommended at the age of 11 or 12)

- **15 years of age or older at initial vaccination:** 3-dose series HPV vaccine at 0, 1 to 2, 6 months (minimum intervals: 4 weeks between doses 1 and 2, 12 weeks between doses 2 and 3, 5 months between doses 1 and 3; repeat dose if administered too soon)

- **Between 9 and 14 years of age at initial vaccination and received 1 dose, or 2 doses less than 5 months apart:** 1 dose HPV vaccine

- **Between 9 and 14 years of age at initial vaccination and received 2 doses at least 5 months apart:** HPV vaccination complete, no additional dose needed

- If completed valid vaccination series with any HPV vaccine, no additional doses needed

Special Situations

- **Immunocompromising conditions (including HIV infection) up to 26 years of age:** 3-dose series HPV vaccine at 0, 1 to 2, 6 months as above

- **Men who have sex with men and transgender persons up to 26 years of age:** 2- or 3-dose series HPV vaccine depending on age at initial vaccination as above

- **Pregnancy through 26 years of age:** HPV vaccination not recommended until after pregnancy; no intervention needed if vaccinated while pregnant; pregnancy testing not needed before vaccination

Influenza Vaccination
Routine Vaccination

Persons six months of age or older: one dose IIV, routine influenza vaccination (RIV), or live, attenuated flu vaccine (LAIV) appropriate for age and health status annually

Special Situations

- **Egg allergy, hives only:** one dose IIV, RIV, or LAIV appropriate for age and health status annually

- **Egg allergy more severe than hives (e.g., angioedema, respiratory distress):** one dose IIV, RIV, or LAIV appropriate for age and health status annually in a medical setting under the supervision of healthcare provider who can recognize and manage severe allergic conditions

- Immunocompromising conditions (including HIV infection), anatomical or functional asplenia, pregnant women, close contacts and caregivers of severely immunocompromised persons in protected environment, use of influenza antiviral medications in the previous 48 hours, with cerebrospinal fluid leak or cochlear implant: 1 dose IIV or RIV annually (LAIV not recommended)

- **History of Guillain-Barré syndrome within six weeks of previous dose of influenza vaccine:** Generally should not be vaccinated

Measles, Mumps, and Rubella Vaccination
Routine Vaccination

- No evidence of immunity to measles, mumps, or rubella: one dose measles, mumps, and rubella (MMR)

  - **Evidence of immunity:** Born before 1957 (except healthcare personnel), documentation of receipt of MMR, laboratory evidence of immunity or disease (diagnosis of disease without laboratory confirmation is not evidence of immunity)

Special Situations

- **Pregnancy with no evidence of immunity to rubella:** MMR contraindicated during pregnancy; after pregnancy (before discharge from a healthcare facility), 1 dose MMR

- **Nonpregnant women of childbearing age with no evidence of immunity to rubella:** 1 dose MMR

- **HIV infection with a cluster of differentiation 4 (CD4) count greater than or equal to 200 cells/μL for at least 6 months and no evidence of immunity to measles, mumps, or rubella:** 2-dose series MMR at least 4 weeks apart; MMR contraindicated in HIV infection with a CD4 count less than 200 cells/μL

- **Severe immunocompromising conditions:** MMR contraindicated

- **Students in postsecondary educational institutions, international travelers, and household or close personal contacts of immunocompromised persons with no evidence of immunity to measles, mumps, or rubella:** 1 dose

MMR if previously received 1 dose MMR, or 2-dose series MMR at least 4 weeks apart if previously did not receive any MMR

- **Healthcare personnel born in 1957 or later with no evidence of immunity to measles, mumps, or rubella:** 2-dose series MMR at least 4 weeks apart for measles or mumps, or at least 1 dose MMR for rubella; if born before 1957, consider 2-dose series MMR at least 4 weeks apart for measles or mumps, or 1 dose MMR for rubella

Meningococcal Vaccination
Special Situations for MenACWY

- **Anatomical or functional asplenia, including sickle cell disease, HIV infection, persistent complement component deficiency, eculizumab use:** 2-dose series MenACWY (Menactra, Menveo) at least 8 weeks apart and revaccinate every 5 years if risk remains

- **Travel in countries with hyperendemic or epidemic meningococcal disease, microbiologists routinely exposed to *Neisseria meningitidis*:** 1 dose MenACWY and revaccinate every 5 years if risk remains

- **First-year college students who live in residential housing (if not previously vaccinated at age 16 years or older) and military recruits:** 1 dose MenACWY

Special Situations for MenB

- **Anatomical or functional asplenia, including sickle cell disease, persistent complement component deficiency, eculizumab use, microbiologists routinely exposed to *Neisseria meningitidis*:** 2-dose series MenB-4C (Bexsero) at least 1 month apart, or 3-dose series MenB-FHbp (Trumenba) at 0, 1 to 2, 6 months (if dose 2 was administered at least 6 months after dose 1, dose 3 not needed); MenB-4C and MenB-FHbp are not interchangeable (use same product for all doses in series)

- **Pregnancy:** Delay MenB until after pregnancy unless at increased risk and vaccination benefit outweighs potential risks

- **Healthy adolescents and young adults between 16 and 23 years of age (age 16 through 18 years preferred) not**

at increased risk for meningococcal disease: Based on individual clinical decision, may receive 2-dose series MenB-4C at least 1 month apart, or 2-dose series MenB-FHbp at 0, 6 months (if dose 2 was administered less than 6 months after dose 1, administer dose 3 at least 4 months after dose 2); MenB-4C and MenB-FHbp are not interchangeable (use the same product for all doses in the series)

Pneumococcal Vaccination
Routine Vaccination

- **65 years of age or older (immunocompetent):** 1 dose pneumococcal vaccination (PCV) 13 if previously did not receive PCV13, followed by 1 dose PPSV23 at least 1 year after PCV13 and at least 5 years after last dose PPSV23

  - Previously received PPSV23 but not PCV13 at 65 years of age or older: 1 dose PCV13 at least 1 year after PPSV23

  - When both PCV13 and PPSV23 are indicated, administer PCV13 first (PCV13 and PPSV23 should not be administered during the same visit)

Special Situations

- **Between 19 and 64 years of age with chronic medical conditions (chronic heart [excluding hypertension], lung, or liver disease; diabetes), alcoholism, or cigarette smoking:** 1 dose PPSV23

- **19 years of age or older with immunocompromising conditions (congenital or acquired immunodeficiency [including B- and T-lymphocyte deficiency, complement deficiencies, phagocytic disorders, HIV infection], chronic renal failure, nephrotic syndrome, leukemia, lymphoma, Hodgkin disease, generalized malignancy, iatrogenic immunosuppression [e.g., drug or radiation therapy], solid organ transplant, multiple myeloma) or anatomical or functional asplenia (including sickle cell disease and other hemoglobinopathies):** 1 dose PCV13 followed by 1 dose PPSV23 at least 8 weeks later, then another dose PPSV23 at least 5 years after previous PPSV23; at age 65 years or older, administer 1 dose PPSV23 at least 5 years after most recent PPSV23 (note: only 1 dose PPSV23 recommended at age 65 years or older)

- **19 years of age or older with a cerebrospinal fluid leak or cochlear implant:** 1 dose PCV13 followed by 1 dose PPSV23 at least 8 weeks later; at age 65 years or older, administer another dose PPSV23 at least 5 years after PPSV23 (note: only 1 dose PPSV23 recommended at age 65 years or older)

Tetanus, Diphtheria, and Pertussis Vaccination
Routine Vaccination

Previously did not receive Tdap at or after the age of 11: 1 dose Tdap, then Td booster every 10 years

Special Situations

- **Previously did not receive primary vaccination series for tetanus, diphtheria, and pertussis:** 1 dose Tdap followed by 1 dose Td at least 4 weeks after Tdap, and another dose Td 6 to 12 months after last Td (Tdap can be substituted for any Td dose, but preferred as the first dose); Td booster every 10 years thereafter

- **Pregnancy:** 1 dose Tdap during each pregnancy, preferably in the early part of gestational weeks 27 to 36

Varicella Vaccination
Routine Vaccination

- **No evidence of immunity to varicella:** 2-dose series varicella routine vaccination (VAR) 4 to 8 weeks apart if previously did not receive the varicella-containing vaccine (VAR or MMRV [measles-mumps-rubella-varicella vaccine] for children); if previously received 1 dose varicella-containing vaccine: 1 dose VAR at least 4 weeks after the first dose

  - **Evidence of immunity:** U.S.-born before 1980 (except for pregnant women and healthcare personnel [see below]), documentation of 2 doses varicella-containing vaccine at least 4 weeks apart, diagnosis or verification of a history of varicella or herpes zoster by a healthcare provider, laboratory evidence of immunity or disease

Special Situations

- **Pregnancy with no evidence of immunity to varicella:**
  VAR contraindicated during pregnancy; after pregnancy (before
  discharge from a healthcare facility), 1 dose VAR if previously
  received 1 dose varicella-containing vaccine, or dose 1 of 2-dose
  series VAR (dose 2: 4 to 8 weeks later) if previously did not
  receive any varicella-containing vaccine, regardless of whether
  U.S.-born before 1980

- **Healthcare personnel with no evidence of immunity
  to varicella:** 1 dose VAR if previously received 1 dose
  varicella-containing vaccine, or 2-dose series VAR
  4 to 8 weeks apart if previously did not receive any
  varicella-containing vaccine, regardless of whether U.S.-born
  before 1980

- **HIV infection with a CD4 count greater than or equal to
  200 cells/μL with no evidence of immunity:** Consider 2-dose
  series VAR 3 months apart based on individual clinical decision;
  VAR contraindicated in HIV infection with a CD4 count less
  than 200 cells/μL

- **Severe immunocompromising conditions:** VAR
  contraindicated

Zoster Vaccination
Routine Vaccination

- **50 years of age or older:** 2-dose series routine zoster
  vaccination (RZV) 2 to 6 months apart (minimum interval:
  4 weeks; repeat dose if administered too soon) regardless of
  previous herpes zoster or previously received live- attenuated
  herpes zoster vaccine (ZVL) (administer RZV at least 2 months
  after ZVL)

- **60 years of age or older:** 2-dose series RZV 26 months apart
  (minimum interval: 4 weeks; repeat dose if administered too
  soon) or 1 dose ZVL if not previously vaccinated (if previously
  received ZVL, administer RZV at least 2 months after ZVL); RZV
  preferred over ZVL

Special Situations

- **Pregnancy:** ZVL contraindicated; consider delaying RZV until after pregnancy if RZV indicated

- **Severe immunocompromising conditions (including HIV infection with a CD4 count less than 200 cells/μL):** ZVL contraindicated; recommended use of RZV under review.

Chapter 79

Possible Side Effects from Vaccines

Any vaccine can cause side effects. For the most part, these are minor (for example, a sore arm or low-grade fever) and go away within a few days. Listed below are vaccines licensed in the United States and side effects that have been associated with each of them. This information is copied directly from the Centers for Disease Control and Prevention (CDC) Vaccine Information Statements, which are derived from the Advisory Committee on Immunization Practices (ACIP) recommendations for each vaccine.

Remember, vaccines are continually monitored for safety, and as with any medication, vaccines can cause side effects. However, a decision not to immunize a child also involves risk and could put the child and others who come into contact with her or him at risk of contracting a potentially deadly disease.

Diphtheria, Tetanus, and Acellular Pertussis Vaccine Side Effects
What Are the Risks from This Vaccine?

- Redness, soreness, swelling, and tenderness where the shot is given are common after the Diphtheria, Tetanus, and Acellular Pertussis (DTaP) vaccine.

This chapter includes text excerpted from "Possible Side-Effects from Vaccines," Centers for Disease Control and Prevention (CDC), July 12, 2018.

- Fever, fussiness, tiredness, poor appetite, and vomiting sometimes happen one to three days after DTaP vaccination.

- More serious reactions, such as seizures, nonstop crying for three hours or more, or high fever (over 105°F), after DTaP vaccination happen much less often. Rarely, the vaccine is followed by swelling of the entire arm or leg, especially in older children when they receive their fourth or fifth dose.

- Long-term seizures, coma, lowered consciousness, or permanent brain damage happens extremely rarely after DTaP vaccination.

As with any medicine, there is a very remote chance of a vaccine causing a severe allergic reaction, other serious injuries, or death.

Hepatitis A Vaccine Side Effects
What Are the Risks from Hepatitis A Vaccine?

With any medicine, including vaccines, there is a chance of side effects. These are usually mild and go away on their own, but serious reactions are also possible.

Most people who get the hepatitis A vaccine do not have any problems with it.

Minor problems following hepatitis A vaccine include:

- Soreness or redness where the shot was given

- Low-grade fever

- Headache

- Tiredness

If these problems occur, they usually begin soon after the shot and last one or two days.

Your doctor can tell you more about these reactions.

Other problems that could happen after this vaccine:

- People sometimes faint after a medical procedure, including vaccination. Sitting or lying down for about 15 minutes can help prevent fainting and injuries caused by a fall. Tell your provider if you feel dizzy or have vision changes or ringing in the ears.

- Some people get shoulder pain that can be more severe and last longer than the more routine soreness that can follow injections. This happens very rarely.

- Any medication can cause a severe allergic reaction. Such reactions from a vaccine are very rare, estimated at about one in a million doses, and would happen within a few minutes to a few hours after the vaccination.

As with any medicine, there is a very remote chance of a vaccine causing a serious injury or death.

Hepatitis B Vaccine Side Effects
What Are the Risks from Hepatitis B Vaccine?

With any medicine, including vaccines, there is a chance of side effects. These are usually mild and go away on their own, but serious reactions are also possible.

Most people who get hepatitis B vaccine do not have any problems with it.

Minor problems following hepatitis B vaccine include:

- Soreness where the shot was given

- Temperature of 99.9°F or higher

If these problems occur, they usually begin soon after the shot and last one or two days.

Your doctor can tell you more about these reactions.

Other problems that could happen after this vaccine:

- People sometimes faint after a medical procedure, including vaccination. Sitting or lying down for about 15 minutes can help prevent fainting and injuries caused by a fall. Tell your provider if you feel dizzy or have vision changes or ringing in the ears.

- Some people get shoulder pain that can be more severe and last longer than the more routine soreness that can follow injections. This happens very rarely.

- Any medication can cause a severe allergic reaction. Such reactions from a vaccine are very rare, estimated at about one in a million doses, and would happen within a few minutes to a few hours after the vaccination.

As with any medicine, there is a very remote chance of a vaccine causing a serious injury or death.

Haemophilus Influenzae *Type B Vaccine Side Effects*
What Are the Risk from Haemophilus Influenzae *Type B Vaccine?*

With any medicine, including vaccines, there is a chance of side effects. These are usually mild and go away on their own. Serious reactions are also possible but are rare.

Most people who get the *Haemophilus influenzae* type B (Hib) vaccine do not have any problems with it.

Mild problems following Hib vaccine:

- Redness, warmth, or swelling where the shot was given

- Fever

These problems are uncommon. If they occur, they usually begin soon after the shot and last two or three days.

Problems that could happen after any vaccine:

- Any medication can cause a severe allergic reaction. Such reactions from a vaccine are very rare, estimated at fewer than one in a million doses, and would happen within a few minutes to a few hours after the vaccination.

As with any medicine, there is a very remote chance of a vaccine causing a serious injury or death.

Older children, adolescents, and adults might also experience these problems after any vaccine:

- People sometimes faint after a medical procedure, including vaccination. Sitting or lying down for about 15 minutes can help prevent fainting and injuries caused by a fall. Tell your doctor if you feel dizzy or have vision changes or ringing in the ears.

- Some people get severe pain in the shoulder and have difficulty moving the arm where the shot was given. This happens very rarely.

Human-Papillomavirus Gardasil-9 Vaccine Side Effects
What Are the Risks from This Vaccine?

With any medicine, including vaccines, there is a chance of side effects. These are usually mild and go away on their own, but serious reactions are also possible.

Most people who get the HPV vaccine do not have any serious problems with it.

Mild or moderate problems following HPV vaccine:

- Reactions in the arm where the shot was given:
  - Soreness (about 9 people in 10)
  - Redness or swelling (about 1 person in 3)
- Fever:
  - Mild (100°F) (about 1 person in 10)
  - Moderate (102°F) (about 1 person in 65)
- Other problems:
  - Headache (about 1 person in 3)

Problems that could happen after any injected vaccine:

- People sometimes faint after a medical procedure, including vaccination. Sitting or lying down for about 15 minutes can help prevent fainting and injuries caused by a fall. Tell your doctor if you feel dizzy or have vision changes or ringing in the ears.
- Some people get severe pain in the shoulder and have difficulty moving the arm where the shot was given. This happens very rarely.
- Any medication can cause a severe allergic reaction. Such reactions from a vaccine are very rare, estimated at about one in a million doses, and would happen within a few minutes to a few hours after the vaccination.

As with any medicine, there is a very remote chance of a vaccine causing a serious injury or death.

Inactivated Influenza Vaccine Side Effects
What Are the Risks from Inactivated Influenza Vaccine?

With any medicine, including vaccines, there is a chance of reactions. These are usually mild and go away on their own, but serious reactions are also possible.

Most people who get a flu shot do not have any problems with it.

Minor problems following a flu shot include:

- Soreness, redness, or swelling where the shot was given
- Hoarseness
- Sore, red or itchy eyes
- Cough
- Fever
- Aches
- Headache
- Itching
- Fatigue

If these problems occur, they usually begin soon after the shot and last one or two days.

More serious problems following a flu shot can include the following:

- There may be a small increased risk of Guillain-Barré Syndrome (GBS) after the inactivated flu vaccine. This risk has been estimated at one or two additional cases per million people vaccinated. This is much lower than the risk of severe complications from flu, which can be prevented by flu vaccine.

- Young children who get the flu shot along with the pneumococcal vaccine (PCV13), and/or the DTaP vaccine at the same time might be slightly more likely to have a seizure caused by fever. Ask your doctor for more information. Tell your doctor if a child who is getting a flu vaccine has ever had a seizure.

Problems that could happen after any injected vaccine:

- People sometimes faint after a medical procedure, including vaccination. Sitting or lying down for about 15 minutes can help prevent fainting and injuries caused by a fall. Tell your doctor if you feel dizzy or have vision changes or ringing in the ears.

- Some people get severe pain in the shoulder and have difficulty moving the arm where the shot was given. This happens very rarely.

- Any medication can cause a severe allergic reaction. Such reactions from a vaccine are very rare, estimated at about one in a million doses, and would happen within a few minutes to a few hours after the vaccination.

As with any medicine, there is a very remote chance of a vaccine causing a serious injury or death.

Live Influenza Vaccine Side Effects
What Are the Risks from Live Attenuated Influenza Vaccine?

With any medicine, including vaccines, there is a chance of reactions. These are usually mild and go away on their own, but serious reactions are also possible.

Most people who get the live attenuated influenza vaccine (LAIV) do not have any problems with it. Reactions to LAIV may resemble a very mild case of flu.

Problems that have been reported following LAIV: Children and adolescents between 2 and 17 years of age:

- Runny nose/nasal congestion

- Cough

- Fever

- Headache and muscle aches

- Wheezing

- Abdominal pain, vomiting, or diarrhea

Adults between 18 and 49 years of age:

- Runny nose/nasal congestion

- Sore throat

- Cough

- Chills

- Tiredness/weakness

- Headache

Problems that could happen after any vaccine:

- Any medication can cause a severe allergic reaction. Such reactions from a vaccine are very rare, estimated at about one in

651

a million doses, and would happen within a few minutes to a few hours after the vaccination.

As with any medicine, there is a very small chance of a vaccine causing a serious injury or death.

Measles, Mumps, and Rubella Vaccine Side Effects
What Are the Risks from the Measles, Mumps, and Rubella Vaccine?

With any medicine, including vaccines, there is a chance of reactions. These are usually mild and go away on their own, but serious reactions are also possible.

Getting the measles, mumps, and rubella (MMR) vaccine is much safer than getting measles, mumps, or rubella disease. Most people who get MMR vaccine do not have any problems with it.

After MMR vaccination, a person might experience:

Minor events:

• Sore arm from the injection

• Fever

• Redness or rash at the injection site

• Swelling of glands in the cheeks or neck

If these events happen, they usually begin within two weeks after the shot. They occur less often after the second dose.

Moderate events:

• Seizure (jerking or staring) often associated with fever

• Temporary pain and stiffness in the joints, mostly in teenage or adult women

• Temporary low platelet count, which can cause unusual bleeding or bruising

• Rash all over the body

Severe events occur very rarely:

• Deafness

• Long-term seizures, coma, or lowered consciousness

• Brain damage

Other things that could happen after this vaccine:

- People sometimes faint after medical procedures, including vaccination. Sitting or lying down for about 15 minutes can help prevent fainting and injuries caused by a fall. Tell your provider if you feel dizzy or have vision changes or ringing in the ears.

- Some people get shoulder pain that can be more severe and last longer than routine soreness that can follow injections. This happens very rarely.

- Any medication can cause a severe allergic reaction. Such reactions to a vaccine are estimated at about one in a million doses, and would happen within a few minutes to a few hours after the vaccination.

As with any medicine, there is a very remote chance of a vaccine causing a serious injury or death.

Measles, Mumps, Rubella, and Varicella Vaccine Side Effects

What Are the Risks from Measles, Mumps, Rubella, and Varicella Vaccine?

With any medicine, including vaccines, there is a chance of reactions. These are usually mild and go away on their own, but serious reactions are also possible.

Getting the measles, mumps, rubella, and varicella (MMRV) vaccine is much safer than getting measles, mumps, rubella, or chickenpox disease. Most children who get the MMRV vaccine do not have any problems with it.

After MMRV vaccination, a child might experience:

Minor events:

- Sore arm from the injection

- Fever

- Redness or rash at the injection site

- Swelling of glands in the cheeks or neck

If these events happen, they usually begin within two weeks after the shot. They occur less often after the second dose.

Moderate events:

- Seizure often associated with fever

- The risk of these seizures is higher after MMRV than after separate MMR and chickenpox vaccines when given as the first dose of the series. Your doctor can advise you about the appropriate vaccines for your child.

- Temporary low platelet count, which can cause unusual bleeding or bruising

- Infection of the lungs (pneumonia) or the brain and spinal cord coverings (encephalitis, meningitis)

- Rash all over the body

If your child gets a rash after vaccination, it might be related to the varicella component of the vaccine. A child who has a rash after the MMRV vaccination might be able to spread the varicella vaccine virus to an unprotected person. Even though this happens very rarely, children who develop a rash should stay away from people with weakened immune systems and unvaccinated infants until the rash goes away.

Severe events have very rarely been reported following MMR vaccination and might also happen after MMRV. These include:

- Deafness

- Long-term seizures, coma, lowered consciousness

- Brain damage

Other things that could happen after this vaccine:

- People sometimes faint after medical procedures, including vaccination. Sitting or lying down for about 15 minutes can help prevent fainting and injuries caused by a fall. Tell your provider if you feel dizzy or have vision changes or ringing in the ears.

- Some people get shoulder pain that can be more severe and last longer than routine soreness that can follow injections. This happens very rarely.

- Any medication can cause a severe allergic reaction. Such reactions to a vaccine are estimated at about one in a million doses, and would happen a few minutes to a few hours after the vaccination.

As with any medicine, there is a very remote chance of a vaccine causing a serious injury or death.

Meningococcal ACWY Vaccine Side Effects
What Are the Risks from Meningococcal Vaccines?

With any medicine, including vaccines, there is a chance of side effects. These are usually mild and go away on their own within a few days, but serious reactions are also possible.

As many as half of the people who get meningococcal ACWY vaccine have mild problems following vaccination, such as redness or soreness where the shot was given. If these problems occur, they usually last for one or two days.

A small percentage of people who receive the vaccine experience muscle or joint pains.

Problems That Could Happen after Any Injected Vaccine

- People sometimes faint after a medical procedure, including vaccination. Sitting or lying down for about 15 minutes can help prevent fainting, and injuries caused by a fall. Tell your doctor if you feel dizzy or light-headed or have vision changes.

- Some people get severe pain in the shoulder and have difficulty moving the arm where the shot was given. This happens very rarely.

- Any medication can cause a severe allergic reaction. Such reactions from a vaccine are very rare, estimated at about 1 in a million doses, and would happen within a few minutes to a few hours after the vaccination.

As with any medicine, there is a very remote chance of a vaccine causing a serious injury or death.

Pneumococcal Conjugate Vaccine Side Effects
What Are the Risks from Pneumococcal Conjugate Vaccine?

With any medicine, including vaccines, there is a chance of reactions. These are usually mild and go away on their own, but serious reactions are also possible.

Problems reported following pneumococcal conjugate vaccine (PCV13) varied by age and dose in the series. The most common problems reported among children were:

- About half became drowsy after the shot, had a temporary loss of appetite, or had redness or tenderness where the shot was given.

- About 1 out of 3 had swelling where the shot was given.

- About 1 out of 3 had a mild fever, and about 1 in 20 had a fever over 102.2°F.

- Up to about 8 out of 10 became fussy or irritable.

Adults have reported pain, redness, and swelling where the shot was given, as well as mild fever, fatigue, headache, chills, or muscle pain.

Young children who get PCV13 along with the inactivated flu vaccine at the same time may be at an increased risk for seizures caused by fever. Ask your doctor for more information.

Problems that could happen after any vaccine:

- People sometimes faint after a medical procedure, including vaccination. Sitting or lying down for about 15 minutes can help prevent fainting and injuries caused by a fall. Tell your doctor if you feel dizzy or have vision changes or ringing in the ears.

- Some older children and adults get severe pain in the shoulder and have difficulty moving the arm where the shot was given. This happens very rarely.

- Any medication can cause a severe allergic reaction. Such reactions from a vaccine are very rare, estimated at about one in a million doses, and would happen within a few minutes to a few hours after the vaccination.

As with any medicine, there is a very small chance of a vaccine causing a serious injury or death.

Pneumococcal Polysaccharide Vaccine Side Effects
What Are the Risks from Pneumococcal Polysaccharide?

With any medicine, including vaccines, there is a chance of side effects. These are usually mild and go away on their own, but serious reactions are also possible.

About half of people who get the pneumococcal polysaccharide vaccine (PPSV) have mild side effects, such as redness or pain where the shot is given, which go away within about two days.

Less than 1 out of 100 people develop a fever, muscle aches, or more severe local reactions.

Problems that could happen after any vaccine:

- People sometimes faint after a medical procedure, including vaccination. Sitting or lying down for about 15 minutes can help prevent fainting and injuries caused by a fall. Tell your doctor if you feel dizzy or have vision changes or ringing in the ears.

- Some people get severe pain in the shoulder and have difficulty moving the arm where the shot was given. This happens very rarely.

- Any medication can cause a severe allergic reaction. Such reactions from a vaccine are very rare, estimated at about one in a million doses, and would happen within a few minutes to a few hours after the vaccination.

As with any medicine, there is a very remote chance of a vaccine causing a serious injury or death.

Polio Vaccine Side Effects

With any medicine, including vaccines, there is a chance of side effects. These are usually mild and go away on their own, but serious reactions are also possible.

Some people who get inactivated polio vaccine (IPV) get a sore spot where the shot was given. IPV has not been known to cause serious problems, and most people do not have any problems with it.

Other problems that could happen after this vaccine:

- People sometimes faint after a medical procedure, including vaccination. Sitting or lying down for about 15 minutes can help prevent fainting and injuries caused by a fall. Tell your provider if you feel dizzy or have vision changes or ringing in the ears.

- Some people get shoulder pain that can be more severe and last longer than the more routine soreness that can follow injections. This happens very rarely.

- Any medication can cause a severe allergic reaction. Such reactions from a vaccine are very rare, estimated at about one in a million doses, and would happen within a few minutes to a few hours after the vaccination.

- As with any medicine, there is a very remote chance of a vaccine causing a serious injury or death.

657

Rabies Vaccine Side Effects
What Are the Risks from Rabies Vaccine?

A vaccine, as with any medicine, is capable of causing serious problems, such as severe allergic reactions. The risk of a vaccine causing serious harm or death is extremely small. Serious problems from rabies vaccine are very rare.

Mild problems:

- Soreness, redness, swelling, or itching where the shot was given (30 to 74%)
- Headache, nausea, abdominal pain, muscle aches, dizziness (5 to 40%)

Moderate problems:

- Pain in the joints, fever (about 6 percent of booster doses)

Other nervous system disorders, such as Guillain Barré syndrome (GBS), have been reported after rabies vaccine, but this happens so rarely that it is not known whether they are related to the vaccine.

Rotavirus Vaccine Side Effects
What Are the Risks from Rotavirus Vaccine?

With a vaccine, as with any medicine, there is a chance of side effects. These are usually mild and go away on their own. Serious side effects are also possible but are rare.

Most babies who get rotavirus vaccine do not have any problems with it. But, some problems have been associated with rotavirus vaccine:

Mild problems following rotavirus vaccine:

- Babies might become irritable, or have mild, temporary diarrhea or vomiting after getting a dose of rotavirus vaccine.

Serious problems following rotavirus vaccine:

- Intussusception is a type of bowel blockage that is treated in a hospital and could require surgery. It happens naturally in some babies every year in the United States, and usually, there is no known reason for it.

There is also a small risk of intussusception from rotavirus vaccination, usually within a week after the first or second vaccine dose. This additional risk is estimated to range from about 1 in 20,000 to 1 in 100,000 U.S. infants who get rotavirus vaccine. Your doctor can give you more information.

Problems that could happen after any vaccine:

- Any medication can cause a severe allergic reaction. Such reactions from a vaccine are very rare, estimated at fewer than one in a million doses, and usually happen within a few minutes to a few hours after the vaccination.

As with any medicine, there is a very remote chance of a vaccine causing a serious injury or death.

Adult Tetanus and Diphtheria Vaccine
What Are the Risks from Adult Tetanus and Diphtheria Vaccine?

With any medicine, including vaccines, there is a chance of side effects. These are usually mild and go away on their own. Serious reactions are also possible but are rare.

Most people who get an adult tetanus and diphtheria (Td) vaccine do not have any problems with it.

Mild problems following Td vaccine:
(Did not interfere with activities)

- Pain where the shot was given (about 8 people in 10)

- Redness or swelling where the shot was given (about 1 person in 4)

- Mild fever (rare)

- Headache (about 1 person in 4)

- Tiredness (about 1 person in 4)

Moderate problems following Td vaccine:
(Interfered with activities, but did not require medical attention)

- Fever over 102°F (rare)

Severe problems following Td vaccine:
(Unable to perform usual activities; required medical attention)

- Swelling, severe pain, bleeding and/or redness in the arm where the shot was given (rare).

Problems that could happen after any vaccine:

- People sometimes faint after a medical procedure, including vaccination. Sitting or lying down for about 15 minutes can help prevent fainting and injuries caused by a fall. Tell your doctor if you feel dizzy or have vision changes or ringing in the ears.

- Some people get severe pain in the shoulder and have difficulty moving the arm where the shot was given. This happens very rarely.

- Any medication can cause a severe allergic reaction. Such reactions from a vaccine are very rare, estimated at fewer than one in a million doses, and would happen within a few minutes to a few hours after the vaccination.

As with any medicine, there is a very remote chance of a vaccine causing a serious injury or death.

Combined Tetanus, Diphtheria, and Pertussis Vaccine
What Are the Risks from the Combined Tetanus, Diphtheria, and Pertussis Vaccine?

With any medicine, including vaccines, there is a chance of side effects. These are usually mild and go away on their own. Serious reactions are also possible but are rare.

Most people who get the combined tetanus, diphtheria, and pertussis (Tdap) vaccine do not have any problems with it.

Mild problems following Tdap:
(Did not interfere with activities)

- Pain where the shot was given (about 3 in 4 adolescents or 2 in 3 adults)

- Redness or swelling where the shot was given (about 1 person in 5)

- Mild fever of at least 100.4°F (up to about 1 in 25 adolescents or 1 in 100 adults)

- Headache (about 3 or 4 people in 10)

- Tiredness (about 1 person in 3 or 4)

- Nausea, vomiting, diarrhea, stomach ache (up to 1 in 4 adolescents or 1 in 10 adults)

- Chills, sore joints (about 1 person in 10)

- Body aches (about 1 person in 3 or 4)

- Rash, swollen glands (uncommon)

Moderate problems following Tdap:
(Interfered with activities, but did not require medical attention)

- Pain where the shot was given (up to 1 in 5 or 6)

- Redness or swelling where the shot was given (up to about 1 in 16 adolescents or 1 in 12 adults)

- Fever over 102°F (about 1 in 100 adolescents or 1 in 250 adults)

- Headache (about 1 in 7 adolescents or 1 in 10 adults)

- Nausea, vomiting, diarrhea, stomach ache (up to 1 or 3 people in 100)

- Swelling of the entire arm where the shot was given (up to about 1 in 500).

Severe problems following Tdap:
(Unable to perform usual activities; required medical attention)

- Swelling, severe pain, bleeding, and redness in the arm where the shot was given (rare)

Problems that could happen after any vaccine:

- People sometimes faint after a medical procedure, including vaccination. Sitting or lying down for about 15 minutes can help prevent fainting and injuries caused by a fall. Tell your doctor if you feel dizzy or have vision changes or ringing in the ears.

- Some people get severe pain in the shoulder and have difficulty moving the arm where the shot was given. This happens very rarely.

- Any medication can cause a severe allergic reaction. Such reactions from a vaccine are very rare, estimated at fewer than one in a million doses, and would happen within a few minutes to a few hours after the vaccination.

As with any medicine, there is a very remote chance of a vaccine causing a serious injury or death.

The safety of vaccines is always being monitored. With any medicine, including vaccines, there is a chance of side effects. These are usually mild and go away on their own. Serious reactions are also possible but are rare.

Most people who get Td vaccine do not have any problems with it.

Mild problems following Td vaccine:
(Did not interfere with activities)

- Pain where the shot was given (about 8 people in 10)

- Redness or swelling where the shot was given (about 1 person in 4)

- Mild fever (rare)

- Headache (about 1 person in 4)

- Tiredness (about 1 person in 4)

Moderate problems following Td vaccine:
(Interfered with activities, but did not require medical attention)

- Fever over 102°F (rare)

Severe problems following Td vaccine:
(Unable to perform usual activities; required medical attention)

- Swelling, severe pain, bleeding and/or redness in the arm where the shot was given (rare)

Problems that could happen after any vaccine:

- People sometimes faint after a medical procedure, including vaccination. Sitting or lying down for about 15 minutes can help prevent fainting and injuries caused by a fall. Tell your doctor if you feel dizzy or have vision changes or ringing in the ears.

- Some people get severe pain in the shoulder and have difficulty moving the arm where the shot was given. This happens very rarely.

- Any medication can cause a severe allergic reaction. Such reactions from a vaccine are very rare, estimated at fewer than one in a million doses, and would happen within a few minutes to a few hours after the vaccination.

As with any medicine, there is a very remote chance of a vaccine causing a serious injury or death.

Varicella Vaccine Side Effects
What Are the Risks from the Varicella Vaccine?

With any medicine, including vaccines, there is a chance of reactions. These are usually mild and go away on their own, but serious reactions are also possible.

Getting the chickenpox vaccine is much safer than getting chickenpox disease. Most people who get the chickenpox vaccine do not have any problems with it.

After chickenpox vaccination, a person might experience:

Minor events:

- Sore arm from the injection

- Fever

- Redness or rash at the injection site

If these events happen, they usually begin within two weeks after the shot. They occur less often after the second dose.

More serious events following chickenpox vaccination are rare. They can include:

- Seizure often associated with fever

- Infection of the lungs or the brain and spinal cord coverings (meningitis)

- Rash all over the body

A person who develops a rash after chickenpox vaccination might be able to spread the varicella vaccine virus to an unprotected person. Even though this happens very rarely, anyone who gets a rash should stay away from people with weakened immune systems and unvaccinated infants until the rash goes away. Talk with your healthcare provider to learn more.

Other things that could happen after this vaccine:

- People sometimes faint after medical procedures, including vaccination. Sitting or lying down for about 15 minutes can help prevent fainting and injuries caused by a fall. Tell your doctor if you feel dizzy or have vision changes or ringing in the ears.

- Some people get shoulder pain that can be more severe and last longer than routine soreness that can follow injections. This happens very rarely.

- Any medication can cause a severe allergic reaction. Such reactions to a vaccine are estimated at about one in a million doses, and would happen within a few minutes to a few hours after the vaccination.

As with any medicine, there is a very remote chance of a vaccine causing a serious injury or death.

Chapter 80

Vaccine Adverse Event Reporting System

About Vaccine Adverse Event Reporting System

The Vaccine Adverse Event Reporting System (VAERS) is a national vaccine safety surveillance program run by the Centers for Disease Control and Prevention (CDC) and the U.S. Food and Drug Administration (FDA). The VAERS serves as an early warning system to detect possible safety issues with U.S. vaccines by collecting information about adverse events (possible side effects or health problems) that occur after vaccination.

The VAERS was created in 1990 in response to the National Childhood Vaccine Injury Act. If any health problem happens after vaccination, anyone—doctors, nurses, vaccine manufacturers, and any member of the general public—can submit a report to the VAERS.

How the Vaccine Adverse Event Reporting System Is Used

The VAERS is used to detect possible safety problems—called "signals"—that may be related to vaccination. If a vaccine safety signal is identified through the VAERS, scientists may conduct further studies to find out if the signal represents an actual risk.

This chapter includes text excerpted from "Vaccine Adverse Event Reporting System (VAERS)," Centers for Disease Control and Prevention (CDC), August 28, 2015. Reviewed July 2019.

665

The main goals of the VAERS are to:

- Detect new, unusual, or rare adverse events that happen after vaccination

- Monitor increases in known side effects, such as arm soreness where the shot was given

- Identify potential patient risk factors for particular types of health problems related to vaccines

- Assess the safety of newly licensed vaccines

- Watch for unexpected or unusual patterns in adverse event reports

- Serve as a monitoring system in public health emergencies

What to Report to the Vaccine Adverse Event Reporting System

Anyone who gives or receives a licensed vaccine in the United States is encouraged to report any significant health problem that occurs after vaccination. An adverse event can be reported even if it is uncertain or unlikely that the vaccine caused it. Reporting to the VAERS helps scientists at the CDC and the FDA better understand the safety of vaccines.

What Happens after a Vaccine Adverse Event Reporting System Report Is Submitted

Each VAERS report is assigned a VAERS identification number. This number can be used to provide additional information to the VAERS if necessary. The CDC or the FDA scientists follow up on selected cases of serious adverse events immediately by obtaining medical records to better understand the event. Then, letters are sent one year after vaccination to check the recovery status of the patient for all serious reports that listed recovery status as "not recovered" on the initial report.

What We Can Learn from Vaccine Adverse Event Reporting System Data

Approximately 30,000 VAERS reports are filed each year. About 85 to 90 percent of the reports describe mild side effects, such as fever, arm soreness, and crying or mild irritability. The remaining reports are classified as serious, which means that the adverse event resulted in permanent disability, hospitalization, life-threatening illness, or death. While these problems happen after vaccination, they are rarely caused by the vaccine.

The VAERS form collects information about:

- The type of vaccine received

- The timing of the vaccination

- The onset of the adverse event

- Current illnesses or medication

- Past history of adverse events following vaccination

- Demographic information

The FDA and the CDC use VAERS data to monitor vaccine safety and conduct research studies.

Strengths and Limitations of Vaccine Adverse Event Reporting System Data

When evaluating the VAERS data, it is important to understand the strengths and limitations. The VAERS data contain both coincidental events and those truly caused by vaccines.

Table 80.1. Strengths and Limitations of Vaccine Adverse Event Reporting System Data

Strengths	Limitations
VAERS collects national data from all U.S. states and territories.	It is generally not possible to find out from VAERS data if a vaccine caused the adverse event.
VAERS accepts reports from anyone.	Reports submitted to VAERS often lack details and sometimes contain errors.
The VAERS form collects information about the vaccine, the person vaccinated, and the adverse event.	Serious adverse events are more likely to be reported than mild side effects.
Data are publicly available.	Rate of reports may increase in response to media attention and increased public awareness.
VAERS can be used as an early warning system to identify rare adverse events.	It is not possible to use VAERS data to calculate how often an adverse event occurs in a population.

Table 80.1. Continued

Strengths	Limitations
It is possible to follow up with patients to obtain health records, when necessary.	

How to Access Vaccine Adverse Event Reporting System Data

The VAERS data (without patient information) are publicly available online through a system called "VAERS WONDER" (wonder.cdc. gov/vaers.html).

Chapter 81

Vaccination Records

Adult Vaccination Records

Your vaccination record (sometimes called "your immunization record") provides a history of all the vaccines you received as a child and adult. This record may be required for certain jobs, travel abroad, or school registration.

How to Locate Your Vaccination Records

Unfortunately, there is no national organization that maintains vaccination records. The Centers for Disease Control and Prevention (CDC) does not have this information. The records that exist are the ones you or your parents were given when the vaccines were administered and the ones in the medical record of the doctor or clinic where the vaccines were given.

If you need official copies of vaccination records, or if you need to update your personal records, there are several places you can look:

- Ask your parents or other caregivers if they have records of your childhood immunizations.

This chapter contains text excerpted from the following sources: Text under the heading "Adult Vaccination Records" is excerpted from "Keeping Your Vaccine Records Up to Date," Centers for Disease Control and Prevention (CDC), May 2, 2016; Text under the heading "Vaccination Records for Kids" is excerpted from "For Parents: Vaccines for Your Children," Centers for Disease Control and Prevention (CDC), May 17, 2019.

- Try looking through baby books or other saved documents from your childhood.

- Check with your high school and/or college health services for dates of any immunizations. Keep in mind that generally records are kept only for one to two years after students leave the system.

- Check with previous employers (including the military) that may have required immunizations.

- Check with your doctor or public health clinic. Keep in mind that vaccination records are maintained at the doctor's office for a limited number of years.

- Contact your state's health department. Some states have registries (Immunization Information Systems) that include adult vaccines.

What to Do If You Cannot Find Your Records

If you cannot find your personal records or records from the doctor, you may need to get some of the vaccines again. While this is not ideal, it is safe to repeat vaccines. The doctor can also sometimes do blood tests to see if you are immune to certain vaccine-preventable diseases.

Tools to Record Your Vaccinations

People move, travel, and change healthcare providers more than previous generations. Finding old immunization information can be difficult and time-consuming. Therefore, it is critical that you keep an accurate and up-to-date record of the vaccinations you have received. Keeping an immunization record and storing it with other important documents (or in a safe place) will save you time and unnecessary hassle.

Ask your doctor, pharmacist, or another vaccine provider for an immunization record. Bring this record with you to health visits, and ask your vaccine provider to sign and date the form for each vaccine you receive. That way, you can be sure that the immunization information is current and correct.

If your vaccine provider participates in an immunization registry, ask that your vaccines be documented there as well.

Vaccination Records for Kids

It's extremely important for you to track your child's vaccination records, especially if your state requires certain vaccines for child care or school.

Saving Your Child's Vaccination Records

Good record-keeping begins with good record-taking. Start tracking your child's vaccination records as soon as your child gets his or her first shot when he or she is born. You can keep track of your child's records by:

- Getting a vaccination tracking card from your child's doctor or your state health department.
- Printing and using the CDC's birth-6 years well-visit immunization and developmental tracker (www.cdc.gov/vaccines/parents/downloads/milestones-tracker.pdf).
- Asking your doctor to enter the vaccines your child has received in your state's immunization information system (IIS). An IIS is a statewide immunization registry doctors and public health clinics use to save and update vaccination records.

When you maintain a copy of your child's vaccination record:

- Keep the record in a safe place where you can easily locate it.
- Bring it to each of your child's doctor visits.
- Ask the doctor or nurse to jot down the vaccine given, date, and dosage on your child's vaccination record.
- Write down the name of the doctor's office or clinic where your child got the shot so you know where to get official records when you need them.

It is important for you to save and update your child's vaccine records, since you will likely be required to provide them when you register your child for school, child care, summer camp, or an athletic team. You may also need up-to-date records when your child travels internationally.

Finding Official Vaccination Records

If you do not have a copy of your child's vaccine records or can't find them, you may be able to retrieve an official copy by contacting your:

- Child's doctor or clinic

  - Doctors and public health clinics usually track any shots they give to your child.

  - If your child has had more than one doctor or clinic give him or her shots, call or visit each one to get the records.

  - Keep in mind doctors and clinics may only save vaccination records for a few years.

- States' immunization registry

  - Your state's immunization registry may have most, if not all, of your child's records.

  - Contact your state's registry to request an official copy.

  - Please be aware that the process for requesting records can vary greatly across states and can take some time to complete.

  - Additionally, if your state does not automatically opt-in its residents or you requested to opt out your child from the registry, then the vaccination records won't be available.

- Child's school

  - Most K–12 schools, colleges, and universities keep on file the vaccination records of its students.

  - Take into account that schools generally keep these records for only a year or two after the student graduates, transfers to another school, or leaves the school system. If you need records from a college or university, contact the corresponding medical services or student health department.

What If You Cannot Find Your Child's Records

Your child should be considered susceptible to disease and should be vaccinated (or revaccinated) if you cannot find his or her records or their records are incomplete. It is safe for your child to receive a vaccine, even if he or she may have already received it. Alternatively, your child could also have their blood tested for antibodies to determine his or her immunity to certain diseases. However, these tests may not always be accurate and doctors may prefer to revaccinate your child for best protection. Talk to your child's doctor to determine what vaccines your child needs for protection against vaccine-preventable diseases.

Chapter 82

Vaccine Misinformation May Have Tragic Consequences

Vaccines

Vaccines are generally made from weakened strains of disease-causing microbes that are not virulent enough to cause an infection. When they are introduced to the body, the immune system learns to produce cells that can defeat the infection, thus making the body capable of resisting the disease in the future.

The Success of Vaccination

Immunization programs have been very successful at controlling infectious diseases. More than 200 years ago, British physician Edward Jenner pioneered the smallpox vaccine. Smallpox has since been eradicated worldwide, and it is estimated that five million lives are saved annually as a result of the smallpox vaccine. This achievement should be compelling evidence that vaccines work, and do so astonishingly well.

In total, the United Nations International Children's Emergency Fund (UNICEF) estimates that immunization saves approximately nine million lives annually the world over. In addition to smallpox, vaccination has brought under control such diseases as diphtheria, tetanus, yellow fever, whooping cough, polio, and measles.

Misinformation about Vaccines

A report by the Centers for Disease Control and Prevention (CDC) estimated that 77 percent of U.S. children between 19 and 35 months of age were being fully immunized with the recommended vaccinations. Reasons for the remaining 33 percent being either not immunized or under-immunized include limited healthcare access, financial barriers, and misconceptions about vaccinations and vaccine safety.

Misinformation about vaccines has existed as long as vaccines themselves. Parents who delay or refuse vaccination because of misinformation can place their own children, as well as other children, at risk of contracting preventable diseases.

The anti-vaccine debate increased in intensity with the publication of a study by Dr. Andrew Wakefield in the scientific journal Lancet in 1998, which concluded that autism was linked to the measles, mumps, and rubella vaccine (MMR). This led to ripples in the medical community and spread panic among some parents, celebrities, and politicians, with a resultant drop in vaccination rates. The study was later declared a fraud, and Wakefield was stripped of his medical license.

Why Would Parents Willingly Put Their Children at Risk of Vaccine-Preventable Diseases?

- The absence of societal fear is one factor. For centuries, people lived in terror of communicable diseases, but immunization resulted in lower incidences of such illnesses, and subsequent generations have not been exposed to such diseases as polio, rubella, and diphtheria. The absence of disease visibility has resulted in a lack of community fear, so in a sense the immunization program has become a victim of its own success. But, fortunately, the majority of parents have continued to realize that vaccination is essential for the safety of their children and the benefit of community health.

- The timing of vaccinations makes them scapegoats for various disorders that may occur around the same time as immunization. Children of vaccination age are often subject to a number of minor illnesses, but just because a disorder is detected at the time of vaccination does not necessarily indicate that vaccination caused the disorder. Additionally, fever is a common side effect of vaccination, but life-threatening reactions are very rare, and most medical professionals advise that this and other minor side effects should not be a deterrent to the protection offered by immunization.

- Uninformed people may disseminate misinformation. Parents rely on multiple resources for information about vaccines, including websites, family members, friends, and celebrities, some of whom could be seriously misinformed.

- A person often perceives risk based on his or her limited experiences and knowledge. Someone who has come across the child of a family member or friend who had an adverse reaction to vaccination might perceive it as overly risky. People also tend to tolerate natural risks (infectious diseases) more easily than man-made risks (vaccination side effects). Risks that have clear benefits associated with them are generally tolerated better than risks with benefits that are not immediate or not understood well.

Vaccination in the United States

All 50 U.S. states mandate that children be vaccinated against certain diseases before they enter school. Children who have health conditions that could be exacerbated by vaccination can seek to be exempted. And, except for Mississippi, all states allow religious exemptions, while exemptions based on personal and moral beliefs are allowed in 20 states.

The Consequences of Misinformation

Vaccination rates are still high in the United States, but requests for exemptions have increased. Since the chances of contracting a vaccine-preventable infection is quite small in the United States, what is the risk?

The danger lies in clusters of communities in which like-minded anti-vaccination parents live. In 1991, a measles outbreak occurred in Philadelphia in schools run by fundamentalist churches. About 350 children attending these schools were not immunized, and the infection spread to 1,500 children, leading to nine fatalities.

Pockets of unvaccinated children exist around the nation, particularly in the states of California, Utah, Oregon, and Washington. Vaccine exemptions are particularly high in Washington, where some elementary schools have an exemption rate of 43 percent. Nevertheless, overall vaccination rates in these states remain relatively high.

Measles was declared to have been eliminated in the United States in the year 2000. But in 2015, a measles outbreak occurred at Disneyland in California. It turned into a large-scale outbreak that spread to 13 states across the country and affected 147 people. The disease was determined to have been primarily carried by unvaccinated children whose parents put them and other children at risk by taking them to a crowded public place.

That the outbreak was contained serves as testament to the success of vaccination programs. It also demonstrates that science by itself cannot totally overcome the detrimental effects of virulent misinformation. The risks of immunization are very negligible, while the advantages are great and the repercussions of not vaccinating are extremely high. Vaccines are backed by more than a century of scientific research and safeguards. They are rigorously tested, and effective systems ensure potency, purity, and safety.

Children need to be protected against preventable diseases by ensuring vaccination. And this seems to be possible only if we inoculate ourselves with facts.

References

1. Patel, Kavita and Hart, Rio. "What the Anti-Vaxxers Are Getting Dangerously Wrong," Brookings, February 6, 2015.

2. Myers, Martin G., and Pineda, Diego. "Misinformation about Vaccines," AutismTruths, n.d.

3. Parker, Laura. "The Anti-Vaccine Generation: How Movement against Shots Got Its Start," National Geographic, February 6, 2015.

4. "Vaccinating Ourselves Against Misinformation," Union of Concerned Scientists, February 2015.

Chapter 83

What Would Happen If We Stopped Vaccinations?

Before the middle of the last century, diseases such as whooping cough, polio, measles, *Haemophilus influenzae*, and rubella struck hundreds of thousands of infants, children, and adults in the United States. Thousands died every year from them. As vaccines were developed and became widely used, rates of these diseases declined, and most of them are nearly gone from our country at present.

- Nearly everyone in the United States got measles before there was a vaccine, and hundreds died from it each year. At present, most doctors have never seen a case of measles.

- More than 15,000 Americans died from diphtheria in 1921, before there was a vaccine. Only 2 cases of diphtheria have been reported to the Centers for Disease Control and Prevention (CDC) between 2004 and 2014.

- An epidemic of rubella (German measles) in 1964 to 1965 infected 12½ million Americans, killed 2,000 babies, and caused 11,000 miscarriages. Since 2012, 15 cases of rubella were reported to the CDC.

This chapter includes text excerpted from "What Would Happen If We Stopped Vaccinations?" Centers for Disease Control and Prevention (CDC), June 29, 2018.

Given successes like these, it might seem reasonable to ask, "Why should we keep vaccinating against diseases that we will probably never see?" Here is why:

Vaccines Do Not Just Protect Yourself

Most vaccine-preventable diseases are spread from person to person. If one person in a community gets an infectious disease, she or he can spread it to others who are not immune. But, a person who is immune to a disease because she or he has been vaccinated cannot get that disease and cannot spread it to others. The more people who are vaccinated, the fewer opportunities a disease has to spread.

If one or two cases of the disease are introduced into a community where most people are not vaccinated, outbreaks will occur. In 2013, for example, several measles outbreaks occurred around the country, including large outbreaks in New York City and Texas—mainly among groups with low vaccination rates. If vaccination rates dropped to low levels nationally, diseases could become as common as they were before vaccines.

Diseases Have Not Disappeared

The United States has very low rates of vaccine-preventable diseases, but this is not true everywhere in the world. Only one disease—smallpox—has been totally erased from the planet. Polio is close to being eliminated, but it still exists in several countries. More than 350,000 cases of measles were reported from around the world in 2011, with outbreaks in the Pacific, Asia, Africa, and Europe. In that same year, 90 percent of measles cases in the United States were associated with cases imported from another country. Only the fact that most Americans are vaccinated against measles prevented these clusters of cases from becoming epidemics.

Disease rates are low in the United States. But, if we let ourselves become vulnerable by not vaccinating, a case that could touch off an outbreak of some disease that is under control is just a plane ride away.

A Final Example: What Could Happen

We know that a disease that is apparently under control can suddenly return because we have seen it happen in countries such as Japan, Australia, and Sweden. Here is an example from Japan. In 1974, about 80 percent of Japanese children were getting pertussis (whooping cough) vaccine. That year, there were only 393 cases of whooping cough in the entire country and not a single pertussis-related death. Then immunization rates began to drop, until only about 10 percent of children were being vaccinated. In 1979, more than 13,000 people got whooping cough, and 41 died. When routine vaccination was resumed, the disease numbers dropped again.

The chances of your child getting a case of measles, chickenpox, or whooping cough might be quite low at present. But, vaccinations are not just for protecting ourselves and are not just for today. They also protect the people around us (some of whom may be unable to get certain vaccines, might have failed to respond to a vaccine, or might be susceptible for other reasons). And they also protect our children's children and their children by keeping diseases that we have almost defeated from making a comeback. What would happen if we stopped vaccinations? We could soon find ourselves battling epidemics of diseases we thought we had conquered decades ago.

Chapter 84

Preventing Transmission of Infections in Hospitals and Nursing Homes

Chapter Contents

Section 84.1—Tips for Patients to Prevent
Healthcare-Associated Infections 682

Section 84.2—Prevention and Control of Influenza
in Healthcare Settings 683

Section 84.1

Tips for Patients to Prevent Healthcare-Associated Infections

This section includes text excerpted from "Patient Safety: What You Can Do to Be a Safe Patient," Centers for Disease Control and Prevention (CDC), March 26, 2014. Reviewed July 2019.

Every day, patients get infections in healthcare facilities while they are being treated for something else. These infections can have devastating emotional, financial, and medical effects. Worst of all, they can be deadly.

Healthcare procedures can leave you vulnerable to germs that cause healthcare-associated infections (HAIs). These germs can be spread in healthcare settings from patient to patient on unclean hands of healthcare personnel or through the improper use or reuse of equipment.

These infections are not limited to hospitals. For example, in the past 10 years alone, there have been more than 30 outbreaks of hepatitis B and hepatitis C in nonhospital healthcare settings, such as outpatient clinics, dialysis centers, and long-term care facilities.

What Patients Can Do

1. **Speak up.**

   Talk to your doctor about all questions or worries you have. Ask them what they are doing to protect you.

   • If you have a catheter, ask each day if it is necessary.

   • Ask your doctor how she or he prevents surgical site infections (SSIs). Also, ask how you can prepare for surgery to reduce your infection risk.

2. **Keep hands clean.**

   Be sure everyone cleans their hands before touching you.

3. **Get smart.**

   Ask if tests will be done to make sure the right antibiotic is prescribed.

4. **Know the signs and symptoms of infection.**

   Some skin infections, such as methicillin-resistant *Staphylococcus aureus* (MRSA), appear as redness, pain, or drainage at an IV catheter site or surgery site. Often, these symptoms come with a fever. Tell your doctor if you have these symptoms.

5. **Watch out for deadly diarrhea (*C. difficile*).**

    Tell your doctor if you have 3 or more diarrhea episodes in 24 hours, especially if you have been taking an antibiotic.

6. **Protect yourself.**

    Get vaccinated against the flu and other infections to avoid complications.

Section 84.2

Prevention and Control of Influenza in Healthcare Settings

This section includes text excerpted from "Prevention Strategies for Seasonal Influenza in Healthcare Settings," Centers for Disease Control and Prevention (CDC), October 30, 2018.

Influenza is primarily a community-based infection that is transmitted in households and community settings. Each year, 5 to 20 percent of the U.S. residents acquire an influenza virus infection, and many will seek medical care in ambulatory healthcare settings (e.g., pediatricians' offices, urgent-care clinics). In addition, more than 200,000 persons, on average, are hospitalized each year for influenza-related complications. Healthcare-associated influenza infections can occur in any healthcare setting and are most common when influenza is also circulating in the community. Therefore, the influenza prevention measures outlined in this section should be implemented in all healthcare settings. Supplemental measures may need to be implemented during influenza season if outbreaks of healthcare-associated influenza occur within certain facilities, such as long-term care facilities and hospitals.

Influenza Modes of Transmission

Traditionally, influenza viruses have been thought to spread from person to person primarily through large-particle respiratory droplet transmission (e.g., when an infected person coughs or sneezes near a susceptible person). Transmission via large-particle droplets requires close contact between source and recipient persons, because droplets generally travel only short distances (approximately six feet or less) through the air. Indirect contact transmission via hand transfer of influenza virus from virus-contaminated surfaces or objects to mucosal surfaces of the face (e.g., nose, mouth) may also occur. Airborne transmission via small particle aerosols in the vicinity of the infectious individual may also occur; however, the relative contribution of the different modes of influenza transmission is unclear. Airborne transmission over longer distances, such as from one patient room to another, has not been documented and is thought not to occur. All respiratory secretions and bodily fluids, including diarrheal stools, of patients with influenza are considered to be potentially infectious; however, the risk may vary by strain. Detection of influenza virus in blood or stool in influenza-infected patients is very uncommon.

Fundamental Elements to Prevent Influenza Transmission

Preventing the transmission of influenza virus and other infectious agents within healthcare settings requires a multi-faceted approach. The spread of the influenza virus can occur among patients, healthcare personnel (HCP), and visitors; in addition, HCP may acquire influenza from persons in their household or community. The core prevention strategies include:

- Administration of influenza vaccine
- Implementation of respiratory hygiene and cough etiquette
- Appropriate management of ill HCP
- Adherence to infection control precautions for all patient-care activities and aerosol-generating procedures
- Implementing environmental and engineering infection control measures.

Successful implementation of many, if not all, of these strategies, is dependent on the presence of clear administrative policies and organizational leadership that promote and facilitate adherence to these recommendations among the various people within the health-care setting, including patients, visitors, and HCP. These administrative measures are included within each recommendation where appropriate. Furthermore, this guidance should be implemented in the context of a comprehensive infection prevention program to prevent transmission of all infectious agents among patients and HCP.

Recommendations
Promote and Administer Seasonal Influenza Vaccine

Annual vaccination is the most important measure to prevent seasonal influenza infection. Achieving high influenza vaccination rates of HCP and patients is a critical step in preventing healthcare transmission of influenza from HCP to patients and from patients to HCP. According to current national guidelines, unless contraindicated, vaccinate all people six months of age and older, including HCP, patients, and residents of long-term care facilities.

Systematic strategies employed by some institutions to improve HCP vaccination rates have included providing incentives, providing vaccine at no cost to HCP, improving access (e.g., offering vaccination at work and during work hours), requiring personnel to sign declination forms to acknowledge that they have been educated about the benefits and risks of vaccination, and mandating influenza vaccination for all HCP without contraindication. Many of these approaches have been shown to increase vaccination rates; tracking influenza vaccination coverage among HCP can be an important component of a systematic approach to protecting patients and HCP. Regardless of the strategy used, strong organizational leadership and infrastructure for clear and timely communication and education, and for program implementation, have been common elements in successful programs.

Take Steps to Minimize Potential Exposures

A range of administrative policies and practices can be used to minimize influenza exposures before arrival, upon arrival, and throughout the duration of the visit to the healthcare setting. Measures include screening and triage of symptomatic patients and the implementation of respiratory hygiene and cough etiquette. Respiratory hygiene and cough etiquette are measures designed to minimize potential exposures of all respiratory pathogens, including influenza virus, in healthcare settings and should be adhered to by everyone?—patients, visitors, and HCP?—upon entry and continued for the entire duration of stay in healthcare settings.

Before Arrival at a Healthcare Setting

- When scheduling appointments, instruct patients and persons who accompany them to inform HCP upon arrival if they have symptoms of any respiratory infection (e.g., cough, runny nose, fever) and to take appropriate preventive actions (e.g., wear a face mask upon entry, follow triage procedure).

- During periods of increased influenza activity:

  - Take steps to minimize elective visits by patients with suspected or confirmed influenza. For example, consider establishing procedures to minimize visits by patients seeking care for mild influenza-like illness who are not at an increased risk for complications from influenza (e.g., provide telephone consultation to patients with mild respiratory illness to determine if there is a medical need to visit the facility).

Upon Entry and during Visit to a Healthcare Setting

- Take steps to ensure that all persons with symptoms of a respiratory infection adhere to respiratory hygiene, cough etiquette, hand hygiene, and triage procedures throughout the duration of the visit. These might include:

  - Posting visual alerts (e.g., signs, posters) at the entrance and in strategic places (e.g., waiting areas, elevators, cafeterias) to provide patients and HCP with instructions (in appropriate languages) about respiratory hygiene and cough etiquette, especially during periods when influenza virus is circulating in the community. Instructions should include:

  - How to use face masks or tissues to cover nose and mouth when coughing or sneezing and to dispose of contaminated items in waste receptacles

  - How and when to perform hand hygiene

  - Implementing procedures during patient registration that facilitate adherence to appropriate precautions (e.g., at the time of patient check-in, inquire about the presence of symptoms of a respiratory infection, and if present, provide instructions).

- Provide face masks to patients with signs and symptoms of respiratory infection.

- Provide supplies to perform hand hygiene to all patients upon arrival to a facility (e.g., at the entrance of a facility, waiting rooms, at patient check-in) and throughout the entire duration of the visit to the healthcare setting.

- Provide space and encourage persons with symptoms of respiratory infections to sit as far away from others as possible. If available, facilities may wish to place these patients in a separate area while waiting for care.

- During periods of increased community influenza activity, facilities should consider setting up triage stations that facilitate rapid screening of patients for symptoms of influenza and separation from other patients.

Monitor and Manage Ill Healthcare Personnel

Healthcare personnel who develop fever and respiratory symptoms should be:

- Instructed not to report to work, or if at work, to stop patient-care activities, don a face mask, and promptly notify their supervisor and infection control personnel/occupational health before leaving work

- Reminded that adherence to respiratory hygiene and cough etiquette after returning to work is always important. If symptoms such as cough and sneezing are still present, HCP should wear a face mask during patient-care activities. The importance of performing frequent hand hygiene (especially before and after each patient contact and contact with respiratory secretions) should be reinforced.

- Excluded from work until at least 24 hours after they no longer have a fever (without the use of fever-reducing medicines such as acetaminophen). Those with ongoing respiratory symptoms should be considered for evaluation by occupational health to determine the appropriateness of contact with patients.

- Considered for temporary reassignment or exclusion from work for seven days from symptom onset or until the resolution of symptoms, whichever is longer, if returning to care for patients in a protective environment (PE), such as hematopoietic stem cell transplant patients (HSCT).

- Patients in these environments are severely immunocompromised, and infection with the influenza virus can lead to severe disease. Furthermore, once infected, these patients can have prolonged viral shedding despite antiviral treatment and expose other patients to influenza virus infection. Prolonged shedding also increases the chance of developing and spreading antiviral-resistant influenza strains; clusters of influenza antiviral resistance cases have been found among severely immunocompromised persons exposed to a common source or healthcare setting.

- Healthcare personnel with influenza or many other infections may not have fever or may have fever alone as an initial symptom or sign. Thus, it can be very difficult to distinguish influenza from many other causes, especially early in a person's illness. HCP with fever alone should follow workplace policy for HCP with fever until a more specific cause of fever is identified or until fever resolves.

Healthcare personnel who develop acute respiratory symptoms without fever may still have influenza infection and should be:

- Considered for evaluation by occupational health to determine the appropriateness of contact with patients. HCP suspected of having influenza may benefit from influenza antiviral treatment.

- Reminded that adherence to respiratory hygiene and cough etiquette after returning to work is always important. If symptoms such as cough and sneezing are still present, HCP should wear a face mask during patient-care activities. The importance of performing frequent hand hygiene (especially before and after each patient contact) should be reinforced.

- Allowed to continue or return to work unless assigned to care for patients requiring a PE such as HSCT; this HCP should be considered for temporary reassignment or considered for exclusion from work for seven days from symptom onset or until the resolution of all noncough symptoms, whichever is longer.

Facilities and organizations providing healthcare services should:

- Develop sick leave policies for HCP that are nonpunitive, flexible, and consistent with public health guidance to allow and encourage HCP with suspected or confirmed influenza to stay home.

  - Policies and procedures should enhance the exclusion of HCPs who develop a fever and respiratory symptoms from work for at least 24 hours after they no longer have a fever, without the use of fever-reducing medicines.

- Ensure that all HCP, including staff who are not directly employed by the healthcare facility but provide essential daily services, are aware of the sick leave policies.

- Employee health services should establish procedures for tracking absences; reviewing job tasks and ensuring that personnel known to be at a higher risk for exposure to those with suspected or confirmed influenza are given priority for vaccination; ensuring that employees have prompt access, including via telephone to medical consultation and, if necessary, early treatment; and promptly identifying individuals with possible influenza. HCP should self-assess for symptoms of febrile respiratory illness. In most cases, decisions about work restrictions and assignments for personnel with respiratory illness should be guided by clinical signs and symptoms rather than by laboratory testing for influenza because laboratory testing may result in delays in diagnosis, false-negative test results, or both.

Adhere to Standard Precautions

During the care of any patient, all HCP in every healthcare setting should adhere to standard precautions, which are the foundation for preventing transmission of infectious agents in all healthcare settings. Standard precautions assume that every person is potentially infected or colonized with a pathogen that could be transmitted in the health-care setting. Elements of standard precautions that apply to patients with respiratory infections, including those caused by the influenza virus, are summarized below. All aspects of standard precautions (e.g., injection safety) are not emphasized in this section but can be found in the Centers for Disease Control and Prevention (CDC) Healthcare Infection Control Practices Advisory Committee (HICPAC) guideline titled Guideline for Isolation Precautions: Preventing Transmission of Infectious Agents in Healthcare Settings, Guidelines for Preventing

Healthcare-Associated Pneumonia and Guidelines for Hand Hygiene in Healthcare Settings Published 2002.

Hand Hygiene

- Healthcare personnel should perform hand hygiene frequently, including before and after all patient contact; contact with potentially infectious material; and before putting on and upon removal of personal protective equipment, including gloves. Hand hygiene in healthcare settings can be performed by washing with soap and water or using alcohol-based hand rubs. If hands are visibly soiled, use soap and water, not alcohol-based hand rubs.

- Healthcare facilities should ensure that supplies for performing hand hygiene are available.

Gloves

- Wear gloves for any contact with potentially infectious material. Remove gloves after contact, followed by hand hygiene. Do not wear the same pair of gloves for the care of more than one patient. Do not wash gloves for the purpose of reuse.

Gowns

- Wear gowns for any patient-care activity when contact with blood, bodily fluids, secretions (including respiratory), or excretions is anticipated. Remove gown, and perform hand hygiene before leaving the patient's environment. Do not wear the same gown for the care of more than one patient.

Adhere to Droplet Precautions

- Droplet precautions should be implemented for patients with suspected or confirmed influenza for 7 days after illness onset or until 24 hours after the resolution of fever and respiratory symptoms, whichever is longer, while a patient is in a healthcare facility. In some cases, facilities may choose to apply droplet precautions for longer periods based on clinical judgment, such as in the case of young children or severely immunocompromised patients, who may shed influenza virus for longer periods of time.

- Place patients with suspected or confirmed influenza in a private room or area. When a single patient room is not available, consultation with infection control personnel is recommended to assess the risks associated with other patient placement options (e.g., cohorting [i.e., grouping patients infected with the same infectious agents together to confine their care to one area and prevent contact with susceptible patients], keeping the patient with an existing roommate).

- Healthcare personnel should don a face mask when entering the room of a patient with suspected or confirmed influenza. Remove the face mask when leaving the patient's room, dispose of the face mask in a waste container, and perform hand hygiene.

  - If some facilities and organizations opt to provide employees with alternative personal protective equipment, this equipment should provide the same protection of the nose and mouth from splashes and sprays provided by face masks (e.g., face shields and N95 respirators or powered air purifying respirators).

- If a patient under droplet precautions requires movement or transport outside of the room:

  - Have the patient wear a face mask, if possible, and follow respiratory hygiene and cough etiquette and hand hygiene.

  - Communicate information about patients with suspected, probable, or confirmed influenza to appropriate personnel before transferring them to other departments in the facility (e.g., radiology, laboratory) or to other facilities.

Patients under droplet precautions should be discharged from medical care when clinically appropriate, not based on the period of potential virus shedding or recommended duration of droplet precautions. Before discharge, communicate the patient's diagnosis and current precautions with posthospital care providers (e.g., home-healthcare agencies, long-term care facilities) as well as transporting personnel.

Use Caution when Performing Aerosol-Generating Procedures

Some procedures performed on patients with suspected or confirmed influenza infection may be more likely to generate higher

691

concentrations of infectious respiratory aerosols than coughing, sneezing, talking, or breathing. These procedures potentially put HCP at an increased risk for influenza exposure. Although there are limited data available on influenza transmission related to such aerosols, many authorities recommend that additional precautions be used when such procedures are performed. These include some procedures that are usually planned ahead of time, such as bronchoscopy, sputum induction, elective intubation, and extubation, and autopsies; and some procedures that often occur in unplanned, emergent settings and can be lifesaving, such as cardiopulmonary resuscitation, emergent intubation, and open suctioning of airways. Ideally, a combination of measures should be used to reduce exposures from these aerosol-generating procedures when performed on patients with suspected or confirmed influenza. However, it is appropriate to take feasibility into account, especially in challenging emergent situations, where timeliness in performing a procedure can be critical to achieving a good patient outcome. Precautions for aerosol-generating procedures include:

- Only performing these procedures on patients with suspected or confirmed influenza if they are medically necessary and cannot be postponed.

- Limiting the number of HCP present during the procedure to only those essential for patient care and support. As is the case for all HCP, ensure that HCP whose duties require them to perform or be present during these procedures are offered influenza vaccination.

- Conducting the procedures in an airborne infection isolation room (AIIR) when feasible. This will not be feasible for unplanned, emergent procedures unless the patient is already in an AIIR. Such rooms are designed to reduce the concentration of infectious aerosols and prevent their escape into adjacent areas using controlled air exchanges and directional airflow. They are single patient rooms at negative pressure relative to the surrounding areas and with a minimum of 6 air changes per hour (12 air changes per hour are recommended for new construction or renovation). Air from these rooms should be exhausted directly to the outside or be filtered through a high-efficiency particulate air (HEPA) filter before recirculation. Room doors should be kept closed except when entering or leaving the room, and entry and exit should be minimized during and shortly after the procedure. Facilities should monitor and document the proper negative-pressure function of these rooms.

- Considering the use of portable HEPA filtration units to further reduce the concentration of contaminants in the air. Some of these units can connect to local exhaust ventilation systems (e.g., hoods, booths, tents) or have inlet designs that allow close placement to the patient to assist with source control; however, these units do not eliminate the need for respiratory protection for individuals entering the room because they may not entrain all of the room air. Information on air flow/air entrainment performance should be evaluated for such devices.

- Healthcare personnel should adhere to standard precautions, including wearing gloves, a gown, and either a face shield that fully covers the front and sides of the face or goggles.

- Healthcare personnel should wear respiratory protection equivalent to a fitted N95 filtering facepiece respirator or equivalent N95 respirator (e.g., powered air purifying respirator, elastomeric) during aerosol-generating procedures. When respiratory protection is required in an occupational setting, respirators must be used in the context of a comprehensive respiratory protection program that includes fit-testing and training as required under the Occupational Safety and Health Administration's (OSHA) Respiratory Protection Standard.

- Unprotected HCP should not be allowed in a room where an aerosol-generating procedure has been conducted until sufficient time has elapsed to remove potentially infectious particles.

- Conduct environmental surface cleaning following procedures.

Manage Visitor Access and Movement within the Facility

Limit visitors for patients in isolation for influenza to persons who are necessary for the patient's emotional well-being and care. Visitors who have been in contact with the patient before and during hospitalization are a possible source of influenza for other patients, visitors, and staff.

For persons with acute respiratory symptoms, facilities should develop visitor restriction policies that consider the location of a patient being visited (e.g., oncology units) and circumstances, such

693

as end-of-life situations, where exemptions to the restriction may be considered at the discretion of the facility.

Visits to patients in isolation for influenza should be scheduled and controlled to allow for:

- Screening visitors for symptoms of acute respiratory illness before entering the hospital

- Facilities should provide instruction, before visitors enter patients' rooms, on hand hygiene, limiting surfaces touched, and use of personal protective equipment (PPE) according to current facility policy while in the patient's room.

- Visitors should not be present during aerosol-generating procedures.

- Visitors should be instructed to limit their movement within the facility.

- If consistent with facility policy, visitors can be advised to contact their healthcare provider for information about influenza vaccination.

Monitor Influenza Activity

Healthcare settings should establish mechanisms and policies by which HCP are promptly alerted about increased influenza activity in the community or if an outbreak occurs within the facility and when a collection of clinical specimens for viral culture may help to inform public health efforts. Close communication and collaboration with local and state health authorities are recommended. Policies should include designations of specific persons within the healthcare facility who are responsible for communication with public health officials and dissemination of information to HCP.

Implement Environmental Infection Control

Standard cleaning and disinfection procedures (e.g., using cleaners and water to clean surfaces prior to applying disinfectants to frequently touched surfaces or objects for indicated contact times) are adequate for influenza virus environmental control in all settings within the healthcare facility, including those patient-care areas in which aerosol-generating procedures are performed. Management of laundry, food service utensils, and medical waste should also be performed in accordance with standard procedures. There are no data suggesting that these items are associated with influenza virus transmission when these items are properly managed. Laundry and food service utensils should first be cleaned, then sanitized as appropriate. Some medical waste may be designated as regulated or biohazardous waste and require special handling and disposal methods approved by the state authorities.

Implement Engineering Controls

Consider designing and installing engineering controls to reduce or eliminate exposures by shielding HCP and other patients from infected individuals. Examples of engineering controls include installing physical barriers, such as partitions in triage areas or curtains that are drawn between patients in shared areas. Engineering controls may also be important to reduce exposures related to specific procedures, such as using closed suctioning systems for airways suction in intubated patients. Another important engineering control is ensuring that appropriate air-handling systems are installed and maintained in healthcare facilities.

Train and Educate Healthcare Personnel

Healthcare administrators should ensure that all HCP receive job- or task-specific education and training on preventing transmission of infectious agents, including influenza, associated with healthcare during orientation to the healthcare setting. This information should be updated periodically during ongoing education and training programs. Competency should be documented initially and repeatedly, as appropriate, for the specific staff positions. A system should be in place to ensure that HCP employed by outside employers meet these education and training requirements through programs offered by the outside employer or by participation in the healthcare facility's program.

- Key aspects of influenza and its prevention that should be emphasized to all HCP include:

  - Influenza signs, symptoms, complications, and risk factors for complications. HCP should be made aware that, if they have conditions that place them at a higher risk of complications, they should inform their healthcare provider immediately if they become ill with an influenza-like illness so they can receive early treatment if indicated.

- The central role of administrative controls, such as vaccination, respiratory hygiene, and cough etiquette, sick policies, and precautions during aerosol-generating procedures

- Appropriate use of personal protective equipment including respirator fit testing and fit checks

- Use of engineering controls and work practices, including infection control procedures to reduce exposure

Administer Antiviral Treatment and Chemoprophylaxis of Patients and Healthcare Personnel when Appropriate

Refer to the CDC website for the most current recommendations on the use of antiviral agents for treatment and chemoprophylaxis. Both HCP and patients should be reminded that persons treated with influenza antiviral medications continue to shed influenza virus while on treatment. Thus, hand hygiene, respiratory hygiene, and cough etiquette practices should continue while on treatment.

Considerations for Healthcare Personnel at a Higher Risk for Complications of Influenza

Healthcare personnel at a higher risk for complications from influenza infection include pregnant women and women up to 2 weeks postpartum; persons 65 years of age and older; and persons with chronic diseases, such as asthma, heart disease, diabetes, diseases that suppress the immune system, certain other chronic medical conditions, and morbid obesity. Vaccination and early treatment with antiviral medications are very important for HCP at higher risk for influenza complications because they can decrease the risk of hospitalizations and deaths. HCP at a higher risk for complications should check with their healthcare provider if they become ill so that they can receive early treatment.

Some HCP may identify themselves as being at a higher risk of complications, and express concerns about their risks. These concerns should be discussed and the importance of careful adherence to these guidelines should be emphasized. Work accommodations to avoid potentially high-risk exposure scenarios, such as performing or assisting with aerosol-generating procedures on patients with suspected or confirmed influenza, may be considered in some settings, particularly for HCP with more severe or unstable underlying disease.

Chapter 85

Legal Authorities for Isolation and Quarantine to Control the Spread of Contagious Diseases

Isolation and Quarantine

Isolation and quarantine help protect the public by preventing exposure to people who have or may have a contagious disease.

- Isolation separates sick people with a contagious disease from people who are not sick.

- Quarantine separates and restricts the movement of people who were exposed to a contagious disease to see if they become sick.

In addition to serving as medical functions, isolation and quarantine also are "police power" functions, derived from the right of the state to take action affecting individuals for the benefit of society.

This chapter includes text excerpted from "Legal Authorities for Isolation and Quarantine," Centers for Disease Control and Prevention (CDC), October 8, 2014. Reviewed July 2019.

Federal Law

The federal government derives its authority for isolation and quarantine from the Commerce Clause of the U.S. Constitution.

Under section 361 of the Public Health Service Act (42 U.S. Code § 264), the U.S. Secretary of Health and Human Services is authorized to take measures to prevent the entry and spread of communicable diseases from foreign countries into the United States and between states.

The authority for carrying out these functions on a daily basis has been delegated to the Centers for Disease Control and Prevention (CDC).

Centers for Disease Control and Prevention's Role

Under 42 Code of Federal Regulations parts 70 and 71, the CDC is authorized to detain, medically examine, and release persons arriving into the United States and traveling between states who are suspected of carrying these communicable diseases.

As part of its federal authority, the CDC routinely monitors persons arriving at the U.S. land border crossings and passengers and crew arriving at the U.S. ports of entry for signs or symptoms of communicable diseases.

When alerted about an ill passenger or crew member by the pilot of a plane or captain of a ship, the CDC may detain passengers and crew as necessary to investigate whether the cause of the illness on board is a communicable disease.

State, Local, and Tribal Law

States have police power functions to protect the health, safety, and welfare of persons within their borders. To control the spread of disease within their borders, states have laws to enforce the use of isolation and quarantine.

These laws can vary from state to state, and they can be specific or broad. In some states, local health authorities implement state law. In most states, breaking a quarantine order is a criminal misdemeanor.

Tribes also have police power authority to take actions that promote the health, safety, and welfare of their own tribal members. Tribal health authorities may enforce their own isolation and quarantine laws within tribal lands if such laws exist.

Who Is in Charge?
The Federal Government

- Acts to prevent the entry of communicable diseases into the United States. Quarantine and isolation may be used at the U.S. ports of entry
- Is authorized to take measures to prevent the spread of communicable diseases between states
- May accept state and local assistance in enforcing the federal quarantine
- May assist state and local authorities in preventing the spread of communicable diseases

State, Local, and Tribal Authorities

- Enforce isolation and quarantine within their borders

It is possible for federal, state, local, and tribal health authorities to have and use all at the same time separate but coexisting legal quarantine power in certain events. In the event of a conflict, federal law is supreme.

Enforcement

If a quarantinable disease is suspected or identified, the CDC may issue a federal isolation or quarantine order.

Public health authorities at the federal, state, local, and tribal levels may sometimes seek help from police or other law enforcement officers to enforce a public health order.

U.S. Customs and Border Protection (CBP) officers and U.S. Coast Guard (USCG) officers are authorized to help enforce federal quarantine orders.

Breaking a federal quarantine order is punishable by fines and imprisonment.

Federal law allows the conditional release of persons from quarantine if they comply with medical monitoring and surveillance.

Federal Quarantine Rarely Used

Large-scale isolation and quarantine were last enforced during the influenza ("Spanish Flu") pandemic from 1918 to 1919. In history, only a few public health events have prompted federal isolation or quarantine orders.

Chapter 86

U.S. Nationally Notifiable Infectious Diseases: Protecting the Public Health

To protect Americans from serious disease, the National Notifiable Diseases Surveillance System (NNDSS) helps public health departments monitor, control, and prevent about 120 diseases. These diseases are important to monitor nationwide and include infectious diseases, such as Zika; foodborne outbreaks, such as *Escherichia coli* (*E. coli*); and noninfectious conditions, such as lead poisoning. About 3,000 public health departments gather and use data on these diseases to protect their local communities. Through the NNDSS, the Centers for Disease Control and Prevention (CDC) receives and uses these data to keep people healthy and defend America from health threats.

The National Notifiable Diseases Surveillance System is a multi-faceted program that includes the surveillance system for the collection, analysis, and sharing of health data. It also includes policies; laws; electronic messaging standards; people; partners; information systems; processes; and resources at the local, state, territorial, and national levels.

This chapter includes text excerpted from "National Notifiable Diseases Surveillance System (NNDSS)," Centers for Disease Control and Prevention (CDC), March 13, 2019.

Supporting Public Health Surveillance in Jurisdictions and at the Centers for Disease Control and Prevention

Notifiable disease surveillance begins at the level of local, state, and territorial public health departments (also known as "jurisdictions"). Jurisdictional laws and regulations mandate the reporting of cases of specified infectious and noninfectious conditions to health departments. The health departments work with healthcare providers, laboratories, hospitals, and other partners to obtain the information needed to monitor, control, and prevent the occurrence and spread of these health conditions.

The CDC Division of Health Informatics and Surveillance (DHIS) supports the NNDSS by receiving, securing, processing, and providing nationally notifiable infectious diseases data to disease-specific CDC programs. The DHIS also supports local, state, and territorial public health departments in helping them collect, manage, and submit case notification data to the CDC for the NNDSS. The DHIS provides this support through funding; health information exchange standards and frameworks; electronic health information systems; and technical support through the NNDSS website, tools, and training. The DHIS and CDC programs publish statistical data based on the NNDSS to support recognition of outbreaks, monitoring of shifts in disease patterns, and evaluation of disease control activities.

These programs collaborate with the Council of State and Territorial Epidemiologists (CSTE) to determine which conditions reported to local, state, and territorial public health departments are nationally notifiable. The CDC programs, in collaboration with subject matter experts in the CSTE and in health departments, determine what data elements are included in national notifications. Health departments participating in the NNDSS voluntarily submit case notification data to the DHIS and also submit some data directly to the CDC programs.

National Notifiable Diseases Surveillance System Modernization Initiative

With the evolution of technology and data and exchange standards, the CDC is strengthening and modernizing the infrastructure supporting the NNDSS. As part of the CDC Surveillance Strategy, the NNDSS Modernization Initiative (NMI) is enhancing the system's ability to provide more comprehensive, timely, and higher quality data than ever before for public health decision-making.

Through this multi-year initiative, the CDC is increasing the robustness of the NNDSS technological infrastructure so that it is based on interoperable, standardized data and exchange mechanisms.

Chapter 87

Countering Bioterrorism and Emerging Infectious Diseases

Facilitating the Development of Medical Countermeasures

The U.S. government's efforts to counter bioterrorism is comprised of a number of essential elements for which the Center for Biologics Evaluation and Research (CBER) plays an integral role. One such element is the expeditious development and licensing of products to diagnose, treat, or prevent disease following exposure to pathogens that have been identified as bioterrorism agents. These products must be reviewed and approved prior to the large-scale productions necessary to create and maintain a stockpile. Staff must guide the products through the regulatory process, including the manufacturing, preclinical testing, clinical trials, and the licensing and approval processes. Experts in these areas are needed to expedite the licensing

This chapter includes text excerpted from the following sources: Text under the heading "Facilitating the Development of Medical Countermeasures" is excerpted from "Countering Bioterrorism and Emerging Infectious Diseases," U.S. Food and Drug Administration (FDA), March 23, 2018; Text under the heading "Countering Bioterrorism Questions and Answers" is excerpted from "Countering Bioterrorism Questions and Answers," U.S. Food and Drug Administration (FDA), January 31, 2018.

and approval process for these products. This process is extremely complex and early involvement by staff is crucial to the success of the expedited review process.

The CBER works with other federal agencies and industries through the Public Health Emergency Medical Countermeasure Enterprise (PHEMCE) on a broad array of projects aimed at making our nation better prepared for chemical, biological, radiological, and nuclear (CBRN) threats and emerging infectious diseases through the development of new countermeasures.

In addition, the CBER also monitors the impact of emergencies or outbreaks of disease on the safety and availability of the blood supply.

Preparedness for and response to an attack involving biological agents are complicated by a large number of potential agents (most of which are rarely encountered naturally), their sometimes long incubation periods and consequent delayed onset of disease, and their potential for secondary transmission. In addition to naturally occurring pathogens, agents used by bioterrorists may be genetically engineered to resist current therapies and evade vaccine-induced immunity. Pathogens that have been identified as potential biological warfare agents include those that cause anthrax, botulism, plague, smallpox, tularemia, and the hemorrhagic fevers, among others.

The CBER's regulatory science and research programs focus on developing a comprehensive approach to rapid pathogen detection, enhancing preparedness for seasonal and influenza vaccines, and facilitating licensure of medical countermeasures for treating or preventing diseases due to bioterrorist attacks. The purpose of the regulatory science program is to provide both proactive solutions to fill gaps in scientific data, tools, or approaches needed to perform a regulatory review, while also providing a cadre of scientific experts that are available to be responsive to public health emergencies that may require a laboratory response.

Countering Bioterrorism Questions and Answers
Has the Center for Biologics Evaluation and Research Had Any Involvement in Countering Bioterrorism?

The CBER continues to be very active in supporting the U.S. government's initiatives to develop medical countermeasures and counter bioterrorism and emerging infectious diseases, including pandemic influenza. The CBER staff have participated in numerous meetings, briefings, and conferences representing the FDA with staff from the U.S. Department of Defense, the U.S. Department of Health and

Human Services (DHHS), U.S. Department of Homeland Security, and the Office of Management and Budget (OMB), as well as other DHHS Agencies, including the Biomedical Advanced Research and Development Authority (BARDA), National Institutes of Health (NIH), and the Centers for Disease Control and Prevention (CDC). The Center has also engaged in the development of new regulatory models to accommodate the need for preparedness in the case of an emergency attack. Procedures and protocols have been developed to enable the use of investigational new drugs in a highly controlled, safe manner for particular emergency situations, such as responding to a bioterrorist attack that exposes individuals to the agents that cause anthrax, smallpox, and botulism.

What Types of Medical Countermeasures Are Currently Available in the Event of a Terrorist Attack?

The CBER has licensed vaccines for both anthrax and smallpox. In addition, there is a licensed treatment for complications from smallpox vaccination. Since 9/11 and the anthrax attacks of late 2001, the CBER has worked with numerous manufacturers to develop and bring to licensure countermeasures against many potential biological agents. There are products in development that include new vaccines or treatments for anthrax, smallpox, botulism, plague, and others.

What Regulations or Guidance Documents Exist That Would Help with the Development of Safe and Effective New Products That Might Be Used in Countering Bioterrorism?

In May 2002, the FDA published "Approval of Biological Products when Human Efficacy Studies are not Ethical or Feasible" [21 CFR 601 Subpart H, as well as 21 CFR 314 Subpart I for New Drugs]. This rule, known simply as the "Animal Rule," was designed to permit approval or licensing of drugs and biologics that are intended to reduce or prevent serious or life-threatening conditions caused by exposure to biological, chemical, radiological, or nuclear substances. This rule amends the new drug and biological product regulations to identify the information needed to provide substantial evidence of the efficacy of a new drug and biological products only when human efficacy studies are not ethical and field trials are not feasible. The new rule does not address the need for safety data which still must be established through human clinical trials.

In January 2009, a draft guidance called "Animal Models—Essential Elements to Address Efficacy Under the Animal Rule" was published. After opening the docket for comments twice and holding a public meeting to hear comments on the guidance, this document is under revision by a CDER/CBER team and will be republished as draft guidance for comment in the future.

In December 2007, an interim final rule was published "Exceptions or Alternatives to Labeling Requirements for Products Held by the Strategic National Stockpile" to permit FDA Center Directors to grant exceptions or alternatives to certain regulatory labeling requirements applicable to human drugs, biological products, or medical devices that are or will be held in the Strategic National Stockpile (SNS). This rule was issued to facilitate the safety, effectiveness, and availability of appropriate medical countermeasures stored in the SNS in the event of a public health emergency. In February 2012, the final rule was published in the federal register without change from the interim final rule.

Has the Center for Biologics Evaluation and Research Approved Any New Biologics under the Animal Rule so Far?

The CBER has not approved any new products under the Animal Rule to date. However, several products in development and on the licensure path are moving toward approval through this mechanism. The Center for Drugs Evaluation and Research (CDER) has approved two products to date using the Animal Rule: Pyridostigmine Bromide, and Cyanokit.

Part Eight

Additional Help and Information

Chapter 88

Glossary of Terms Related to Contagious Diseases

acute: A short-term, intense health effect.

adjuvant: A substance sometimes included in a vaccine formulation to enhance the immune-stimulating properties of the vaccine.

adverse events: Undesirable experiences occurring after immunization that may or may not be related to the vaccine.

antibiotics: Medicines that damage or kill bacteria and are used to treat some bacterial diseases.

antibodies: Molecules (also called immunoglobulins) produced by a B cell in response to an antigen. When an antibody attaches to an antigen, it destroys the antigen.

antigen: A substance or molecule that is recognized by the immune system. The molecule can come from foreign materials such as bacteria or viruses.

antitoxin: Antibodies capable of destroying toxins generated by micro-organisms including viruses and bacteria.

artificially acquired immunity: Immunity provided by vaccines, as opposed to naturally acquired immunity, which is acquired from exposure to a disease-causing organism.

This glossary contains terms excerpted from documents produced by several sources deemed reliable.

asthma: A chronic medical condition where the bronchial tubes (in the lungs) become easily irritated.

attenuated vaccine: A vaccine in which live virus is weakened through chemical or physical processes in order to produce an immune response without causing the severe effects of the disease.

B cells: Small white blood cells crucial to the immune defenses. Also known as B lymphocytes.

bone marrow: A soft tissue located within bones that produce all blood cells, including the ones that fight infection.

booster shot: Supplementary dose of a vaccine, usually smaller than the first dose, that is given to maintain immunity.

cell: The smallest unit of life.

chronic health condition: A health-related state that lasts for a long period of time (e.g., cancer, asthma).

communicable disease: An infectious disease that is contagious and which can be transmitted from one source to another by infectious bacteria or viral organisms.

computed tomography (CT): A procedure for taking X-ray images from many different angles and then assembling them into a cross-section of the body. This technique is generally used to visualize bone.

conjugate vaccine: A vaccine in which proteins that are easily recognizable to the immune system are linked to the molecules that form the outer coat of disease-causing bacteria to promote an immune response.

contagious disease: A very communicable disease capable of spreading rapidly from one person to another by contact or close proximity.

contraindication: A condition in a recipient which is likely to result in a life-threatening problem if a vaccine were given.

diphtheria: A bacterial disease marked by the formation of a false membrane, especially in the throat, which can cause death.

disease: A state in which a function or part of the body is no longer in a healthy condition.

DNA (deoxyribonucleic acid): A complex molecule found in the cell nucleus that contains an organism's genetic information.

DNA vaccine: A vaccine that uses a microbe's genetic material, rather than the whole organism or its parts, to stimulate an immune response.

encephalitis: Inflammation of the brain caused by a virus. Encephalitis can result in permanent brain damage or death.

encephalopathy: A general term describing brain dysfunction.

endemic: The continual, low-level presence of disease in a community.

epidemic: A disease outbreak that affects many people in a region at the same time.

exposure: Contact with infectious agents (bacteria or viruses) in a manner that promotes transmission and increases the likelihood of disease.

genes: Units of genetic material (DNA) that carry the directions a cell uses to perform a specific function.

genetic material: Molecules of DNA (deoxyribonucleic acid) or RNA (ribonucleic acid) that carry the directions that cells or viruses use to perform a specific function, such as making a particular protein molecule.

genomes: All of an organism's genetic material. A genome is organized into specific functional units called genes.

herpes zoster: A disease characterized by painful skin lesions that occur mainly on the trunk (back and stomach) of the body but which can also develop on the face and in the mouth. Also known as the shingles.

hives: The eruption of red marks on the skin that are usually accompanied by itching.

immune globulin: A protein found in the blood that fights infection. Also known as gamma globulin.

immune response: Reaction of the immune system to foreign invaders such as microbes.

immune system: A complex network of specialized cells, tissues, and organs that defends the body against attacks by disease-causing microbes.

immunity: Protection from germs.

inactivated vaccine or killed vaccine: A vaccine made from a whole virus or bacteria inactivated with chemicals or heat.

incubation period: The time from contact with infectious agents (bacteria or viruses) to onset of disease.

infection: A state in which disease-causing microbes have invaded or multiplied in body tissues.

infectious agents: Organisms capable of spreading disease (e.g., bacteria or viruses).

intussusception: A type of bowel blockage that happens when one portion of the bowel slides into the next, much like the pieces of a telescope.

jaundice: Yellowing of the skin and eyes. This condition is often a symptom of hepatitis infection.

lesion: An abnormal change in the structure of an organ, due to injury or disease.

live, attenuated vaccine: A vaccine made from microbes that have been weakened in the laboratory so that they cannot cause disease.

lupus: A disease characterized by inflammation of the connective tissue (which supports and connects all parts of the body).

lymph node: A small bean-shaped organ of the immune system, distributed widely throughout the body and linked by lymphatic vessels.

lymphocyte: A white blood cell central to the immune system's response to foreign microbes. B cells and T cells are lymphocytes.

macrophage: A large and versatile immune cell that devours and kills invading microbes and other intruders.

magnetic resonance imaging (MRI): A noninvasive procedure that uses magnetic fields and radio waves to produce three-dimensional computerized images of areas inside the body.

memory cells: A group of cells that help the body defend itself against disease by remembering prior exposure to specific organisms (e.g., viruses or bacteria). Therefore, these cells are able to respond quickly when these organisms repeatedly threaten the body.

molecule: A building block of a cell. Some examples are proteins, fats, and carbohydrates.

mutate: To change a gene or unit of hereditary material that results in a new inheritable characteristic.

naturally acquired immunity: Immunity produced by antibodies passed from mother to fetus (passive), or by the body's own antibody and cellular immune response to a disease-causing organism (active).

orchitis: A complication of mumps infection occurring in males (who are beyond puberty).

otitis media: A viral or bacterial infection that leads to inflammation of the middle ear.

outbreak: Sudden appearance of a disease in a specific geographic area (e.g., neighborhood or community) or population (e.g., adolescents).

pandemic: An epidemic occurring over a very large geographic area.

parasites: Plants or animals that live, grow, and feed on or within another living organism.

pathogens: Organisms (e.g., bacteria, viruses, parasites and fungi) that cause disease in human beings.

petechiae: A tiny reddish or purplish spot on the skin or mucous membrane, commonly part of infectious diseases such as typhoid fever.

placebo: A substance or treatment that has no effect on human beings.

pneumonia: Inflammation of the lungs characterized by fever, chills, muscle stiffness, chest pain, cough, shortness of breath, rapid heart rate, and difficulty breathing.

polysaccharide: A long, chain-like molecule made up of a linked sugar molecule. The outer coats of some bacteria are made of polysaccharides.

potency: A measure of strength.

quarantine: The isolation of a person or animal who has a disease (or is suspected of having a disease) in order to prevent further spread of the disease.

recombinant: Of or resulting from new combinations of genetic material or cells.

Reye syndrome: Encephalopathy (general brain disorder) in children following an acute illness such as, influenza or chickenpox. Symptoms include vomiting, agitation, and lethargy. This condition may result in coma or death.

serology: Measurement of antibodies, and other immunological properties, in the blood serum.

strain: A specific version of an organism. Many diseases, including human immunodeficiency virus (HIV)/acquired immune deficiency syndrome (AIDS) and hepatitis, have multiple strains.

subunit vaccine: A vaccine that uses one or more components of a disease-causing organism, rather than the whole, to stimulate an immune response.

T cell or T lymphocyte: A white blood cell that directs or participates in immune defenses.

tetanus: A toxin-producing bacterial disease marked by painful muscle spasms.

thimerosal: A mercury-containing preservative used in some vaccines and other products since the 1930s.

tissue: A group of similar cells joined to perform the same function.

titer: The detection of antibodies in blood through a laboratory test.

toxin: Agent produced by plants and bacteria, normally very damaging to cells.

toxoid: A toxin, such as those produced by certain bacteria, that has been treated by chemical means, heat or irradiation and is no longer capable of causing disease.

toxoid vaccine: A vaccine containing a toxoid, used to protect against toxins produced by certain bacteria.

vaccine: A product made from very small amounts of weak or dead germs that can cause diseases—for example, viruses, bacteria, or toxins. It prepares your body to fight the disease faster and more effectively so you won't get sick. Vaccines are administered through needle injections, by mouth, and by aerosol.

virus: A tiny organism that multiplies within cells and causes disease such as chickenpox, measles, mumps, rubella, pertussis, and hepatitis. Viruses are not affected by antibiotics, the drugs used to kill bacteria.

X-ray: A type of radiation used in the diagnosis and treatment of cancer and other diseases. In low doses, X-rays are used to diagnose diseases by making pictures of the inside of the body.

Chapter 89

Directory of Organizations with Information about Contagious Diseases

Government Agencies That Provide Information about Contagious Diseases

Agency for Healthcare Research and Quality (AHRQ)
Office of Communications and Knowledge Transfer (OCKT)
5600 Fishers Ln.
Seventh Fl.
Rockville, MD 20857
Phone: 301-427-1104
Website: www.ahrq.gov

Centers for Disease Control and Prevention (CDC)
1600 Clifton Rd.
Atlanta, GA 30329-4027
Toll-Free: 800-CDC-INFO
(800-232-4636)
Toll-Free TTY: 888-232-6348
Website: www.cdc.gov
E-mail: cdcinfo@cdc.gov

Resources in this chapter were compiled from several sources deemed reliable; all contact information was verified and updated in July 2019.

Division of STD Prevention (DSTDP)
Centers for Disease Control and Prevention (CDC)
1600 Clifton Rd.
Atlanta, GA 30329-4027
Toll-Free: 800-CDC-INFO
(800-232-4636)
Toll-Free TTY: 888-232-6348
Website: www.cdc.gov/std

Division of Viral Hepatitis (DVH)
National Center for HIV/AIDS, Viral Hepatitis, STD, and TB Prevention
1600 Clifton Rd. N.E.
MS G-37
Atlanta, GA 30329-4018
Toll-Free: 800-CDC-INFO
(800-232-4636)
Toll-Free TTY: 888-232-6348
Website: www.cdc.gov/hepatitis

Eunice Kennedy Shriver *National Institute of Child Health and Human Development (NICHD)*
Information Resource Center (IRC)
P.O. Box 3006
Rockville, MD 20847
Toll-Free: 800-370-2943
Toll-Free TTY: 888-320-6942
Toll-Free Fax: 866-760-5947
Website: www.nichd.nih.gov
E-mail: NICHDInformation
ResourceCenter@mail.nih.gov

Federal Trade Commission (FTC)
600 Pennsylvania Ave. N.W.
Washington, DC 20580
Toll-Free: 877-FTC-HELP
(877-382-4357)
Phone: 202-326-2222
Website: www.ftc.gov

Genetics Home Reference (GHR)
8600 Rockville Pike
Bethesda, MD 20894
Website: ghr.nlm.nih.gov

Health Resources and Services Administration (HRSA)
5600 Fishers Ln.
Rockville, MD 20857
Toll-Free: 800-221-9393
Toll-Free TTY: 877-897-9910
Website: www.hrsa.gov

Healthfinder®
U. S. Department of Health and Human Services (HHS)
1101 Wootton Pkwy
Rockville, MD 20852
Website: www.healthfinder.gov
E-mail: healthfinder@hhs.gov

MedlinePlus
U.S. National Library of Medicine (NLM)
8600 Rockville Pike
Bethesda, MD 20894
Toll-Free: 888-FIND-NLM
(888-346-3656)
Phone: 301-594-5983
Website: www.medlineplus.gov

718

MedWatch
U.S. Food and Drug
Administration (FDA)
10903 New Hampshire Ave.
Silver Spring, MD 20993-0002
Toll-Free: 888-INFO-FDA
(888-463-6332)
Phone: 301-796-8240
Website: www.fda.gov/Safety/
MedWatch/default.htm

*National Cancer Institute
(NCI)*
Cancer Information Service
(CIS)
9609 Medical Center Dr.
BG 9609 MSC 9760
Bethesda, MD 20892
Toll-Free: 800-4-CANCER
(800-422-6237)
Toll-Free TTY: 800-332-8615
Website: www.cancer.gov
E-mail: cancergovstaff@mail.nih.
gov

*National Center for
Complementary and
Integrative Health (NCCIH)*
9000 Rockville Pike
Bethesda, MD 20892
Toll-Free: 888-644-6226
Toll-Free TTY: 866-464-3615
Toll-Free Fax: 866-464-3616
Website: nccih.nih.gov
E-mail: info@nccih.nih.gov

*National Diabetes
Information Clearinghouse
(NDIC)*
National Institute of Diabetes
and Digestive and Kidney
Diseases (NIDDK) Health
Information Center (HIC)
Toll-Free: 800-860-8747
Toll-Free TTY: 866-569-1162
Website: www.diabetes.niddk.
nih.gov
E-mail: healthinfo@niddk.nih.
gov

*National Health Information
Center (NHIC)*
U. S. Department of Health and
Human Services (HHS)
1101 Wootton Pkwy
Ste. LL 100
Rockville, MD 20852
Toll-Free: 800-336-4797
Phone: 301-565-4167
Fax: 240-453-8282
Website: www.health.gov/NHIC
E-mail: odphpinfo@hhs.gov

*National Heart, Lung, and
Blood Institute (NHLBI)*
Health Information Center
(HIC)
P.O. Box 30105
Bethesda, MD 20824-0105
Phone: 301-592-8573
TTY: 240-629-3255
Website: www.nhlbi.nih.gov
E-mail: nhlbiinfo@nhlbi.nih.gov

National Institute of Allergy and Infectious Diseases (NIAID)
Office of Communications and Government Relations (OCGR)
5601 Fishers Ln. MSC 9806
Bethesda, MD 20892-9806
Toll-Free: 866-284-4107
Phone: 301-496-5717
Toll-Free TDD: 800-877-8339
Fax: 301-402-3573
Website: www.niaid.nih.gov
E-mail: ocpostoffice@niaid.nih.gov

National Institute of Diabetes and Digestive and Kidney Diseases (NIDDK)
Health Information Center (HIC)
Toll-Free: 800-860-8747
Toll-Free TTY: 866-569-1162
Website: www.niddk.nih.gov
E-mail: healthinfo@niddk.nih.gov

National Institute of Neurological Disorders and Stroke (NINDS)
National Institutes of Health (NIH) Neurological Institute
P.O. Box 5801
Bethesda, MD 20824
Toll-Free: 800-352-9424
Website: www.ninds.nih.gov

National Institute on Aging (NIA)
Information Center
31 Center Dr. MSC 2292
Bldg. 31 Rm. 5C27
Bethesda, MD 20892
Toll-Free: 800-222-2225
Toll-Free TTY: 800-222-4225
Website: www.nia.nih.gov
E-mail: niaic@nia.nih.gov

National Institutes of Health (NIH)
9000 Rockville Pike
Bethesda, MD 20892
Phone: 301-496-4000
TTY: 301-402-9612
Website: www.nih.gov

National Prevention Information Network (NPIN)
Centers for Disease Control and Prevention (CDC)
P.O. Box 6003
Rockville, MD 20849-6003
Website: npin.cdc.gov
E-mail: NPIN-Info@cdc.gov

National Vaccine Injury Compensation Program (NVCIP)
Health Resources and Services Administration (HRSA)
5600 Fishers Ln.
Rockville, MD 20857
Toll-Free: 800-221-9393
Toll-Free TTY: 877-897-9910
Website: www.hrsa.gov/vaccinecompensation

National Women's Health Information Center (NWHIC)
Office on Women's Health (OWH)
200 Independence Ave. S.W.
Rm. 712E
Washington, DC 20201
Toll-Free: 800-994-9662
Phone: 202-690-7650
Fax: 202-205-2631
Website: www.womenshealth.gov

Office of Dietary Supplements (ODS)
National Institutes of Health (NIH)
6100 Executive Blvd.
Rm. 3B01. MSC 7517
Bethesda, MD 20852
Phone: 301-435-2920
Fax: 301-480-1845
Website: dietary-supplements.info.nih.gov
E-mail: ods@nih.gov

Office of the Assistant Secretary for Preparedness and Response (ASPR)
U.S. Department of Health and Human Services (HHS)
200 Independence Ave., S.W.
Rm. 638G
Washington, DC 20201
Website: www.phe.gov

U.S. Department of Health and Human Services (HHS)
200 Independence Ave. S.W.
Hubert H. Humphrey Bldg.
Washington, DC 20201
Toll-Free: 877-696-6775
Website: www.hhs.gov

U.S. Environmental Protection Agency (EPA)
1200 Pennsylvania Ave. N.W.
Washington, DC 20460
Website: www.epa.gov

U.S. Food and Drug Administration (FDA)
10903 New Hampshire Ave.
Silver Spring, MD 20993-0002

U.S. National Library of Medicine (NLM)
8600 Rockville Pike
Bethesda, MD 20894
Toll-Free: 888-FIND-NLM
(888-346-3656)
Phone: 301-594-5983
Website: www.nlm.nih.gov

Vaccine Adverse Event Reporting System (VAERS)
P.O. Box 1100
Rockville, MD 20849-1100
Toll-Free: 800-822-7967
Toll-Free Fax: 877-721-0366
Website: www.vaers.hhs.gov
E-mail: info@vaers.org

Vaccines and Immunizations
Centers for Disease Control and Prevention (CDC)
1600 Clifton Rd.
Atlanta, GA 30329-4027
Toll-Free: 800-CDC-INFO
(800-232-4636)
Toll-Free TTY: 888-232-6348
Website: www.cdc.gov/vaccines

Private Agencies That Provide Information about Contagious Diseases

American Academy of Allergy, Asthma, & Immunology (AAAAI)
555 E. Wells St.
Ste. 1100
Milwaukee, WI 53202-3823
Phone: 414-272-6071
Website: www.aaaai.org
E-mail: info@aaaai.org

American Academy of Family Physicians (AAFP)
11400 Tomahawk Creek Pkwy
Leawood, KS 66211-2680
Toll-Free: 800-274-2237
Phone: 913-906-6000
Fax: 913-906-6075
Website: www.aafp.org
E-mail: aafp@aafp.org

American Association of Blood Banks (AABB)
4550 Montgomery Ave.
N. Tower Ste. 700
Bethesda, MD 20814
Phone: 301-907-6977

American Cancer Society (ACS)
250 Williams St. N.W.
Atlanta, GA 30303
Toll-Free: 800-227-2345
Toll-Free TTY: 866-228-4327
Website: www.cancer.org

American Liver Foundation (ALF)
National Office
39 Bdwy.
Ste. 2700
New York, NY 10006
Toll-Free: 800-465-4837
Phone: 212-668-1000
Website: www.liverfoundation.org

American Lung Association (ALA)
National Office
55 W. Wacker Dr.
Ste. 1150
Chicago, IL 60601
Toll-Free: 800-LUNGUSA (800-586-4872)
Website: www.lung.org
E-mail: info@lung.org

American Medical Association (AMA)
AMA Plaza 330 N. Wabash Ave.
Ste. 39300
Chicago, IL 60611-5885
Toll-Free: 800-262-3211
Phone: 312-464-4782
Website: www.ama-assn.org

American Sexual Health Association (ASHA)
P.O. Box 13827
Research Triangle Park, NC 27709
Phone: 919-361-8400
Fax: 919-361-8425
Website: www.ashasexualhealth.org
E-mail: info@ashasexualhealth.org

Hepatitis Foundation International (HFI)
8121 Georgia Ave.
Ste. 350
Silver Spring, MD 20910
Toll-Free: 800-891-0707
Phone: 301-565-9410
Website: www.hepatitisfoundation.org

Immunization Safety Review Committee (ISR)
500 Fifth St. N.W.
Washington, DC 20001
Phone: 202-334-2352
Fax: 202-334-1412
Website: www.iom.edu/imsafety
E-mail: iowww@nas.edu

National Foundation for Infectious Diseases (NFID)
7201 Wisconsin Ave.
Ste. 750
Bethesda, MD 20814
Phone: 301-656-0003
Fax: 301-907-0878
Website: www.nfid.org

National Network for Immunization Information (NNii)
World Health Organization (WHO)
Fax: 409-772-5208
Website: www.who.int/vaccine_safety/initiative/communication/network/NNii/en

National Patient Advocate Foundation (NPAF)
Phone: 202-347-8009
Website: www.npaf.org
E-mail: action@npaf.org

The Nemours Foundation / KidsHealth®
1600 Rockland Rd.
Wilmington, DE 19803
Phone: 302-651-4046
Website: www.kidshealth.org
E-mail: info@kidshealth.org

World Health Organization (WHO)
Ave. Appia 20
1211 Geneva
Switzerland
Phone: 41-22-791-2111
Website: www.who.int
E-mail: erecruit@who.int

Index

Index

Page numbers followed by 'n' indicate a footnote. Page numbers in *italics* indicate a table or illustration.

A

AAAAI *see* American Academy of Allergy, Asthma, & Immunology
AABB *see* American Association of Blood Banks
AAFP *see* American Academy of Family Physicians
"About Chickenpox" (CDC) 93n
"About Diphtheria" (CDC) 277n
"About Flu" (CDC) 176n
"About Norovirus" (CDC) 213n
"About Pneumococcal Disease" (CDC) 350n
"About Ringworm" (CDC) 451n
"About Zika" (CDC) 237n
abstinence, sexually transmitted diseases (STDs) 45
acetaminophen
   chickenpox 96
   flu and cold medication 473, 503
   OTC medications 498
   Zika 243
acne, OTC medications 496

acquired immunodeficiency syndrome (AIDS)
   home tests 557
   microbial diseases 16
   overview 161–8
   pneumonia 307
   risks of blood transfusion 52
   trichomoniasis 461
   tuberculosis (TB) 372
ACS *see* American Cancer Society
acute, defined 711
acute infections, microbes 8
acute respiratory distress, Avian influenza 90
acyclovir
   herpes 141
   immunodeficiency diseases 36
   microbial diseases 18
   prescription medicines 564
adaptive immunity, immune response 25
adefovir dipivoxil, hepatitis B 158
adenoviruses
   conjunctivitis 108
   overview 85–7
   viral hepatitis 160
"Adenoviruses" (CDC) 85n
adjuvants
   defined 711

adjuvants, *continued*
  vaccination 26
  vaccine ingredients 603
adolescents
  chickenpox 94
  chlamydia 256
  immunization 629
  vaccines side effects 661
adoption, screening for infectious
  diseases 68
adult immunization, overview 633–43
adverse events
  defined 711
  drug–drug interactions 508
  Vaccine Adverse Event Reporting
    System (VAERS) 665
  vaccine safety 604
Advil (ibuprofen)
  chickenpox 96
  drug interactions 507
  fever 485
  respiratory syncytial virus
    (RSV) 224
aerobic bacteria, microbes 5
Agency for Healthcare Research and
  Quality (AHRQ), contact 717
AHRQ *see* Agency for Healthcare
  Research and Quality
AIDS *see* acquired immunodeficiency
  syndrome
airplanes
  contagious disease transmission 54
  microbes 41
air travel
  contagious disease transmission 54
  tuberculosis (TB) 375
"Air Travel" (CDC) 54n
ALA *see* American Lung Association
aldactone (spironolactone), drug
  interactions 506
ALF *see* American Liver Foundation
allergic conjunctivitis *see*
  conjunctivitis
allergic reactions
  body lice 419
  herbal supplements 523
  immune cells 26
  vaccine ingredients 611
  vaccines side effects 647

allergic rhinitis, probiotics 520
allergies
  bioterrorism 80
  cold and flu 471, 516
  sexually transmitted diseases
    (STDs) 45
aloe latex, herbal supplements 529
aloe vera, herbal supplements 530
alpha interferon, hepatitis 158
alveoli, pneumonia 307
AMA *see* American Medical
  Association
amantadine
  antiviral drugs 568
  drug resistance 584
  immunodeficiency diseases 36
Ambien (zolpidem), drug
  interactions 506
amebiasis, overview 405–8
"Amebiasis—General Information"
  (CDC) 405n
amebic dysentery, amebiasis 406
amebic meningitis, overview 433–5
American Academy of Allergy,
  Asthma, & Immunology (AAAAI),
  contact 722
American Academy of Family
  Physicians (AAFP), contact 722
American Association of Blood Banks
  (AABB), contact 722
American Cancer Society (ACS),
  contact 722
American ginseng, flu and
  colds 512
American Liver Foundation (ALF),
  contact 722
American Lung Association (ALA),
  contact 722
American Medical Association (AMA),
  contact 722
American Sexual Health Association
  (ASHA), contact 723
amiodarone, drug interactions 508
amoxicillin
  infectious mononucleosis 128
  scarlet fever 346
  staph infection 332
  strep throat testing and
    treatment 554

ampicillin
  drug resistance 582
  group B strep (GBS) 359
  infectious mononucleosis 128
anaerobic bacteria, microbes 5
anal sex
  chlamydia 253
  cryptosporidiosis 415
  Ebola virus disease (EVD) 118
  gonorrhea 146
  HIV and AIDS 163
  pelvic inflammatory disease
    (PID) 386
  trichomoniasis 459
anemia
  blood transfusion 47
  fifth disease 132
  herbal supplements 527
  immunodeficiency diseases 35
anthrax
  bioterrorism 72
  countering bioterrorism 706
  preparedness of the United
    States 79
"Anthrax—Preparedness" (CDC) 79n
antibiotic resistance
  antibiotic safety 572
  handwashing 595
  Hansen disease 285
  microbial diseases 18
antibiotics
  antibiotic safety and drug
    resistance 573
  bioterrorism 79
  chlamydia 257
  Clostridium difficile infection 269
  conjunctivitis 112
  fever 484
  Hansen disease 285
  methicillin-resistant *Staphylococcus
    aureus* 303
  microbes 18
  overview 562–3
  pelvic inflammatory disease
    (PID) 385
  pneumonia 317
  staph infections 330
  Streptococcus pneumoniae 355
  trichomoniasis 461

antibiotics, *continued*
  vaccine ingredients 611
  vancomycin-resistant enterococci
    (VRE) 392
"Antibiotics, Antivirals, and
  Other Prescription Medicines"
  (Omnigraphics) 561n
"Antibiotics Aren't Always the
  Answer" (CDC) 572n
antibodies
  defined 711
  genital herpes 139
  home tests for HIV 557
  immune system response to
    infection 28
  immunizations 622
  immunodeficiency 34
  influenza 189
  syphilis 365
antifungal medications
  microbial diseases 19
  prescription medicines 565
  ringworm 456
antigen-presenting cell (APC),
  immune system response to
  infection 27
antigens
  defined 711
  immune system response to
    infection 30
  immunizations 622
  influenza 550
  vaccine types 607
  vaccines 598
antihistamines
  cold or flu symptoms 470
  drug interactions 508
antimicrobial resistance
  chancroid 248
  gonorrhea 146
  methicillin-resistant *Staphylococcus
    aureus* 302
  overview 575–9
antiretroviral therapy (ART)
  HIV and AIDS 161
  microbial diseases 18
antitoxin, defined 711
"Antiviral Drugs for Seasonal
  Influenza: Additional Links and
  Resources" (CDC) 567n

729

antiviral medications
  avian flu 91
  Ebola virus disease (EVD) 122
  flu 181
  hepatitis B 158
  pandemic flu 186
  prescription medicines 564
antiviral therapy, genital
  herpes 137
APC *see* antigen-presenting cell
ART *see* antiretroviral therapy
artificial immunity, preventing
  microbial diseases 14
artificially acquired immunity,
  defined 711
ASHA *see* American Sexual Health
  Association
Aspergillus fumigatus, microbes 6
aspirin
  chickenpox 96
  fever 485
ASPR *see* Office of the Assistant
  Secretary for Preparedness and
  Response
asthma
  adolescent immunization 631
  common colds 105
  defined 712
  flu 180
  pneumonia 311
athlete's foot
  emerging and reemerging
    microbes 10
  tinea infections 451
atopic dermatitis, probiotics 520
attenuated vaccine
  defined 712
  vaccine types 605
autoimmune disorders
  immunodeficiency diseases 35
  mouth sores 490
Avian influenza A virus,
  overview 89–92
"Avian Influenza A Virus Infections in
  Humans" (CDC) 89n
"Avoiding Drug Interactions"
  (FDA) 505n
azithromycin
  chancroid 248

azithromycin, *continued*
  lymphogranuloma venereum
    (LGV) 260
  strep throat testing and
    treatment 554

B

B-cell receptors (BCRS), immune
  system response to infection 25
B cells
  defined 712
  immunodeficiency diseases 34
bacteremia
  pneumonia 314
  Streptococcus pneumoniae 350
bacteria
  blood transfusion 48
  conjunctivitis 108
  diphtheria 278
  drug resistance 573
  Hib disease 287
  microbes 4
  microbial diseases 18
  prescription medicines 562
  strep throat 482
  transmission of microbes 41
  tuberculosis (TB) 373
bacterial infections
  drug resistance 574
  immunodeficiency diseases 35
  pandemic flu 186
bacterial meningitis
  overview 295–9
  preventing microbial diseases 13
"Bacterial Meningitis" (CDC) 295n
bacterial toxins, microbes 5
bacterial vaginosis (BV),
  overview 381–4
"Bacterial Vaginosis"
  (OWH) 381n
BARDA *see* biomedical advanced
  research and development
  authority
BCRS *see* B-cell receptors
beta-lactams
  group B strep (GBS) 359
  methicillin-resistant *Staphylococcus
    aureus* 304

biomedical advanced research and
development authority (BARDA)
bioterrorism 707
pandemic flu 185
biopsy
diagnostic tests for contagious
diseases 545
Hansen disease 285
immunodeficiency diseases 36
microbial diseases 16
bioterrorism, overview 72–81
"Bioterrorism" (CDC) 72n
bird flu *see* avian influenza
blisters
chickenpox 93
childhood immunizations 614
hand, foot, and mouth disease
(HFMD) 149
impetigo 291
mouth sores 490
shingles 100
blood
amebiasis 407
drug interactions 507
hepatitis C 536
immune system 23
immunodeficiency diseases 35
microbial diseases 16
tuberculosis (TB) 373
blood culture
medical tests 544
pneumonia 315
blood tests
fifth disease 133
immunodeficiency diseases 36
medical tests 544
syphilis 364
"Blood Transfusion" (NHLBI) 46n
blood transfusions
infectious mononucleosis 128
risk of infectious disease 46
Zika 240
body lice
overview 418–20
pubic lice 427
"Body Lice—Frequently Asked
Questions (FAQs)" (CDC) 418n
bone marrow
defined 712

bone marrow, *continued*
fever 487
immune system 23
medical tests 545
booster shot
adolescent immunization 630
defined 712
vaccine types 607
Bordetella pertussis
microbes 5
whooping cough 395
Borrelia burgdorferi, microbes 42
botulism
bioterrorism 707
honey 515
microbes 5
breastfeeding
cholera 265
HIV and AIDS 163
trichomoniasis 462
Zika 239
breast milk
Ebola virus disease (EVD) 119
HIV and AIDS 163
immunizations 626
Zika 239
bronchiectasis, pneumonia 311
bronchitis
adenovirus 85
antibiotic safety 574
common colds 104
fever 484
buboes
chancroid 249
lymphogranuloma venereum
(LGV) 259
bugs (germs) *see* microbes
buspar (buspirone), drug
interactions 506
BV *see* bacterial vaginosis

C

CAM *see* complementary and
alternative medicine
cancers
donor tissue or organ
transplantation 32
human papillomavirus (HPV) 169
turmeric 528

Candida, vaginal yeast infection 387

canker sores, mouth sores 491

carbatrol (carbamazepine), seizures 507

catheters
  sepsis 335
  vancomycin-resistant enterococci (VRE) 391

CBER *see* center for biologics evaluation and research

CDC *see* Centers for Disease Control and Prevention

CDER *see* Center for Drugs Evaluation and Research

ceftriaxone
  chancroid 248
  HIV infection 250
  syphilis 367

cell
  defined 712
  immune system 22
  vaccination 26

cellulitis
  fever 484
  staph infection 329

center for biologics evaluation and research (CBER), bioterrorism 706

Center for Drugs Evaluation and Research (CDER), bioterrorism 706

Centers for Disease Control and Prevention (CDC)
  contact 717
  publications
    adenoviruses 85n
    air travel 54n
    amebiasis 405n
    anthrax 79n
    antibiotics 572n
    antimicrobial drug resistance 580n
    antiviral drugs for seasonal influenza 567n
    avian influenza A virus infections 89n
    bacterial meningitis 295n
    bioterrorism 72n
    body lice 418n
    chancroid 247n
    chickenpox 93n

Centers for Disease Control and Prevention (CDC) publications, *continued*
    childhood immunizations 613n
    chlamydia 251n
    cholera 263n
    Clostridioides difficile 269n
    common cold 103n
    conjunctivitis (pink eye) 107n
    contagious diseases on flights 54n
    cruise ship travel 54n
    Cryptosporidium 409n
    diphtheria 277n
    diseases and organisms 46n
    diseases and vaccines 613n
    Ebola virus disease (EVD) 117n
    enterobiasis (pinworm infection) 439n
    Epstein-Barr virus (EBV) and infectious mononucleosis 125n
    flu 176n, 476n
    genital herpes 135n
    genital HPV infection 169n
    gonorrhea 143n
    group A streptococcal (GAS) disease 552n
    group B strep (GBS) 356n
    H1N1 flu (swine flu) 187n
    hand, foot, and mouth disease (HFMD) 149n
    handwashing 591n
    Hansen disease (leprosy) 281n
    head lice 420n
    healthy habits and flu prevention 474n
    Hib disease and vaccine (shot) 287n
    how vaccines work 598n
    hygiene-related diseases 451n
    immunization schedules 633n
    influenza antiviral drug resistance 583n
    influenza testing methods 546n
    international adoption 65n
    legal authorities for isolation and quarantine 697n

Centers for Disease Control and
Prevention (CDC)
publications, *continued*
    lymphogranuloma venereum
      (LGV) 251n
    measles (rubeola) 193n
    meningitis 431n
    mumps 205n
    National Notifiable Diseases
      Surveillance System
      (NNDSS) 701n
    nonpolio enterovirus 209n
    norovirus 213n
    pandemic influenza (flu) 182n
    Parvovirus B19 and fifth
      disease 131n
    patient safety 682n
    pertussis (whooping
      cough) 395n
    pneumococcal disease 350n
    polio 219n
    pubic "crab" lice 425n
    respiratory syncytial virus
      infection (RSV) 223n
    ringworm 451n
    rubella 227n
    scabies 443n
    scarlet fever 344n
    seasonal influenza prevention
      in healthcare settings 683n
    sexually transmitted diseases
      (STDs) prevention 44n
    shigellosis 321n
    smallpox 231n
    sneezing and antibiotics 473n
    sore throat 340n, 479n
    syphilis 361n
    tuberculosis (TB) 369n
    typhoid fever 377n
    vaccination FAQs 621n
    Vaccine Adverse Event
      Reporting System
      (VAERS) 665n
    vaccine decision 601n, 677n
    vaccine records 669n
    vaccines and possible side
      effects 645n
    vaccines for children 669n
    viral meningitis 199n

Centers for Disease Control and
Prevention (CDC)
publications, *continued*
    VISA/VRSA in healthcare
      settings 335n
    VRE in healthcare
      settings 391n
    Zika 237n
cephalosporins
    antibiotics 563
    penicillin allergy 555
cervical cancer
    human papillomavirus
      (HPV) 172, 630
    screening 170
cervical ectopy, chlamydia 253
cervix
    chlamydia 253
    gonorrhea 143
    pelvic inflammatory disease
      (PID) 384
Chagas disease, described 49
chancre, syphilis 362
chancroid, overview 247–50
"Chancroid" (CDC) 247n
chickenpox (varicella)
    children 624
    described 614
    overview 93–98
    latent infection 9
    vaccine-preventable infectious
      diseases 13
    vaccine side effects 663
chikungunya
    described 50
    vector-borne diseases 63
children
    acute pharyngitis 552
    Bacille Calmette-Guérin
      vaccination 375
    chickenpox 9, 95
    Clostridium difficile infection 275
    common colds 103
    conjunctivitis 108
    cough and cold products 503
    cryptosporidiosis 411
    dehydration 214
    diphtheria 279
    fever 486

children, *continued*
  fifth disease 132
  hand, foot, and mouth disease
    (HFMD) 150
  handwashing 594
  head lice 421
  helpful bacterial toxins 5
  hepatitis A vaccine 156
  Hib disease 288
  immunization 69
  influenza 177
  measles 194
  nonpolio enteroviruses 210
  Parvovirus B19 131
  over-the-counter (OTC)
    medicines 499
  pertussis (whooping cough) 396
  pinworm infection 439
  pneumococcal disease 351
  pneumonia 312
  polio 220
  respiratory syncytial virus (RSV)
    infection 226
  ringworm 452
  rotavirus 615
  rubella 228
  scarlet fever 345
  sore throats 479
  vaccine side effects 602
chlamydia, overview 251–8
"Chlamydia—CDC Fact Sheet
  (Detailed)" (CDC) 251n
Chlamydia trachomatis,
  conjunctivitis 108
cholera, overview 263–7
"Cholera—*Vibrio cholerae* infection"
  (CDC) 263n
chronic health condition, defined 712
chronic infections, described 8
cilia, pertussis 395
clindamycin
  methicillin-resistant *Staphylococcus*
    aureus (MRSA) 333
  tabulated *554*
Clostridium botulinum, toxins 5
Clostridioides difficile,
  overview 269–6
"*Clostridioides difficile* (*C. diff*),"
  (CDC) 269n

CMV *see* cytomegalovirus
"Cold, Flu, or Allergy?" (*NIH News in
  Health*) 471n
cold viruses *see* common cold
colitis, *Clostridioides difficile* 269
colloidal silver, hepatitis C 539
coma
  DTaP vaccination 646
  hypoxia 498
  MMR vaccination 652
  Reye syndrome 715
"Combating Antibiotic Resistance"
  (FDA) 572n
combination vaccines
  children 602
  described 624
common colds
  echinacea 522
  overview 103–6
  pertussis 396
  sore throat 480
  vaccination 513
  viral conjunctivitis 111
"Common Colds: Protect Yourself and
  Others" (CDC) 103n
communicable disease
  air travel 54
  defined 712
community-acquired pneumonia,
  described 317
complementary and alternative
  medicine (CAM)
  flu and colds 512
  hepatitis C 536
computed tomography (CT/CAT) scan,
  defined 712
condoms, STD transmission 45
congenital rubella syndrome (CRS),
  serious birth defects 229
conjugate vaccine
  defined 712
  described 608
conjunctivitis
  adenovirus infection 85
  chlamydial pneumonia 252
  nonpolio enterovirus infections 210
  overview 107–15
  pregnant women 225

"Conjunctivitis (Pink Eye)"
(CDC) 107n
contagious diseases, defined 712
contaminated water
cryptosporidiosis 411
hepatitis E virus (HEV) 51
Naegleria fowleri 434
norovirus 215
contamination
cholera 264
crusted scabies 444
cryptosporidiosis 415
contraindication, defined 712
COPD *see* chronic obstructive
pulmonary disease
Cordarone (amiodarone), drug
interactions 508
Corynebacterium diphtheriae,
diphtheria 277
cough medicine, pertussis 399
coughing
acute infections 8
bacterial transmission 297
diphtheria 277
pertussis 395
pneumonia 319
respiratory infections 686
rubella 617
staph infection 332
sore throat 480
tuberculosis (TB) 371
vancomycin-resistant enterococci
(VRE) 392
"Countering Bioterrorism and
Emerging Infectious Diseases"
(FDA) 705n
"Countering Bioterrorism Questions
and Answers" (FDA) 705n
coxsackieviruses, hand, foot, and
mouth disease (HFMD) 150
crab lice *see* pubic lice
CRS *see* congenital rubella syndrome
"Cruise Ship Travel" (CDC) 54n
cruise ships
illnesses and injury aboard 60
respiratory illness outbreak 546
crusted scabies, described 443
Cryptosporidia, microbes 43
cryptosporidiosis, overview 409–15

Cryptosporidium,
cryptosporidiosis 409
"*Cryptosporidium* — General
Information for the Public"
(CDC) 409n
CT scan *see* computed axial
tomography scan
cystic fibrosis, pneumonia 311
cytomegalovirus (CMV), viral
infections 6
cytotoxic T cells, described 28

D

DAMPS *see* danger-associated
molecular patterns
danger-associated molecular
patterns (DAMPS), immune
system 22
decongestants
allergy treatment 473
dextromethorphan (DXM) 496
tabulated *472*
dehydration
chickenpox 95
cholera 264
Clostridium difficile 270
cryptosporidiosis 412
fever 484
hand, foot, and mouth disease
(HFMD) 152
norovirus illness 214
pertussis 399
seeking medical care 481
shigellosis 324
staph infection 331
dendritic cells (DC), immune cell 27
dengue fever (DF), described 51
deoxyribonucleic acid (DNA)
defined 712
gene transfer 577
deoxyribonucleic acid (DNA) vaccines,
described 608
depakote (valproic acid), seizure
control medications 507
dextromethorphan (DXM)
health effects 497
OTC medicines misuse 496
DF *see* dengue fever

DGI *see* disseminated gonococcal
infection
dialysis, mucosal risk for exposure to
blood 636
diaphragm
pelvic inflammatory disease
(PID) 386
trichomoniasis 452
diarrhea
adenovirus infection 85
antibiotics 572
Cryptosporidia 43
ginger 532
handwashing 594
immune system's reaction 17
rotavirus 615
malnutrition 34
milk thistle 537
diarrheal disease
cryptosporidiosis 412
statistics 594
tabulated *10*
dietary supplements
colds and flu 512
drug interactions 507
overview 533–5
probiotics 519
"Dietary Supplements" (NIA) 533n
digoxin, licorice 506
diphenoxylate, shigellosis 324
diphtheria
defined 712
described 614
DTaP 400, 645
overview 277–80
statistics 677
vaccine-preventable infectious
diseases 13
diseases
bacteria 5
defined 712
see also communicable diseases;
contagious diseases; infectious
diseases
"Diseases and Organisms"
(CDC) 46n
disinsection, described 56
disseminated gonococcal infection
(DGI), untreated gonorrhea 145

Division of STD Prevention (DSTDP),
contact 718
Division of Viral Hepatitis (DVH),
contact 718
DNA *see* deoxyribonucleic acid
douche
bacterial vaginosis (BV) 382
pelvic inflammatory disease
(PID) 387
trichomoniasis 463
yeast infections 389
doxycycline
bioterrorism 73
lymphogranuloma venereum
(LGV) 260
methicillin-resistant *Staphylococcus
aureus* (MRSA) 333
syphilis 367
drug interactions, overview 505–9
drug resistance
antibiotic safety 572
antifungal drugs 566
DSTDP *see* Division of STD
Prevention
DTaP; DTP *see* diphtheria tetanus
pertussis vaccine
Dukoral®, cholera 266
DVH *see* Division of Viral Hepatitis
DXM *see* dextromethorphan
dysuria
chlamydia 253
gonorrhea 144

E

Ebola, overview 117–23
Ebola hemorrhagic fever
viral infections 6
see also Ebola
EBV *see* Epstein-Barr virus
echinacea
cold symptoms 514
described 522
flu 513
eczema
allergic conjunctivitis 111
probiotics 520
elevated temperature *see* fever
encephalitis
chickenpox complications 95

encephalitis, *continued*
  defined 713
  hand, foot, and mouth disease
      (HFMD) 150
encephalopathy, defined 713
endemic
  defined 713
  measles 56
  Rocky Mountain spotted fever
      (RMSF) 485
  rubella 227
  vector-borne diseases 63
endocarditis, staphylococcal
  infections 328
Entamoeba dispar, amebiasis 407
Entamoeba histolytica,
  amebiasis 405
entecavir, hepatitis B 158
Enterobius vermicularis see
  pinworm
Environmental Protection Agency
  (EPA) *see* U.S. Environmental
  Protection Agency
epidemic
  adult immunization 639
  body lice 419
  cholera 264
  defined 713
  drug resistance 588
  human immunodeficiency virus
      (HIV) 162
  rubella 227
  vaccination 677
  viral diseases 52
Epstein-Barr virus (EBV)
  hepatitis 155
  overview 125–7
  viral meningitis 200
"Epstein-Barr Virus and Infectious
  Mononucleosis" (CDC) 125n
EPT *see* expedited partner therapy
erythromycin
  chancroid 248
  lymphogranuloma venereum
      (LGV) 260
Escherichia coli
  bacterial meningitis 296
  gram-negative bacteria 48
  tabulated 7

Eunice Kennedy Shriver National
  Institute of Child Health and
  Human Development (NICHD),
  contact 718
EVD *see* Ebola virus disease
expedited partner therapy (EPT),
  chlamydia 258
exposure, defined 713

F

fatigue
  bioterrorism 72
  brucellosis 49
  common colds 106
  Ebola virus disease (EVD) 120
  H1N1 flu virus 188
  infectious mononucleosis 127
  seasonal flu 176
  staph infection 329
  syphilis 363
  tuberculosis (TB) 371
  viral hepatitis 156
febrile seizure, fever 487
Federal Trade Commission (FTC),
  contact 718
fermentation, fungus 6
fever
  adenoviruses 85
  amebiasis 406
  avian flu 90
  bacterial meningitis 297
  bioterrorism 72
  chickenpox 98
  Clostridium difficile infection 272
  colds and flu 468
  conjunctivitis 110
  Ebola virus disease (EVD) 120
  fifth disease 133
  hand, foot, and mouth disease
      (HFMD) 149
  Hib disease 287
  human immunodeficiency virus
      (HIV) 166
  immunodeficiency diseases 35
  lymphogranuloma venereum
      (LGV) 258
  measles 193
  microbial diseases 17

fever, *continued*
  mumps 205
  overview 483–8
  parasitic meningitis 433
  pelvic inflammatory disease
    (PID) 385
  pneumonia 307
  polio 219
  scarlet 344
  seasonal flu 176
  shigellosis 321
  shingles 99
  smallpox 231
  sore throat 480
  staph infection 329
  strep throat 340
  typhoid 377
  vaccines 12
  viral meningitis 201
  whooping cough 396
  Zika virus 237
  see also scarlet fever
"Fever: What You Can Do"
    (Omnigraphics) 483n
fifth disease (*Parvovirus B19*),
    overview 131–4
flu *see* influenza
"Flu and Colds: In Depth"
    (NCCIH) 512n
flu vaccination
  cold and flu 106, 475
  drug resistance 587
  vaccines 600
"Flu: What to Do If You Get Sick"
    (CDC) 476n
fluid-filled blisters
  chickenpox 94
  impetigo 291
  mouth sores 490
fluoroquinolone, lymphogranuloma
    venereum (LGV) 260
foodborne illness, transmission of
    contagious disease 42
food safety
  international adoption 66
  staph infections 330
"For Parents: Vaccines for Your
    Children" (CDC) 669n
formalin, toxoid vaccines 607

FTC *see* Federal Trade Commission
fungal meningitis, overview 435–8
fungus
  conjunctivitis 107
  meningitis 435
  pneumonia 310
  tabulated 7
  tinea infections 451
  vaginal yeast infection 387
fungus ferments, microbes 6

G

gardasil, vaccine antigens 611
GAS disease *see* group A streptococcal
    disease
gastroenteritis, norovirus 214
gastrointestinal illness, transmission
    of communicable diseases 60
GBS *see* group B strep; Guillain-Barré
    syndrome
genes
  antimicrobial resistance 577
  defined 713
  immune cells 30
  microbial diseases 14
  norovirus 213
  pandemic flu 183
  vaccine types 606
  viruses 5
genetic material
  defined 713
  deoxyribonucleic acid (DNA)
    vaccines 608
  seasonal flu 181
Genetics Home Reference (GHR)
  contact 718
  chancroid 247
  latent infections 9
  overview 135–41
  sexually transmitted diseases
    (STDs) 44
"Genital Herpes—CDC Fact Sheet
    (Detailed)" (CDC) 135n
"Genital HPV Infection—Fact Sheet"
    (CDC) 169n
genital HSV-1 infection, genital
    herpes 136
genital HSV-2 infection, genital
    herpes 136

genital warts
human papillomavirus (HPV) 169
see also rubella
genomes
defined 713
recombinant vector vaccines 609
German measles, rubella 227
germs (bugs)
amebiasis 407
Clostridium difficile infection 270
conjunctivitis 110
H1N1 flu 191
handwashing 591
healthcare-associated infections
(HAIs) 682
immune system 622
medical tests 545
pneumonia 309
seasonal flu 180
shigellosis 322
Streptococcus pneumoniae 350
viral meningitis 201
see also microbes
GHR *see* Genetics Home Reference
Giardia lamblia, transmission 41
ginkgo biloba, drug interactions 507
ginseng, drug interactions 507
glycyrrhizin
hepatitis C 538
licorice root 525
goldenseal, described 524
gonorrhea
antimicrobial (drug) resistance 575
lymphogranuloma venereum
(LGV) 260
microbes 41
overview 143–7
pelvic inflammatory disease
(PID) 385
syphilis 361
"Gonorrhea—CDC Fact Sheet
(Detailed Version)" (CDC) 143n
gram-negative bacteria
antimicrobial resistance 576
described 48
gram-positive bacteria, described 48
grapefruit juice, drug interactions 506
green tea, complementary
approaches 518

group A streptococcal infections,
chickenpox 95
"Group A Streptococcal (GAS)
Disease—Pharyngitis (Strep
Throat)" (CDC) 552n
"Group B Strep (GBS)" (CDC) 356n
Guillain-Barré syndrome (GBS), Zika
virus 238
GVHD *see* graft versus host disease

H

HAART *see* highly active
antiretroviral therapy
Haemophilus ducreyi, chancroid 247
Haemophilus influenzae
bacterial conjunctivitis 108
bacterial meningitis 295
Haemophilus influenzae type B (Hib)
bacterial meningitis 296
conjugate vaccines 608
conjunctivitis 115
defined 312
described 617
overview 287–9
vaccine side effects 648
Haemophilus influenzae type B
vaccine, vaccine side effects 648
halcion (triazolam), drug
interactions 506
hand, foot, and mouth disease (HFMD)
nonpolio enteroviruses 210
overview 149–53
"Hand, Foot, and Mouth Disease
(HFMD)" (CDC) 149n
hand hygiene
Clostridium difficile infection 271
described 690
norovirus 216
sore throat 482
vancomycin-intermediate
Staphylococcus aureus
(VISA) 337
whooping cough 400
hand sanitizer
common colds 104
conjunctivitis 113
norovirus 217
methicillin-resistant *Staphylococcus
aureus* (MRSA) 304

handwashing
  adenovirus 87
  amebiasis 408
  common colds 104
  hand, foot, and mouth disease
      (HFMD) 151
  microbial diseases prevention 11
  overview 591–5
  seasonal flu 180
  shigellosis 321
"Handwashing: Clean Hands Save
  Lives" (CDC) 591n
Hansen disease, overview 281–6
hay fever
  conjunctivitis 108
  herbal supplements 524
  probiotics 520
headaches
  brucellosis 49
  chickenpox 94
  common colds 103
  Ebola virus disease (EVD) 120
  fifth disease 131
  hand, foot, and mouth disease
      (HFMD) 150
  hepatitis A vaccine 646
  Hib disease 287
  H1N1 flu virus 188
  mumps 205
  norovirus 214
  parasitic meningitis 432
  rubella 228
  seasonal flu 176
  sore throat 480
  strep throat 341
  Streptococcus pneumoniae 352
  tabulated *473*
  typhoid fever 377
  viral meningitis 201
  whooping cough 399
  Zika virus 237
head lice, overview 420–5
"Head Lice—Frequently Asked
  Questions (FAQs)" (CDC) 420n
Health Resources and Services
  Administration (HRSA), contact 718
Healthfinder®, contact 718
"Healthy Habits to Help Prevent Flu"
  (CDC) 474n

hearing screen, adopted child 67
hemorrhagic rash, chickenpox 97
hepatitis
  milk thistle 526
  overview 155–60
hepatitis A
  adolescent immunization 631
  childhood immunizations 617
  described 156
  vaccine side effects 646
hepatitis B
  antivirals 564
  childhood immunizations 618
  described 157
  subunit vaccines 607
  vaccine side effects 647
hepatitis C
  chronic infections 8
  complementary and alternative
      medicine (CAM) 536
  described 158
  infectious diseases 68
"Hepatitis C: A Focus on Dietary
  Supplements" (NCCIH) 536n
hepatitis D, described 159
hepatitis E, described 160
Hepatitis Foundation International
  (HFI), contact 723
herbal supplements, overview 522–33
"Herbs at a Glance" (NCCIH) 522n
herpes simplex virus (HSV)
  chancroid 248
  genital herpes 135
  human papillomavirus (HPV) 169
  latent infections 9
  mouth sores 490
  viral meningitis 200
herpes zoster (shingles)
  defined 713
  latent infection 9
  varicella vaccination 641
HFI *see* Hepatitis Foundation
  International
HFMD *see* hand, foot, and mouth
  disease
HHS *see* U.S. Department of Health
  and Human Services
Hib *see* *Haemophilus influenzae
  type B*

"Hib Disease and the Vaccine (Shot) to Prevent It" (CDC) 287n
HIV *see* human immunodeficiency virus
hives, defined 713
H1N1 (swine flu)
  influenza antiviral drug resistance 586
  overview 187–91
"H1N1 Flu—2009 H1N1 Flu ("Swine Flu") and You" (CDC) 187n
household pet, microbes 42
"How to Treat Impetigo and Control This Common Skin Infection" (FDA) 291n
"How You Can Prevent Sexually Transmitted Diseases" (CDC) 44n
HPIV *see* human parainfluenza virus
HPV *see* human papillomavirus
HRSA *see* Health Resources and Services Administration
HSV *see* herpes simplex virus
human immunodeficiency virus (HIV)
  chancroid 250
  chickenpox 95
  fifth disease 132
  fungal meningitis 435
  gonorrhea 145
  hepatitis B vaccination 636
  H1N1 flu 190
  overview 161–8
  sexually transmitted diseases (STDs) 44
  shigellosis 322
  Streptococcus pneumoniae 351
  tinea infections 454
  tuberculosis (TB) 371
  viral diseases 52
human papillomavirus (HPV)
  overview 169–73
  sexually transmitted diseases (STDs) 44
human parainfluenza virus (HPIV), pneumonia 310
Hydrodiuril (hydrochlorothiazide), drug interactions 506
"Hygiene-Related Diseases" (CDC) 451n
hyperthermia, fever 483

I

IBD *see* inflammatory bowel disease
ibuprofen
  chickenpox 96
  fever 485
  respiratory syncytial virus (RSV) 224
  tabulated *473*
IgA *see* immunoglobulin A
IgM *see* immunoglobulin M
immigrants
  amebiasis 405
  hepatitis B 157
  malaria 50
immune deficiency disorder, protozoa 7
immune globulin
  defined 713
  hepatitis A 156
  immunodeficiency diseases 36
  measles 56
immune response
  defined 713
  Ebola virus disease (EVD) 120
  probiotics 521
  seasonal flu 181
  staphylococcal infections 328
  strep throat testing 556
immune system
  acquired immunodeficiency syndrome (AIDS) 162
  adenoviruses 86
  bacterial meningitis 299
  chickenpox 93
  conjunctivitis 112
  cryptosporidiosis 412
  defined 713
  dietary supplements 534
  fifth disease 132
  fungal meningitis 435
  measles 196
  microbes 8
  nonpolio enteroviruses 209
  overview 22–4
  pneumonia 309
  probiotics 519
  respiratory syncytial virus (RSV) 225

immune system, *continued*
  tuberculosis (TB) 370
  vaccines 598
  see also immunodeficiency
immunity
  defined 713
  fifth disease 133
  Hansen disease 284
  hepatitis A 156
  nonpolio enteroviruses 209
  overview 22–32
  pandemic flu 183
  tabulated *197*
  varicella vaccination 641
  whooping cough 400
  see also artificially acquired
    immunity; community immunity;
    herd immunity; naturally
    acquired immunity; passive
    immunity
immunization records, adopted
  children 65
Immunization Safety Review
  Committee (ISR), contact 723
"Immunization Schedules"
  (CDC) 633n
"Immunodeficiency and Contagious
  Diseases" (Omnigraphics) 33n
immunodeficiency, overview 33–7
immunoglobulin M (IgM), genital
  herpes 140
Imodium (loperamide), shigellosis 324
impetigo
  methicillin-resistant *Staphylococcus*
    aureus (MRSA) 302
  overview 291–3
  scarlet fever 345
  staph infection 331
inactivated vaccines
  defined 713
  described 606
  see also vaccines
incubation period, defined 713
infected birds, avian flu 89
infections, defined 714
infectious agents, defined 714
infectious disease
  antimicrobial resistance 576
  bacterial meningitis 296

infectious disease, *continued*
  bioterrorism 73
  gonorrhea 143
  microbes 40
  polio 619
  screening 68
  shigellosis 321
  smallpox 231
  strep throat testing 555
infectious mononucleosis
  hepatitis A 155
  overview 127–9
inflammatory muscle disease,
  nonpolio enteroviruses 210
influenza (flu)
  avian flu 89
  conjunctivitis 108
  Ebola virus disease (EVD) 120
  microbial diseases 12
  overview 176–91
  pneumonia 310
  respiratory illnesses 61
  see also seasonal flu
"Influenza Antiviral Drug Resistance"
  (CDC) 583n
influenza vaccine
  pneumonia 311
  side effects 649
  Streptococcus pneumoniae 355
  transmission 62
"Information Regarding the OraQuick
  In-Home HIV Test" (FDA) 556n
innate immune cells, bone marrow 23
insertive partner, human
  immunodeficiency virus (HIV) 165
"International Adoption" (CDC) 65n
intravenous
  antiviral drug resistance 584
  blood transfusion 46
  cholera 265
  Ebola virus disease (EVD) 121
  hand, foot, and mouth disease
    (HFMD) 152
  immunodeficiency diseases 36
  methicillin-resistant *Staphylococcus*
    aureus (MRSA) 304
  norovirus 216
  pneumonia 318
  seasonal flu 181

intravenous, *continued*
  staph infections 330
  syphilis 366
  vancomycin-resistant enterococci
    (VRE) 392
intussusception, defined 714
"Is It a Cold or the Flu? Prevention,
  Symptoms, Treatments" (FDA) 468n
itching
  bacterial vaginosis (BV) 382
  body lice 419
  chickenpox 96
  conjunctivitis 109
  fifth disease 133
  licorice root 526
  scabies 443
  syphilis 363
  trichomoniasis 460

J

Japanese encephalitis, vector-borne
  diseases 63
jaundice
  defined 714
  hepatitis C 537
  viral hepatitis 155
jock itch, tinea infections 451
joint pain
  chikungunya virus 50
  fifth disease 132
  sore throat care 481
  Zika virus 237

K

"Keeping Your Vaccine Records Up to
  Date" (CDC) 669n
"Kids Are Not Just Small Adults—
  Medicines, Children, and the Care
  Every Child Deserves" (FDA) 499n
killed vaccine, defined 713

L

lactobacillus
  probiotics 519
  tabulated 7
lactoferrin, hepatitis C 538
lamivudine, hepatitis B 158

Lanoxin (digoxin), drug
  interactions 506
latex allergies, condom 45
latex condoms
  gonorrhea 147
  hepatitis B 158
  human papillomavirus (HPV) 170
  sexually transmitted diseases
    (STDs) 46
  syphilis 368
"Legal Authorities for Isolation and
  Quarantine" (CDC) 697n
Legionnaires' disease
  described 62
  pneumonia 308
leprosy *see* Hansen disease
lesion, defined 714
LGV *see* lymphogranuloma venereum
ligands, immunity 29
lindane shampoo, pubic lice 427
live, attenuated vaccine, defined 714
lockjaw *see* tetanus vaccine
lozenges, treatment for cold 517
lupus
  defined 714
  immunodeficiency diseases 35
  see also systemic lupus
    erythematosus (SLE)
Lyme disease
  fever 485
  microbes 42
lymph nodes
  biopsy test 545
  defined 714
  Epstein-Barr virus (EBV) 126
  human immunodeficiency virus
    (HIV) 167
  immune system 24
  immunodeficiency diseases 36
  lymphogranuloma venereum
    (LGV) 259
  rubella 228
  sore throat 481
  strep throat 341
lymphadenopathy, chancroid 248
lymphocytes
  bone marrow 23
  defined 714
  infectious mononucleosis 128

lymphogranuloma venereum (LGV),
  overview 258–61
"Lymphogranuloma Venereum (LGV)"
  (CDC) 251n

M

macrophages
  defined 714
  immunity 25
  vaccines 598
magnetic resonance imaging (MRI),
  defined 714
"Making the Vaccine Decision"
  (CDC) 601n
malaria
  adopted children 66
  antiprotozoals 565
  drug interactions 506
  drug resistance 581
  Ebola virus disease (EVD) 120
  fever 485
  microbes 7
  transmission 42
mast cells, immunity 23
mastitis
  mumps 206
  staph infections 334
measles
  conjunctivitis 115
  human papillomavirus (HPV) 638
  overview 193–8
  rubella 227
  transmission 56
  vaccines 12, 606, 677
"Measles (Rubeola)" (CDC) 193n
medical examination, international
  adoptions 67
medical tests *see* tests
"Medical Tests That Diagnose
  Infection" (Omnigraphics) 544n
medications
  chickenpox 97
  chlamydia 257
  drug resistance 588
  Ebola virus disease (EVD) 121
  herpes 140
  human papillomavirus (HPV) 172
  immunizations 621

medications, *continued*
  impetigo 291
  lice 427
  nonpolio enterovirus 211
  shigellosis 324
  stockpile products 74
  tinea infections 457
  transmission of infections 696
  vaccines 645
  whooping cough 396
  see also over-the-counter (OTC)
    medications, complementary and
    alternative medicine (CAM)
MedlinePlus, contact 718
memory cells
  defined 714
  immunity 23
  vaccines 598
meningitis
  drug resistance 579
  genital herpes 137
  tabulated *10*
  transmission of contagious
    disease 42
  varicella vaccine 663
  see also amebic meningitis; bacterial
    meningitis; fungal meningitis;
    parasitic meningitis; viral
    meningitis
"Meningitis" (CDC) 431n
meningococcal disease
  bacterial meningitis 296
  contagious disease transmission 55
  immunization 629
  vaccines 12
methicillin
  drug resistance 582
  healthcare-associated
    infections 682
  Staphylococcus aureus 301
"Methicillin-Resistant *Staphylococcus
  aureus* (MRSA)" (NIAID) 301n
metronidazole
  antiprotozoals 565
  trichomoniasis 461
microbes (germs)
  antimicrobial resistance 575
  bioterrorism 72
  immunity 19

microbes (germs), *continued*
  methicillin-resistant *Staphylococcus aureus* 302
  overview 4–14
  transmission of contagious disease 43
  vaccines 606
  see also bacteria; fungi; protozoa; viruses
microbial infections, prescription medicines 562
microorganisms
  antibiotics 562
  antimicrobial resistance 580
  friendly bacteria 519
  microorganisms 14
  protozoa 7
military recruits, vaccination 639
milk thistle, described 526
mites, scabies 443
MMR *see* measles mumps rubella
MMRV *see* measles mumps rubella varicella vaccine
molecule
  adaptive immunity 25
  antibiotics 562
  defined 714
  Ebola virus disease (EVD) 120
  microbes 5
  vaccine 607
monocytes, bone marrow 23
mosquito bites
  human immunodeficiency virus (HIV) 164
  Zika virus 238
Motrin (ibuprofen)
  chickenpox 96
  fever 485
  respiratory syncytial virus (RSV) 224
  turmeric 528
"Mouth Sores: Causes and Care" (Omnigraphics) 489n
MRI *see* magnetic resonance imaging
MRSA *see* methicillin-resistant *Staphylococcus aureus*
mucosal tissue, immunity 24
mucus
  adenovirus 85

mucus, *continued*
  antibiotics 573
  cold or flu 470
  conjunctivitis 109
  cough and cold 502
  hand, foot, and mouth disease (HFDM) 151
  measles 195
  nonpolio enterovirus 211
  Parvovirus B19 132
  streptococcal infections 351
  whooping cough 398
multidrug therapy, Hansen disease 285
mumps
  adult immunizations 639
  childhood immunizations 615
  measles 56, 193
  overview 205–7
  rubella 227
  vaccine 13, 599, 653
"Mumps" (CDC) 205n
mutate
  antivirals 564
  defined 714
  vaccine 606
Mycobacterium leprae, Hansen disease 281
Mycoplasma pneumoniae, pneumonia 308
Mycobacterium tuberculosis
  antimicrobial resistance 576
  microbial diseases 12
  transmission 55
mycoses, fungus 6
myocarditis
  diphtheria 278
  nonpolio enterovirus 210

N

NAAT *see* nucleic acid amplification testing
nardil (phenelzine), drug interactions 505
nasal rinse, cold and flu 512
National Cancer Institute (NCI), contact 719

National Center for Complementary and Integrative Health (NCCIH)
  contact 719
  publications
    dietary supplements 533n
    flu and colds 512n
    hepatitis A 536n
    herbs 522n
    probiotics 519n
National Diabetes Information Clearinghouse (NDIC),
  contact 719
National Foundation for Infectious Diseases (NFID), contact 723
National Health Information Center (NHIC), contact 719
National Heart, Lung, and Blood Institute (NHLBI)
  contact 719
  publications
    blood transfusion 46n
    pneumonia 307n
National Institute of Allergy and Infectious Diseases (NIAID)
  contact 720
  publications
    antimicrobial (drug) resistance 575n
    immune system 22n, 24n
    methicillin-resistant *Staphylococcus aureus* (MRSA) 301n
    microbes in sickness and in health 4n, 8n, 11n, 15n, 40n
    vaccine types 605n
National Institute of Diabetes and Digestive and Kidney Diseases (NIDDK)
  contact 720
  publication
    viral hepatitis 155n
National Institute of Neurological Disorders and Stroke (NINDS), contact 720
National Institute on Aging (NIA)
  contact 720
  publications
    dietary supplements 533n
    shingles 93n

National Institute on Drug Abuse (NIDA)
  publication
    over-the-counter (OTC) medicines 496n
National Institutes of Health (NIH)
  contact 720
  publications
    sexually transmitted diseases (STDs) 44n
    staphylococcal infections 328n
National Network for Immunization Information (NNii), contact 723
National Notifiable Diseases Surveillance System (NNDSS), public safety 701
"National Notifiable Diseases Surveillance System (NNDSS)" (CDC) 701n
National Patient Advocate Foundation (NPAF), contact 723
National Prevention Information Network (NPIN), contact 720
National Vaccine Injury Compensation Program (NVCIP), contact 720
National Women's Health Information Center (NWHIC), contact 721
natural killer (NK) cells, immune system 23
naturally acquired immunity
  defined 714
  microbes 14
  vaccines 600
NCCIH *see* National Center for Complementary and Integrative Health
NCI *see* National Cancer Institute
NDIC *see* National Diabetes Information Clearinghouse
Neisseria gonorrhoeae, sexually transmitted diseases (STDs) 143
Neisseria meningitidis
  bacterial meningitis 295
  contagious disease transmission 55
  meningococcal vaccination 639
The Nemours Foundation/ KidsHealth®, contact 723

neti pot, complementary and
alternative medicine (CAM) 512
neutralization, adaptive cells 28
neutrophils, Epstein-Barr virus
(EBV) 128
NFID *see* National Foundation for
Infectious Diseases
NHIC *see* National Health
Information Center
NHLBI *see* National Heart, Lung, and
Blood Institute
NIAID *see* National Institute of
Allergy and Infectious Diseases
NIDA *see* National Institute on Drug
Abuse
NIDDK *see* National Institute of
Diabetes and Digestive and Kidney
Diseases
NIH *see* National Institutes of Health
NIH News in Health
publication
cold, flu, or allergy 471n
NINDS *see* National Institute of
Neurological Disorders and Stroke
nitazoxanide, *Cryptosporidium* 413
nits, body lice 418
NK cells *see* natural killer cells
NNDSS *see* National Notifiable
Diseases Surveillance System
NNii *see* National Network for
Immunization Information
"Non-Polio Enterovirus" (CDC) 209n
noroviruses
handwashing 593
overview 213–8
transmission of contagious
disease 60
Norvir (ritonavir), drug
interactions 508
Norwegian scabies, scabies 443
NPAF *see* National Patient Advocate
Foundation
NPIN *see* National Prevention
Information Network
nucleic acid amplification testing
(NAAT)
chlamydia 256
genital herpes 139
influenza virus tests 547

NVCIP *see* National Vaccine Injury
Compensation Program
NWHIC *see* National Women's Health
Information Center
nymphs, body lice 418

O

ODS *see* Office of Dietary
Supplements
Office of Dietary Supplements (ODS),
contact 721
Office of Management and Budget
(OMB), countering bioterrorism 707
Office of the Assistant Secretary for
Preparedness and Response (ASPR)
contact 721
publication
Strategic National Stockpile
(SNS) 74n
Office on Women's Health (OWH)
publications
bacterial vaginosis 381n
pelvic inflammatory disease
(PID) 381n
trichomoniasis 459n
vaginal yeast infections 381n
OMB *see* Office of Management and
Budget
Omnigraphics
publications
antibiotics, antivirals,
and other prescription
medicines 561n
fever 483n
immunodeficiency and
contagious diseases 33n
medical tests and diagnosis of
infection 544n
mouth sores 489n
Staphylococcus aureus and
pregnancy 331n
vaccine misinformation and
tragic consequences 673n
oophoritis, mumps 206
opportunistic infections
human immunodeficiency virus
(HIV) 162
viral diseases 52

OPV *see* oral poliovirus vaccine
oral poliovirus vaccine (OPV),
  polio 221
oral rehydration solution, cholera 265
oral sex
  chlamydia 254
  defined 163
  genital herpes 136
  sexually transmitted diseases
    (STDs) 45
  syphilis 362
orchitis
  defined 715
  mumps 206
oseltamivir
  avian flu 91
  drug resistance 585
  prescription medicines 564
osteomyelitis
  fever 484
  Staphylococcus aureus 336
"OTC Cough and Cold Products: Not
  for Infants and Children under Two
  Years of Age" (FDA) 502n
OTC medications *see* over-the-counter
  medications
otitis media
  defined 715
  infections 350
  international adoption 67
outbreak
  adenovirus 87
  chikungunya virus (CHIKV) 50
  childhood immunizations 614
  cryptosporidiosis 409
  defined 715
  Ebola virus disease (EVD) 122
  flu 475
  genital herpes 136
  hand, foot, and mouth disease
    (HFMD) 150
  impetigo 292
  influenza 181, 456, 546
  lymphogranuloma venereum
    (LGV) 258
  microbes 10
  mouth sores 491
  norovirus 213
  pinworms 442

outbreak, *continued*
  public health 701
  shigellosis 323
  smallpox 233
  transmission of contagious
    disease 61
  vaccine misinformation 675
  viral conjunctivitis 108
over-the-counter (OTC) medications
  antiviral drugs 182
  bacterial vaginosis 383
  chickenpox 96
  cryptosporidiosis 413
  dietary supplements 534
  Epstein-Barr virus (EBV) 127
  fever 485
  hand, foot, and mouth disease
    (HFMD) 152
  human immunodeficiency virus
    (HIV) 556
  impetigo 292
  microbes 19
  nonpolio enterovirus 211
  overview 495–502
  ringworm 455
  see also medications
"Over-the-Counter Medicines"
  (NIDA) 496n
"Overview of Influenza Testing
  Methods" (CDC) 546n
"Overview of the Immune System"
  (NIAID) 22n, 24n
OWH *see* Office on Women's Health
oxacillin, staph infections 303
oxymatrine, complementary and
  alternative medicine (CAM) 538

P

palivizumab, respiratory syncytial
  virus 226
pandemic, defined 715
"Pandemic Influenza (Flu)—Questions
  and Answers" (CDC) 182n
Pap test *see* Papanicolaou test
Papanicolaou test (Pap test), human
  papillomavirus (HPV) 173
parainfluenza virus, common
  cold 106

paralysis
  hand, foot, and mouth disease
    (HFMD) 150
  Hansen disease 283
  nonpolio enterovirus 210
  parasitic meningitis 433
  polio 219
  shingles 100
  syphilis 363
parasites
  amebiasis 406
  antimicrobial resistance 576
  cryptosporidiosis 412
  defined 715
  microbes 7
  parasitic meningitis 432
  risk of infectious disease 49
  trichomoniasis 460
"Parasites—Enterobiasis (Also Known
  as Pinworm Infection)" (CDC) 439n
parasitic meningitis, overview 431
parnate (tranylcypromine), drug
  interactions 505
parotitis, mumps 205
Parvovirus B19 see fifth disease
"*Parvovirus B19* and Fifth Disease—
  Fifth Disease" (CDC) 131n
pathogens
  bioterrorism 705
  defined 715
  immune system response to
    infection 25
  prescription medicines 562
  viral meningitis 201
"Patient Safety: What You Can Do to
  Be a Safe Patient" (CDC) 682n
PCR *see* polymerase chain reaction
peginterferon, hepatitis B 158
pelvic inflammatory disease (PID)
  chlamydia 253
  gonorrhea 144
  immunodeficiency diseases 33
  overview 384–7
"Pelvic Inflammatory Disease"
  (OWH) 381n
penicillin
  methicillin-resistant *Staphylococcus
    aureus* 302
  scarlet fever 346

penicillin, *continued*
  syphilis 364
  strep throat testing and
    treatment 554
  prescription medicines 562
permethrin
  pubic lice 427
  Zika 241
pertussis
  adult immunization
    recommendations 641
  microbes 5
  screening internationally adopted
    children 66
  vaccines side effects 660
  see also whooping cough
pertussis vaccine
  microbes 5
  vaccines side effects 660
  whooping cough 397
"Pertussis (Whooping Cough)"
  (CDC) 395n
petechiae
  defined 715
  strep throat 341, 480
pets
  Ebola virus disease (EVD) 119
  scabies 446
  scarlet fever 345
  tinea infections 454
PHEMCE *see* public-health
  emergency medical countermeasure
  enterprise
PID *see* pelvic inflammatory disease
pink eye *see* conjunctivitis
pinworms, overview 439–42
placebo, defined 715
plague
  bioterrorism 706
  preventing microbial diseases 13
  transmission of microbes 42
plasmodium falciparum, antimicrobial
  (drug) resistance 575
pneumococcal pneumonia
  pneumonia 312
  Streptococcus pneumoniae 354
pneumococcal polysaccharide vaccine
  adolescent immunization 631
  Streptococcus pneumoniae 355

pneumococcal vaccine
  pneumonia 312
  Streptococcus pneumoniae 351
pneumococcus
  pneumonia 317
  Streptococcus pneumoniae 350
Pneumocystis jirovecii, pneumonia 310
pneumonia
  adolescent immunization 631
  antibiotics 573
  childhood immunizations 614
  chlamydia 252
  colds or flu 469
  common colds 104
  defined 715
  diphtheria 278
  fever 484
  flu 180
  Legionnaires' disease 62
  measles 196
  overview 307–19
  respiratory syncytial virus (RSV) 223
  Staphylococcus aureus 302
  streptococcal infections 347
  tabulated *10*
  vaccines 654
  whooping cough 398
"Pneumonia" (NHLBI) 307n
polio
  described 619
  hand, foot, and mouth disease
    (HFMD) 150
  international adoption 66
  microbial diseases 12
  overview 219–21
  vaccine 657
poliomyelitis *see* polio
polymerase chain reaction (PCR)
  chancroid 247
  genital herpes 139
  influenza 547
  syphilis 366
polyneuropathy, diphtheria 278
polysaccharide
  adolescent immunization 631
  conjugate vaccines 608
  defined 715
  streptococcal infections 355
  vaccine side effects 656

"Possible Side-Effects from Vaccines"
  (CDC) 645n
postherpetic neuralgia, shingles 100
postpolio syndrome, polio 220
potency
  defined 715
  immunity 29
  stockpile 76
  vaccine 609
  vaccine misinformation 676
pregnancy
  adult immunization 637
  chlamydia 251
  colds and flu 513
  genital herpes 138
  Hansen disease 283
  herbal supplements 532
  human immunodeficiency virus
    (HIV) 163
  rubella 229
  Staphylococcus aureus 331
  syphilis 364
  trichomoniasis 462
  whooping cough 616
  Zika virus 52
"Prevention Strategies for Seasonal
  Influenza in Healthcare Settings"
  (CDC) 683n
primary immunodeficiency (PID),
  defined 33
prion diseases, described 52
"Probiotics: In Depth" (NCCIH) 519n
protease inhibitor, Lanoxin 508
"Protecting Travelers' Health from
  Airport to Community: Investigating
  Contagious Diseases on Flights"
  (CDC) 54n
protozoa
  described 7
  microbes 19
  prescription medicines 562
  transmission of contagious
    disease 41
psoriasis, aloe vera 529
psychrophiles, bacteria 4
pubic lice, overview 425–9
"Pubic "Crab" Lice—Frequently Asked
  Questions (FAQs)" (CDC) 425n
pyrexia *see* fever

Q

QOL *see* quality of life
quality of life (QOL), complementary and alternative medicine (CAM) 527
quarantine
  defined 715
  legal authorities 697
  transmission of contagious disease 57
quinerva, drugs 506
quinite (quinine), drugs 506
quinolones
  drug resistance 582
  prescription medicines 563

R

RA *see* rheumatoid arthritis
rabies
  microbial diseases 12
  recombinant vector vaccines 609
rapid influenza diagnostic test (RIDT)
  influenza virus tests 547
  seasonal flu 181
Rapivab®, prescription medicines 564
RBCs *see* red blood cells
recombinant, defined 715
recombinant subunit vaccines, subunit vaccines 607
recombinant vector vaccines, described 609
red blood cells (RBCs)
  blood tests 544
  monocytes 27
Reiter syndrome, chlamydial infection 254
Relenza (zanamivir)
  antiviral resistance 584
  prescription medicines 564
respiratory illness
  communicable diseases 60
  handwashing 594
  over-the-counter (OTC) medications 503
  respiratory syncytial virus (RSV) 223
  seasonal flu 176
  whooping cough 401

respiratory syncytial virus (RSV)
  overview 223–6
  pneumonia 310
"Respiratory Syncytial Virus Infection (RSV)" (CDC) 223n
Reston virus, Ebola virus disease (EVD) 117
Reye syndrome
  chickenpox 96
  defined 715
  fever 485
rheumatoid arthritis (RA)
  alternative medicine 532
  fungal meningitis 436
  tuberculosis (TB) 373
rhinorrhea, strep throat 552
rhinoviruses
  common cold 105
  microbes infections 8
ribavirin
  anti-hepatitis 564
  hepatitis C 159
ribonucleic acid (RNA), viruses 5
RIDT *see* rapid influenza diagnostic test
rimantadine
  antivirals 564
  drug resistance 587
ringworm, overview 451–6
ritalin (methylphenidate), drug interactions 506
RNA *see* ribonucleic acid
rotateq vaccine, childhood immunizations 615
rotavirus
  described 615
  immunizations 69
rotavirus vaccine
  immunizations 69
  side effects 658
RSV *see* respiratory syncytial virus
rubella (German measles)
  air travel 58
  vaccinations 677
"Rubella (German Measles, Three-Day Measles)" (CDC) 227n
runny nose
  common colds 103
  fifth disease 131

runny nose, *continued*
  measles 193
  respiratory syncytial virus
    (RSV) 223
  sore throat 480
  strep throat 341
  vaccine side effects 651

S

safety considerations, dietary
  supplements 535
scabies, overview 443–9
"Scabies Frequently Asked Questions
  (FAQs)" (CDC) 443n
scarlatina *see* scarlet fever
scarlet fever
  overview 344–8
  strep throat 341
"Scarlet Fever: All You Need to Know"
  (CDC) 344n
SCD *see* sickle cell disease
schisandra, hepatitis C 538
seasonal flu
  antiviral drugs 567
  healthy habits 474
  overview 176–82
  see also influenza
secondary immunodeficiency (SID),
  described 33
seizure
  amebic meningitis 435
  avian influenza A 90
  bacterial meningitis 298
  ginkgo biloba 507
  syphilis 364
  vaccine side effects 663
sepsis
  bacterial meningitis 295
  chickenpox 95
  gram-negative bacteria 581
  Streptococcus pneumoniae 353
  viral meningitis 201
serology, genital herpes 139
sexually transmitted diseases (STDs)
  chlamydia 251
  genital herpes 140
  lice 427
  syphilis 361
  transmission 44

"Sexually Transmitted Diseases"
  (NIH) 44n
ShanChol®, cholera 266
Shigella, shigellosis 321
"*Shigella*—Shigellosis" (CDC) 321n
shigellosis, overview 321–6
shingles *see* herpes zoster
"Shingles" (NIA) 93n
"Show Me the Science—Why Wash
  Your Hands?" (CDC) 591n
sickle cell disease (SCD)
  influenza 190
  pneumonia 311
SID *see* secondary immunodeficiency
sinusitis
  colds and flu 469
  tabulated *10*
skin diseases
  Hansen disease 285
  tabulated *10*
skin lesions
  diphtheria 277
  microbes 19
smallpox
  antivirals 563
  bioterrorism 72
  microbial diseases 12
  overview 231–5
  vaccination 673
smallpox vaccine
  described 233
  vaccine misinformation 673
smoking
  pneumonia 310
  sore throat 479
sneezing
  adenovirus 87
  colds and flu 468
  group A strep 343
  H1N1 virus 187
  microbes infections 8
  mumps 206
  rubella 617
  sore throat 480
  strep throat 556
sniffles, colds or flu 471
"Sniffle or Sneeze? No Antibiotics
  Please" (CDC) 473n
SNS *see* Strategic National Stockpile

sore throat
  alternative medicine 531
  colds and flu 468
  common colds 103
  respiratory illness 61
  rubella 228
  seasonal flu 176
  strep throat 340
  syphilis 363
"Sore Throat" (CDC) 479n
sore throat care, overview 479–82
spanish flu, federal quarantine 699
spleen
  fever 487
  immune system 24
  infectious mononucleosis 127
  pneumococcal disease 351
  rubella 229
St. John's wort, dietary
  supplements 507
staph infections *see Staphylococcus
  aureus*
"Staphylococcal Infections"
  (NIH) 328n
Staphylococcus aureus
  bacterial conjunctivitis 108
  described 335
  prescription medicines 561
  tabulated 7
"*Staphylococcus aureus* and
  Pregnancy" (Omnigraphics) 331n
Streptococcus pyogenes, impetigo 291
STDs *see* sexually transmitted
  diseases
stool examination, infectious
  diseases 68
strain
  adolescent immunization 631
  anti-influenza 564
  antibiotics 474
  bacterial meningitis 299
  defined 715
  innate immunity 25
  respiratory illness 61
  streptococcal infections 356
  vaccine misinformation 673
Strategic National Stockpile (SNS)
  bioterrorism 708
  overview 74–8

"Strategic National Stockpile"
  (ASPR) 74n
strep throat
  microbial diseases 17
  overview 340–4
  sore throat care 479
  tabulated *11*
  throat culture test 545
"Strep Throat: All You Need to Know"
  (CDC) 340n
Streptococcus pneumoniae
  bacterial meningitis 295
  drug resistance 581
  overview 350–6
Streptococcus salivarius, tabulated 7
"Surveillance for Antimicrobial Drug
  Resistance in Under-Resourced
  Countries" (CDC) 580n
subunit vaccine
  defined 716
  vaccine types 605
swelling
  childhood immunizations 614
  chlamydia 253
  impetigo 293
  measles 193
  microbial diseases 15
  mouth sores 492
  shingles 100
  vaccine side effects 658
  yeast infections 388
syphilis
  chancroid 247
  overview 361–8
  prescription medicines 561
  sexually transmitted diseases
    (STDs) 44
"Syphilis—CDC Fact Sheet (Detailed)"
  (CDC) 361n

T

T cells
  defined 716
  immunodeficiency 34
  microbes 13
  vaccine types 607
T-cell receptors, immune cells

Tamiflu®
anti-influenza 564
antiviral drug resistance 584
Tdap vaccine, adolescent
immunization 630
tegretol, drug interactions 507
telbivudine, hepatitis B 158
temperature *see* fever
tetanus
defined 716
diphtheria 279
microbial diseases 12
toxoid vaccines 608
vaccine misinformation 674
whooping cough 400
tetanus vaccine, childhood
immunizations 619
tetracyclines, prescription
medicines 563
thermophiles, microbes 5
thimerosal
defined 716
tabulated *603*
throat culture, strep throat
testing 342, 553
thymus, immune system 23
thymus extract, alternative
medicine 538
tinea infections, overview 451–7
tinidazole
antiprotozoals 565
trichomoniasis 461
tissue
biopsy test 545
common colds 104
defined 716
diphtheria 278
influenza 191
meningococcal disease 629
microbes 6
pneumonia 314
West Nile virus (WNV) 52
TNF *see* tumor necrosis factor
toll-like receptors (TLRs), innate
immunity 25
tonsils
immunodeficiency 36
papillomavirus 170
sore throat 480

tonsils, *continued*
strep throat 340
toxic shock syndrome (TSS),
staphylococcal infections 328
toxins
defined 716
microbes 5
prescription medicines 562
staphylococcal infections 328
tabulated *603*
whooping cough 395
toxoid vaccines
defined 716
vaccine types 605
Toxoplasma gondii, protozoa 7
transfusion-transmitted infections
(TTIs), blood transfusion 47
transplanted tissues and organs,
immune tolerance 32
Treponema pallidum
chancroid 248
syphilis 361
Trichomonas hominis, tabulated 7
trichomoniasis
overview 459–63
sexually transmitted diseases
(STDs) 44
"Trichomoniasis" (OWH) 459n
trimethoprim-sulfamethoxazole, staph
infections 333
tuberculin skin test (TST), infectious
diseases screening 68
tuberculosis (TB)
microbial diseases 12
overview 369–76
"Tuberculosis—Basic TB Facts"
(CDC) 369n
tumor necrosis factor (TNF), immune
system response 30
Tylenol® (acetaminophen)
fever 485
Zika virus 243
typhoid, adolescent
immunization 632
typhoid fever
Ebola virus disease (EVD) 121
microbial diseases 12
overview 377–9
"Typhoid Fever" (CDC) 377n

U

ultrasound
  pelvic inflammatory disease
    (PID) 385
  Zika virus 242
"Understanding Antimicrobial (Drug)
  Resistance" (NIAID) 575n
"Understanding How Vaccines Work"
  (CDC) 598n
"Understanding Microbes in Sickness
  and in Health" (NIAID) 4n, 8n, 11n,
  15n, 40n
unsanitary conditions
  lice 419
  microbes 10
  polio 220
urinary tract infection (UTI), pelvic
  inflammatory disease (PID) 385
urine test
  microbial diseases 16
  Streptococcus pneumoniae 354
  Zika virus 238
U.S. Department of Health and
  Human Services (HHS)
  contact 721
  publications
      HIV and AIDS 161n
      vaccines for adolescents 629n
U.S. Environmental Protection
  Agency (EPA), contact 721
U.S. Food and Drug Administration
  (FDA)
  contact 721
  publications
      avoiding drug
        interactions 505n
      combating antibiotic
        resistance 572n
      countering bioterrorism
        and emerging infectious
        diseases 705n
      medicines and children 499n
      OraQuick in-home HIV
        test 556n
      OTC cough and cold products
        and infants 502n
      prevention, symptoms,
        treatments of cold or flu 468n
      treating impetigo 291n

U.S. National Library of Medicine
  (NLM), contact 721
"Using Dietary Supplements Wisely"
  (NCCIH) 533n
UTI *see* urinary tract infections

V

"Vaccinate Your Baby for Best
  Protection" (CDC) 613n
vaccination
  flu and colds 513
  group B strep (GBS) 360
  human papillomavirus
    (HPV) 630
  immune response 26
  immune system 599
  records 669
  smallpox 231
"Vaccination FAQs" (CDC) 621n
Vaccine Adverse Event Reporting
  System (VAERS), contact 721
"Vaccine Adverse Event Reporting
  System (VAERS)" (CDC) 665n
"Vaccine Misinformation May
  Have Tragic Consequences"
  (Omnigraphics) 673n
"Vaccine Types" (NIAID) 605n
vaccines
  bacterial meningitis 298
  colds and flu 468
  conjunctivitis 115
  defined 716
  immune system response 26
  microbes 9
  overview 598–604
  pandemic flu 184
  pneumonia 312
  transmission of microbes 42
  tuberculosis (TB) 375
  viral meningitis 202
  whooping cough 400
Vaccines and Immunizations,
  contact 721
VAERS *see* Vaccine Adverse Event
  Reporting System
vaginal discharge
  bacterial vaginosis 382
  gonorrhea 144

vaginal fluids
  Ebola virus disease (EVD) 122
  human immunodeficiency virus
    (HIV) 163
  Zika virus 240
vaginal sex
  chlamydia 255
  gonorrhea 145
  human immunodeficiency virus
    (HIV) 163
  syphilis 367
vaginal swabs, chlamydia 256
vaginal yeast infections, bacterial
  vaginosis (BV) 381
"Vaginal Yeast Infections"
  (OWH) 381n
valacyclovir, genital herpes 141
vancomycin
  Clostridium difficile 272
  Staphylococcus aureus 336
vancomycin-resistant enterococci
  (VRE), antimicrobial resistance 576
vancomycin-resistant *Staphylococcus
  aureus* (VRSA), overview 335–7
variant creutzfeldt-jakob disease
  (vCJD), prion diseases 53
variant flu viruses, influenza 182
varicella *see* chickenpox
varicella-zoster virus (VZV)
  chickenpox 93
  viral meningitis 200
variola virus, smallpox 231
vCJD *see* variant creutzfeldt-jakob
  disease
Vibrio cholerae, vaccine types 606
viral conjunctivitis
  conjunctivitis 108
  nonpolio enteroviruses 210
viral encephalitis, nonpolio
  enteroviruses 210
viral hepatitis *see* hepatitis
"Viral Hepatitis: A through E and
  Beyond" (NIDDK) 155n
viral load, human immunodeficiency
  virus (HIV) 167
viral meningitis
  amebic meningitis 435
  nonpolio enterovirus 210
  overview 199–203

"Viral Meningitis" (CDC) 199n
virion, microbes 6
virus shedding, adenovirus 86
viruses
  common colds 104
  defined 716
  fever 483
  immune system 22
  infectious mononucleosis 127
  influenza 180
  microbes 4
  pneumonia 308
  strep throat 340
  strep throat testing 552
  vaccine types 609
"VISA/VRSA in Healthcare Settings"
  (CDC) 335n
vitamin C, complementary
  approaches 512
vitamin E
  complementary approaches 518
  dietary supplements 507
VRE *see* vancomycin-resistant
  enterococci
"VRE in Healthcare Settings"
  (CDC) 391n
VZV *see* varicella-zoster virus

W

waterborne diseases, communicable
  diseases 59
WBCs *see* white blood cells
West Nile virus (WNV), viral
  diseases 52
"What Are HIV and AIDS?"
  (HHS) 161n
"What Is Ebola Virus Disease?"
  (CDC) 117n
"What Is Hansen Disease?" (CDC) 281n
"What Is Polio?" (CDC) 219n
"What Is Smallpox?" (CDC) 231n
"What Vaccines Do Adolescents
  Need?" (HHS) 629n
"What Would Happen If We Stopped
  Vaccinations?" (CDC) 677n
white blood cells (WBCs)
  blood transfusion 47
  infectious mononucleosis 128
  medical tests 544

whooping cough
  antimicrobial resistance 578
  childhood immunizations 613
  diphtheria 280
  microbes 5
  overview 395–401
  vaccine misinformation 674
WNV *see* West Nile virus
World Health Organization (WHO),
  contact 723

X

X-rays
  defined 716
  fever 485
  group B strep (GBS) 358
  microbial diseases 16
  pneumonia 315
  tuberculosis (TB) 376
Xofluza®, antiviral drugs 568

Y

yeast infections *see* vaginal yeast
  infections

yellow fever
  adolescent immunization 632
  microbes 13
  transmission on cruise
    ships 63
  vaccine misinformation 674
  vaccine types 611
Yersinia pestis, microbes 42
yoga, hepatitis C 536

Z

zanamivir
  anti-influenza 564
  avian flu 91
  drug resistance 584
Zika
  defined 52
  infectious disease 701
  overview 237–44
zinc
  colds 517
  complementary approach 512
  mouth sores 490
zostavax, shingles 101